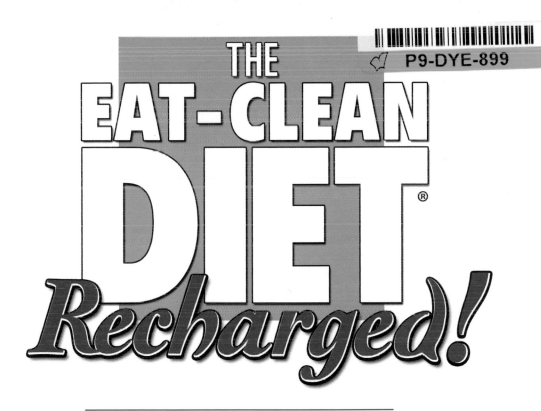

P9-DYE-899

THE EAT-CLEAN DIET® Recharged!

Lasting Fat Loss That's
Better than Ever

TOSCA RENO

RKP ROBERT KENNEDY PUBLISHING

Published by Robert Kennedy Publishing
400 Matheson Blvd. West
Mississauga, ON
L5R 3M1 Canada
Visit us at www.rkpubs.com
and www.toscareno.com

Managing Senior Production Editor: Wendy Morley
Online and Associate Editor: Vinita Persaud
Junior Production Editor: Cali Hoffman
Art Director: Gabriella Caruso Marques
Acting Art Director: Jessica Pensabene
Editorial Designers: Brian Ross and Ellie Jeon
Proofreader: James De Medeiros
Editorial Assistant: Stephanie Maus
Recipe Testers: Ashif Tejani and Terry Snow

Library and Archives Canada Cataloguing in Publication

Reno, Tosca, 1959-
          The eat-clean diet recharged : lasting fat loss
that's better than ever / Tosca Reno.

Includes index.
ISBN 978-1-55210-067-7

          1. Women--Health and hygiene. 2. Physical fitness
for women. 3. Reducing diets. 4. Weight loss. 5. Reducing
diets--Recipes. I. Title.

RM222.2.R462 2009   613'.04244   C2009-905994-0

10 9 8 7 6 5 4 3 2 1

Distributed in Canada by
NBN (National Book Network)
67 Mowat Avenue, Suite 241
Toronto, ON
M6K 3E3

Distributed in USA by
NBN (National Book Network)
15200 NBN Way
Blue Ridge Summit, PA
17214

Printed in Canada

IMPORTANT

The information in this book reflects the author's experiences and opinions and is not intended to replace medical advice.

Before beginning this or any nutritional or exercise regimen, consult your physician to be sure it is appropriate for you. Ask for a physical stress test.

This book is dedicated to the many millions of you who have adopted the Eat-Clean lifestyle. You are intelligent and inspirational, every one of you, and I thank you for your brilliance.

I am indeed always listening!

Tosca Reno

Beet and Arugula Salad
(see page 314)

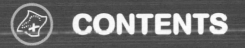

CONTENTS

INTRODUCTION

It is my pleasure to invite you to step into my kitchen and sit at my table. While you settle in and adjust yourself to the hum of this busy room, your nostrils will immediately be bombarded with wonderful, appetite-arousing smells, whether it is a pan full of roasting garlic bulbs drizzled in Mediterranean olive oil, or the aromatic tinge of rosemary-dusted sweet potatoes and bubbling soups and stews overflowing with nourishing fruits of the earth that assault you. Such smells arouse a hunger in you, which I hope to satisfy with the freshest ingredients, grown on healthy soils and infused with fragrant spices. I have prepared these dishes with you in mind.

The information and foods I present here are in keeping with my Eat-Clean philosophy, which is to eat more good food six times a day to achieve a lean, healthy physique. Millions of you have already discovered how powerful Eating Clean is. It works because it satisfies a basic urge in us to eat foods that nourish and rebuild. This is so much more than just stuffing a fast-food greaseburger into our faces! The latter leaves you wanting more, while Eating Clean leaves you happy, content and without the manic cravings that make you head for the refrigerator within minutes of having eaten.

Each chapter of *The Eat-Clean Diet Recharged* has been energized with up-to-date information – much of which has come from our very own readers! I thank you for that. The 50 recipes in this book are brand new and delicious, and you'll enjoy the cooking process from preparation to consumption. I welcome both newcomers and my previous readers to join me at my kitchen table and rediscover eating – eating real food to build your leanest, healthiest and happiest self.

Sincerely,

Tosca Reno

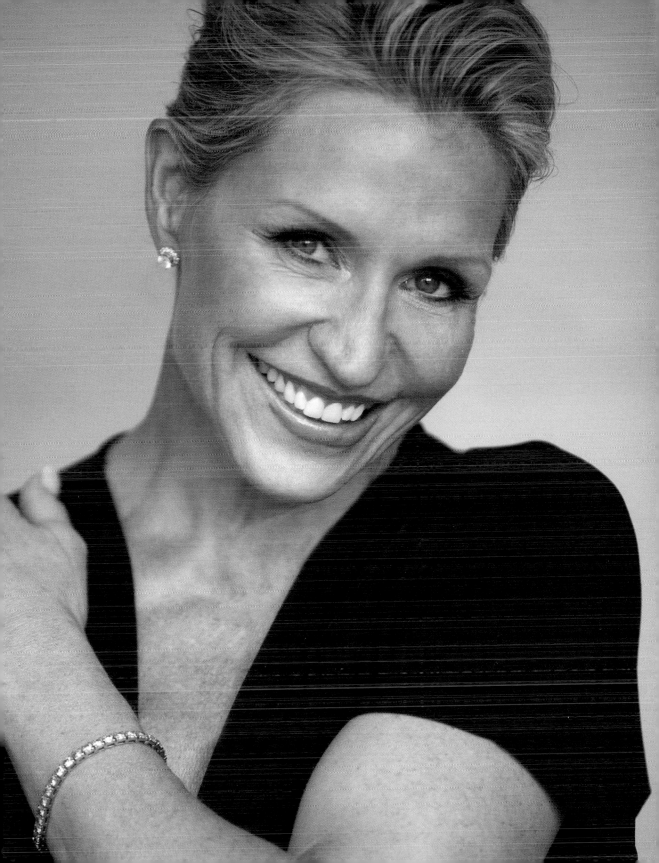

THE EAT-CLEAN PHENOMENON
My invitation for you to enjoy a healthy body.

Welcome to *The Eat-Clean Diet,* a phenomenon that has transformed the way people have eaten for the last several years, and the way fitness and strength athletes have gotten "ripped" for bodybuilding competitions decades before that. How does a diet reach across the landscape of so many different body types? Good question!

At first glance there does not seem to be much connection between the bodies of ordinary folks and those who flex their powerful muscles on stage. Yet

> "It is the food that we eat which is responsible for shaping such a vast array of different body types. Yes, the food!"

marathon runners, bodybuilders, golfers, cyclists, swimmers, gymnasts and high-school-football players all depend on nutrition to give them energy to get through the day and excel at their activity. The common thread between these athletes and regular people is what we all put in our mouths. No matter how extreme, all athletes rely on the best nutrition to give them power and define their physiques. It is the food that we eat which is responsible for shaping such a vast array of body types. Yes, the food!

Should you decide to eat poor quality food, such as what can be purchased at drive-thrus, convenient stores, fast-food establishments and even in some schools across the country, a very different body shape will result. In your busy day today, you may have seen some of these folks. Heavy, misshapen bodies populate every city, town and district in this country and most other countries on Earth. The World Health Organization has coined a new (but aptly descriptive) word called "globesity," which describes what is happening worldwide to the human physique. The word indicates that obesity has become a serious epidemic of global proportions. No one is immune from obesity – it affects everyone from every race, gender and age. For the first time in history, there is a real possibility that children will not outlive their parents as a result of weight-related illnesses and other diseases. There has to be a better way!

This is where *The Eat-Clean Diet* comes in. Several years ago, I began writing about Eating Clean in *Oxygen* magazine. My column, called "Raise the Bar," has helped (and continues to help) many people struggling with weight issues discover a different way to eat and a new way of thinking about food. Readers discovered a powerful and effective way to lose weight at a healthy rate, while eating more. Readers relate to me, which is why my column is so effective.

> "I am a normal woman with everyday issues, just like everyone else, and for a long time, I carried excess weight, too."

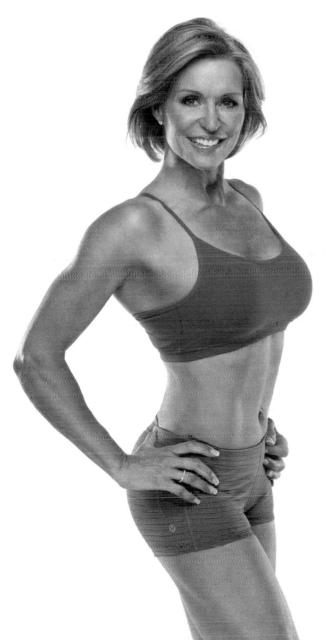

I am a normal woman with everyday issues, just like everyone else, and for a long time, I carried excess weight, too. You will find my story sprinkled throughout the pages of this book. To condense the story slightly, I weighed at my heaviest (204 pounds) at the end of my second year in university. I was 20 years old. It wasn't until the age of 42 that I challenged myself to compete in a bodybuilding competition, and learned about the powerful effects of Eating Clean. My battle with being too heavy, then too skinny, and ultimately a cover model was told paragraphs and columns at a time in "Raise the Bar." You paid attention, wanted more, and here it is.

Years later, hundreds of thousands of you are following the Eat-Clean program, all celebrating your newfound health, happiness and slenderness – congratulations! Eating Clean is a lifestyle, not a diet, and this way of eating is not going away anytime soon. And just in case you missed the latest news, Hollywood has taken notice. Tabloids have reported that celebrities including Halle Berry, Nicole Kidman and Angelina Jolie all live the Eat-Clean lifestyle. I know this won't sway you too much (you will always be the intelligent audience I know you are), but no one is more obsessed with staying in shape than the hotties of Hollywood. Isn't it nice to know you are in good company?

The Eat-Clean phenomenon is your chance to reclaim your life, your health and your wellbeing. No one wants to be heavy. It's a drag to carry excess weight around. I once went scuba diving and had to tie a 14-pound weight belt around my waist so I

> "There is infinite joy to be had in living life with a healthful, lean physique."

could sink down to explore the coral reefs underwater. Just walking to the boat with the added weight hurt my knees and hips. Fortunately, I could simply remove the weight belt and feel the lightness of being myself again. I want you to experience that lightness, too. The human body was meant to walk swiftly through a forest or stroll lightly beside a stream. There is infinite joy to be had in living life with a healthful, lean physique. We will rediscover this joy for you. It is possible starting right now.

I also believe *The Eat-Clean Diet* has been broadly accepted because the timing is right. Many of you have expressed, through your letters and emails to me, that you are simply fed up with what is currently considered "food." You want something better. You are tired of being sick, fat, grumpy, depressed, overlooked, drained of energy, uninterested in sex and a list of other symptoms too long to mention. In the same way that America was tired of an ineffective

government, putting its faith in a new leader with a campaign based on hope and change, I believe Eating Clean has been embraced.

You want and deserve something that promises hope and change for you, too. I can feel the groundswell of change blowing from north to south, and east to west. You are beginning to ask questions about what food really is. We are not all the way there yet, but we are certainly sitting up and paying attention. We need to — the health of our children depends on it. If we don't change the way we eat soon, the consequences will be dire and devastating. It isn't exactly working well now, is it?

Eating Clean is part of a tide of change that will bring health and wellness back to a nation of people who have long done without it. Putting our trust in eating the most nutrient-rich foods to deliver us back to health may sound like a simple, even naive idea. If you doubt the power of Eating Clean, try it for a few weeks and then go back to eating sugar-loaded, over-processed, chemically-charged "food" and tell me how you feel. People report, after trying it, that they can't believe how sick they feel. The bountiful energy they felt while Eating Clean began to disappear with every bite of poisonous food, leaving them wilting and writhing on the couch. Sometimes we don't know how good something is until we give it up!

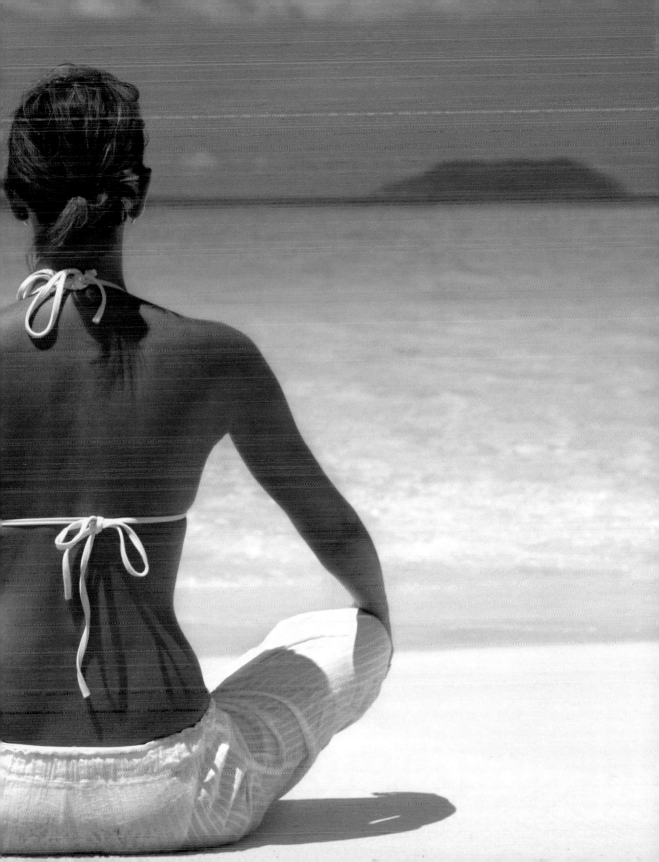

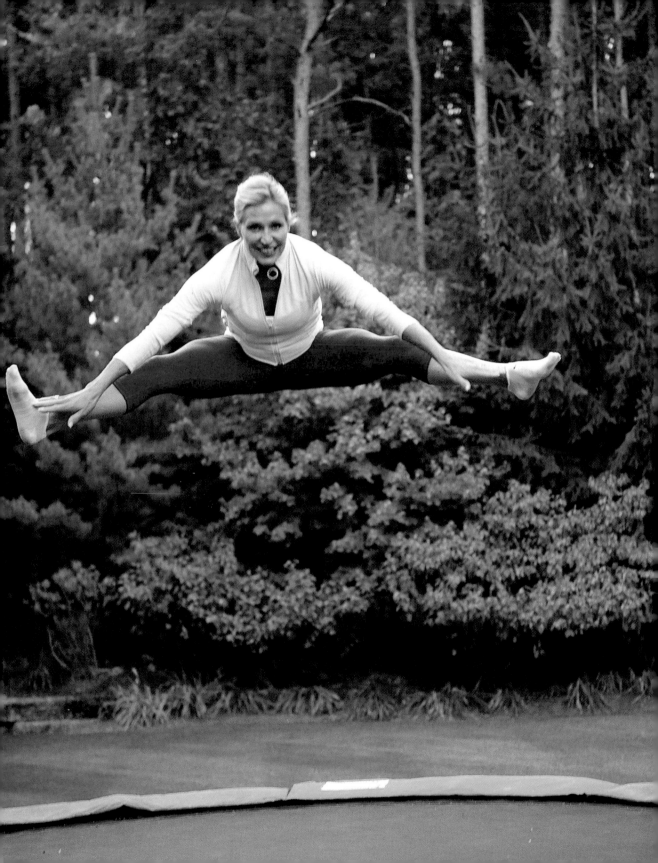

THE EAT-CLEAN DIET PRINCIPLES

1

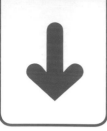

HOW I DISCOVERED EATING CLEAN

Would it surprise you to learn that when Eating Clean you will actually be eating more? I was stunned to discover this fact for myself when I began to prepare for a bodybuilding contest. I admit that I was not particularly interested in becoming a fully flexed out, bodybuilding she-man, but I was curious to see how the preparation would take place and how I might transform my body. I always admired Rachel McLish for her lean and toned physique and wanted one just like it for myself. This was an example of female strength I could live with, even if my own body was not as genetically gifted as hers.

I began the preparations with two simple instructions from my coach: "If you are going to compete, you need to eat more of the right kinds of food and you need to train smart." Those instructions seemed simple enough and I did like food, so eating more seemed like something I could commit to. The reality of those commands issued seriously by my erstwhile coach proved enlightening. The single most important lesson I learned through this process was that the body is not predominantly shaped by exercise, as I had previously believed. Rather, a lean physique is shaped primarily by nutrition – the right kind of nutrition – Clean Nutrition.

"A lean physique is shaped primarily by nutrition – the right kind of nutrition – Clean Nutrition."

I discovered this a few weeks after experimenting with eating more frequently and partnering lean proteins with complex carbohydrates as directed by my coach. While getting dressed for work I tried on a skirt that had been my favorite. It was a denim pencil skirt that I had not been able to wear comfortably for some time – the zipper wouldn't do up by a long shot! I tried that skirt on and it fell to the floor. I had lost enough fat that the skirt just slid over my hips and down even after doing up the zipper. It was one of those crystallizing moments for me. Right there I knew I'd discovered something very powerful about the good food I had been eating (in quantity may I remind you) and weight loss.

The improved food choices I had been making along with moderate amounts of exercise, mostly in the form of strength training, were the catalyst for change. My breakfasts went from toast with peanut butter and jam, followed by a double sugar, double cream coffee to a bowl of oatmeal dressed with flaxseeds and mixed berries, accompanied by four hardboiled egg whites. This was remarkable to me as a newcomer to Eating Clean.

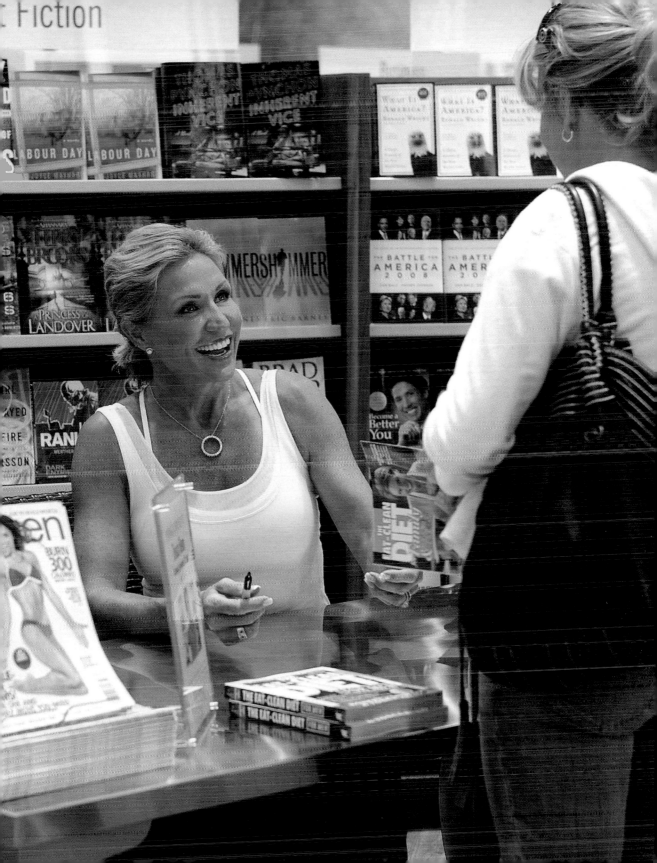

I want to make it clear to you that I did not develop the concept of Clean Eating. The idea is borrowed from the physique industry, where this kind of nutrition is practiced by hundreds of thousands of followers. You can see them in the pages of *Oxygen* and numerous other fitness magazines. Scanning through the pages of publications like these gives you a pretty good idea of how powerful a paradigm shift in eating can be. There are numerous examples of tight, toned physiques, which were created for the most part by practicing Clean Eating. By following a formula I call the Body Beautiful/Body Healthy

Formula, you too can rework your physique to look like those bodies you may already be admiring.

I used this formula to accomplish the daunting (so I thought) task of preparing myself for my physique contest, but it works so well many thousands of you have now learned it too. Here's what my formula means:

BODY BEAUTIFUL/BODY HEALTHY FORMULA

80% NUTRITION + 10% TRAINING + 10% GENETICS = BODY BEAUTIFUL/BODY HEALTHY

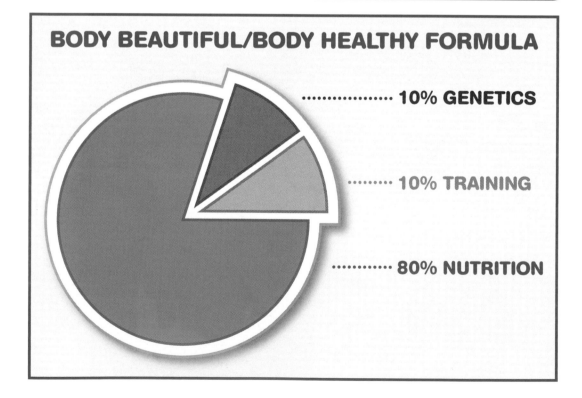

BODY BEAUTIFUL/BODY HEALTHY FORMULA

- 10% GENETICS
- 10% TRAINING
- 80% NUTRITION

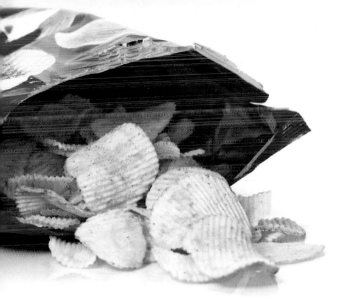

"Nutrition is far more responsible for creating your shape and your health than you ever could have imagined."

If you have been reading correctly you may be wondering if I have made a typo with this formula. 80 percent nutrition shapes a lean healthy body? Really!? I know you are asking yourself this because I have done countless seminars where I have quizzed the audience on what number they would assign to nutrition. Virtually everyone thinks it is 10% nutrition and 80% training. I have to admit that before I discovered Eating Clean I thought that too. I also believed that you had to be genetically gifted to own a killer physique. In some ways you do have to live with the genetic package your parents gave you, but nutrition is far more responsible for creating your shape and your health than you ever could have imagined.

If you have trouble believing food is the primary factor in shaping your physique and consequently your health, let's consider the opposite – the current state

of health and fitness affairs in North America. For the first time in the history of this country, researchers find themselves wondering whether children will lead shorter lives than their parents because of ever-expanding waistlines and the prevalence of what I like to call "anti-foods." Obesity is burgeoning here and in the rest of the world, where it is in fact exploding not only with fat but with disease. There are numerous causes for this problem but the most significant include the quality of the food we consume and the toxic food environment in which we live. Both of these subjects could fill the pages of book after book and I predict they soon will.

The landscape of eating has changed. Food corporations see people like me and you as a free-for-all market of hungry consumers upon whose backs they would like very much to profit. Hence a fast food, drive-thru, get-it-quick, super size it, pull-up-to-the-buffet-and-stuff-yourself attitude toward food. By presenting food at every opportunity, from school cafeterias to hospitals, a toxic food-saturated culture results with no idea of how to stop the madness (as Susan Powter used to say). It's eat, eat, eat, and the more we eat, the better. You can't order a plain black coffee today without the server asking if you are sure, absolutely sure, you don't want sugar and cream. Even when you say, "No thanks, just black," they bring the dreaded sugar and cream anyway! An egg white omelet is, by definition, low fat, and the mere idea of putting cheese on it is laughable if you are already avoiding at least some of the yolks, but a chef hardly knows what to do with himself if you ask for it without, so he loads on the cheddar anyway because heaven forbid you don't get your money's worth!

The quest to eat more food and the biggest size to get the best value possible has brought us partly to the place where we can't see our weight on the scale

"Two out of every three North Americans are overweight or obese and the problem is only getting worse."

anymore. The other problem is the quality of food we are presented with. Our food has literally been doused with chemicals at every stage of its life from seed to consumption – so much so that even at this point (some 40 years after the food explosion began) we still don't have any idea what the results of such chemical "warfare" are or will be. But one thing is certain, at least from the visual standpoint. Two out of every three North Americans are overweight or obese and the problem is only getting worse.

Let's go back to the Body Beautiful/Body Healthy Formula, where I asked you to believe me when I suggest that nutrition is 80 percent responsible for shaping your physique and your health. Good or bad, the proof is all around you. Ask yourself, if you continue what you are doing and continue eating what you are eating, will you look and feel any different five years down the road?

Finally, you have an obligation to be a much more active human being than you are now. If you accept the Eat-Clean lifestyle you will certainly shed unwanted pounds, but you will still be just a leaner version of your current self. A vigorous strength training and moderate cardiovascular exercise program is needed to round out the renovation of your new physique. You will find guidance for implementing the Eat-Clean lifestyle into your home in every page of this book.

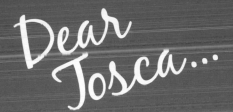

Dear Tosca,

I started off weighing 200 lbs and I was miserable physically and emotionally. I had always been overweight, even as a child. I was wearing women's petite clothes when I was in elementary school. I had always used food as a comfort. My parents divorced when I was young and my dad depended on frozen dinners and fast food to feed us.

Throughout college and grad school, my weight fluctuated. When I graduated and moved to a new town, I didn't know anyone except the pizza deliveryman.

Finally, when I was 28, I made a decision during the Christmas holidays to take my life back and control how I ate. My friend's father had been eating fresh and had huge success so I decided to give it a try. I started out eating a healthy breakfast, and made sure to eat protein and vegetables at every meal with fruit as a snack. I also started to plan out every meal at the beginning of the week, so I was always prepared.

The weight immediately started falling off. I was down 10 lbs in one month. There were some days I would lose 2 lbs in just a day. I weighed myself every day. That scale was my best friend and worst enemy all in one week. It kept me motivated though. I finally had to start looking for new meals to make and that's when I came across your book which helped a lot.

Finally, after a year, I was down 70 lbs. I went from a size 16 to a size 4. I can even wear a size 2 in some pieces of clothing. I have never in my entire life been so small. My mood has improved tremendously, my hair and skin look great, and I have control over my life again. I grew up being made fun of and now I have people telling me how beautiful I am all of the time.

I have never considered this a diet. I have always told people that this is a new way of life, a better way of life. I am now maintaining my current weight of 130 and I have been lifting weights and riding my bike.

Thank you,

Andrea Tuttle

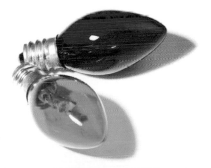

WHAT ARE THE EAT-CLEAN DIET PRINCIPLES?

You now understand that food is a critical factor in your health and wellness. Eat poorly and you become sick and overweight. Eat well and you become a glowing example of health and vibrancy. You will look so good you won't be able to stand yourself! So how then do we get there, and fast? To the right are the eight principles involved in the Eat-Clean lifestyle. Accompanying that is a list of what to eliminate from your current eating habits. Remember, Eating Clean is not about eliminating every tasty item from your diet or being hungry. You need to recognize that some "foods" you are currently eating are things I would rather call "anti-foods" and you must work hard to avoid these, since they are destructive to both excellent health and stunning form.

As you read the following dos and don'ts, try to keep in mind the idea that you may want to go all out (as I did) and jump right off the cliff into Eating Clean full force. That is just the way I am. I have to do it that way or I know I will be too lenient with myself and never get the results I long for. Alternatively, you may want to eliminate just one or two things at a time from your diet to make the transition to Eating Clean easier on yourself. May I recommend that "one thing" be sugar? I helped one young father lose his gut and his sleep apnea headgear simply by asking him to quit drinking the ten (yes, ten!) sodas he was ingesting each day. He hardly had to do any-

thing else! Now that man who couldn't see his feet or make love to his wife is competing in a triathlon. He is reenergized, and there are countless stories just like his.

Approach Eating Clean as the lifestyle it is and make the changes you know you can stick with right now. If you are wired like I am and you must go big or go home, then jump in and feel confident that you will lose weight at a rate of about three pounds per week. If you have to do it in stages, which is equally laudable, then do so, but commit to Eating Clean and begin to add more good practices (good principles) when you are ready.

"Keep in mind the idea that you may want to go all out into Eating Clean full force, or you may want to eliminate just one or two things at a time from your diet."

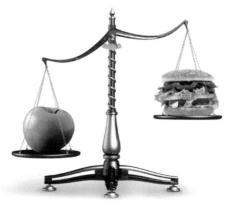

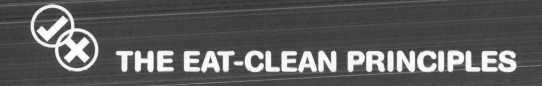

THE EAT-CLEAN PRINCIPLES

WHAT TO DO

- Eat more – eat six small meals each day.

- Eat breakfast every day, within an hour of rising.

- Eat a combination of lean protein and complex carbohydrates at each meal.

- Eat sufficient (two or three servings) healthy fats every day.

- Drink two to three liters of water each day.

- Carry a cooler packed with Clean foods each day.

- Depend on fresh fruits and vegetables for fiber, vitamins, nutrients and enzymes.

- Adhere to proper portion sizes.

WHAT TO AVOID

- Avoid all over-processed foods, particularly white flour and sugar.

- Avoid chemically charged foods.

- Avoid foods containing preservatives.

- Avoid artificial sugars.

- Avoid artificial foods (such as processed cheese slices).

- Avoid saturated and trans fats.

- Avoid sugar-loaded beverages, including colas and juices.

- Avoid (or do your best to limit) alcohol intake.

- Avoid all calorie-dense foods containing little or no nutritional value. I call these anti-foods.

- Avoid super-sizing your meals.

THE EAT-CLEAN DIET PRINCIPLES EXPLAINED

Here is a brief explanation of each of the principles. Try not to let my words bog you down. These principles are as easy to follow as brushing your teeth or combing your hair. If you decide right now to embrace just one of these principles you will be immediately living a healthier lifestyle. That's because each one of these steps is empowering and entirely doable. Imagine what could happen if you cement in your mind that you will accept them all right now! Look out world – here you come!

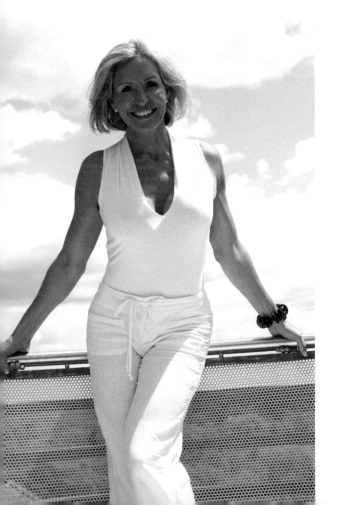

EAT MORE – EAT SIX SMALL MEALS A DAY!

Read those words again. When was the last time someone told you that you would lose weight by eating more? Answer: never! Not a single book or health expert will tell you something that seems so ridiculous at the outset. Yet one of the most effective ways to shed excess pounds is indeed to eat more. Rather than eating three meals each day, or less, as is often the case for those of you who believe in skipping meals, you will now be eating more. Your new goal will be to eat six meals each and every day. How many meals is that per year? 2190! Each one of these meals is essential to your health, critical to your happiness and not to be missed if you want to experience success while Eating Clean. So forget the notion that eating less is the way to lose weight. In fact, eating less is the least effective way to go about it.

Why? I know you are asking yourself how it can be possible to shed unwanted pounds by eating more frequently. I thought the same thing when I started Eating Clean. The answer is two-fold and as simple as understanding that increasing the frequency of your meals causes your metabolism to be stimulated while preventing you from getting too hungry. Think about it. How often does a baby feed? The normal feeding time for a baby is every three hours. These intervals not only keep the baby properly nourished and content, but also the regular receipt of nourishment ensures that all metabolic processes are running efficiently. It is natural for us to require sustenance every three hours, even in adulthood. Once you begin to practice this for yourself you will soon grasp the intelligence of eating more frequently. My only caveat is not to misunderstand eating more frequently as permission to eat everything in sight or in large quantities. You will have to make your portions smaller. The idea is to eat the right kinds of foods often enough in the proper amount to never experience hunger pangs. Each meal becomes an event to fuel the metabolism and should contain the most nutritious foods, also known as Clean foods. Eating must become something that is done with a sense of responsibility to one's health and wellness.

"You will have to make
your portions smaller."

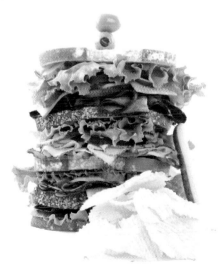

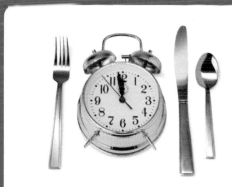

EATING SIX
MEALS A DAY –
THE FRAMEWORK

7:00 AM	MEAL #1	or	BREAKFAST
10:00 AM	MEAL #2	or	MID MORNING
1:00 PM	MEAL #3	or	LUNCH
4:00 PM	MEAL #4	or	MID AFTERNOON
7:00 PM	MEAL #5	or	DINNER
10:00 PM	MEAL #6	or	EVENING

MAKE IT WORK FOR YOU: Adjust your schedule to suit your waking, working and eating time.

HUNGRY? You may want to eat every two-and-a-half hours, depending on how active you are during the day.

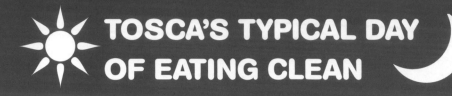

7:00 AM | BREAKFAST

- ½ cup dry oats cooked with 1 cup water, topped with 2 tablespoons each ground flaxseed, wheat germ and bee pollen, and ¼ cup mixed berries
- 4 egg whites, scrambled or hard boiled, and 1 yolk (these are not eaten in the oatmeal)
- 1 cup black coffee or clear green tea
- 1 liter water

10:00 AM | MID MORNING

- 1 apple with 2 tablespoons natural nut butter or 1 scant handful raw unsalted almonds
- 500 ml water

1:00 pm | LUNCH

- 5 oz. water-packed tuna over 2 cups spinach leaves, 1 grated carrot, ½ chopped bell pepper and 1 tomato. Dressed with 1 tablespoon avocado oil, 2 tablespoons lemon or lime juice and 2 tablespoons ground flaxseed
- 500 ml water

3:30 pm | MID AFTERNOON

- 5 oz. grilled boneless skinless chicken breast
- 1 cup steamed mixed vegetables
- 500 ml water

6:30 pm | DINNER

- 5 oz. grilled salmon
- ½ baked sweet potato topped with chopped chives and 1 tablespoon pumpkin oil
- 1 ½ cups steamed mixed vegetables
- 500 ml water
- 1 cup plain green tea

9:30 pm | EVENING

The last meal of the day: I include this meal but if you are not truly hungry there is no need to eat it. Judge for yourself if you are going to need it to get through the night.

- ½ cup kefir with ½ chopped apple or ½ cup mixed berries

    or

- 1 apple with 1 scant handful raw unsalted nuts or 1 tablespoon natural nut butter
- 500 ml water

    and/or

- 1 cup chamomile tea

Good night – and do it all over again tomorrow!

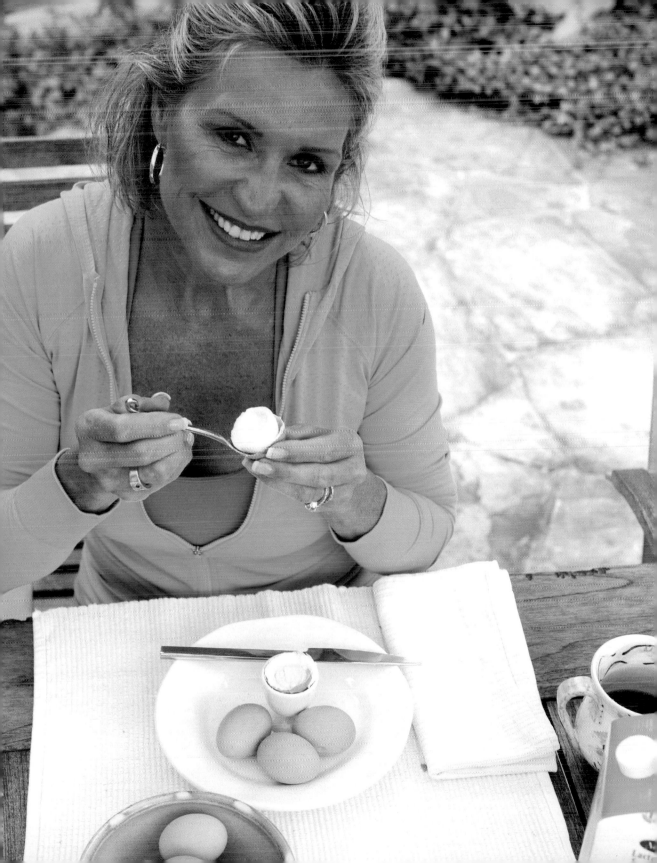

HOW MUCH PROTEIN?

Eating Clean prescribes consuming several small portions of lean protein along with complex carbohydrates each day. Many male and female readers have questioned me on how much protein is sufficient. According to the Institute of Medicine, adults at a healthy weight need a minimum of 0.8 grams of protein for every kilogram of body weight, which is 0.36 grams per pound, to keep from slowly breaking down their own tissues. Beyond that, there's relatively little solid information on how much protein in your diet is ideal, what a healthy target for calories contributed by protein should be, or what kind of protein is best. A good safe starting number is 0.36 grams per pound of body weight, but that does not address what is needed by the active individual – the one who works out more than three times a week, and more specifically, the one who also trains with weights with the same frequency. An active person needs nearly twice as much protein as someone living a sedentary lifestyle. Choose high-quality proteins from nuts, seeds, legumes, quinoa, tofu, poultry, bison, beef, eggs and fish.

EAT BREAKFAST EVERY DAY!

This book has an entire chapter devoted to breakfast (found on page 56), but here are a few words to emphasize the necessity of eating this all-star meal every day. The National Weight Control Registry found that those who shed 30 pounds of weight or more did so with the help of eating breakfast. This morning meal helps us achieve better nutrition and it's also been proven that early eaters consume less saturated fat and cholesterol over the course of the day than someone who skips breakfast.

Similarly, a Nielsen's National Eating Trends Survey revealed that a woman who consumed a cereal-based breakfast regularly weighed on average nine pounds less than her non-cereal-eating counterpart. The study found that cereal-eating men were six pounds lighter than those who didn't bother with a morning meal.

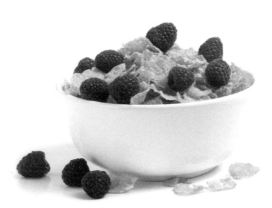

At one time or another each of us has skipped breakfast, thinking that by doing so we would lose weight. At first glance this seems to make sense. By eating fewer calories, you should logically be able to drop pounds. However, humans are not the result of mathematical equations. Each of us is unique and the way our bodies operate varies from one to another. Math alone is not enough to help us shed weight. Looking at it as a numbers-only game would be negating the myriad of factors contributing to how fat is removed from the body and why some fat prefers to stick around – especially in the problem areas. The logic breaks down even further when you discover that people who *do* eat breakfast are many times more likely to be slim than those who *don't*.

Eating breakfast on a regular basis helps keep the body nourished and satisfied while providing abundant energy. This in turn makes for productive human beings – everyone from the schoolchild to the Manhattan businessman. In your case, eating breakfast is the first of many lifestyle changes you can make to shed that annoying five or 105 pounds once and for all.

LEAN PROTEIN PLUS COMPLEX CARBOHYDRATES AT EVERY MEAL!

I hinted that eating more frequently helps us to stay lean and healthy and also prevents us from becoming overly hungry. This won't happen if you make a habit of munching on doughnuts and downing a bucket of soda for breakfast. Just as cars do not operate properly on dirty gas, the human body does not function well on poor fuel. Eating foods devoid of nutrients stimulates your craving for more of them, and there is never a real sense of satisfaction in what you have eaten. You might be able to identify with the fuzzy, exhausted feeling some of us get in the afternoon. It feels like you have hit a wall and don't even have sufficient energy to pick up the phone.

> "Eating breakfast regularly keeps the body nourished."

Contrast that feeling with the sense of abundant energy you reap when you make better food choices – that is when you choose high-grade foods as your fuel of preference. That fuel comes from a combination of lean protein partnered with complex carbohydrates consumed at every sitting. Even without an in-depth knowledge of food chemistry, the average person understands that nutrient-dense foods do make a difference. You can feel it in your increased energy levels, your joy of living and a sense that you are doing right by your body. According to Lee Labrada, fitness guru and author of *The Lean Body Promise*, "By eating protein with your complex carbohydrates, you'll slow down the carb-to-fat conversion process even more." This is why complex carbohydrates should always be eaten with protein.

Macronutrients Defined

A BREAKDOWN OF NUTRIENTS

How much protein, complex carbohydrates and healthy fats should you eat each day? Each day strive to consume:

55% complex carbohydrates + 27% lean proteins + 18% healthy fats = daily total healthy nutrition.

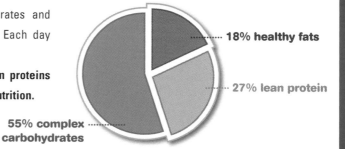

18% healthy fats

27% lean protein

55% complex carbohydrates

....

Note: These numbers are optimal, but not something you need to worry about too much. If you are eating the correct portions of lean protein and complex carbohydrates, these numbers should be reached naturally.

PROTEIN

You should eat six servings of protein each day. Protein is primarily found in meat, poultry, fish and eggs, but is also found in dairy and to some degree in vegetable and grain sources. Tofu, chia seed, quinoa and hemp seed are complete proteins. Other plant sources must be eaten in combination in order to be complete.

....

EXAMPLES OF LEAN PROTEIN

- Beans of all kids
- Beef tenderloin
- Bison
- Canned salmon, packed in water
- Canned tuna, packed in water
- Chicken breasts
- Chickpeas
- Eggs
- Fat-free plain yogurt
- Fresh fish (cod, salmon, tilapia, etc.)
- Kefir

- Lean ground turkey
- Lentils
- Low-fat cottage cheese
- Natural nut butters (almond, cashew, peanut, etc.)
- Non-dairy beverages (fat-free almond, rice or soymilk)
- Pork tenderloin
- Tempeh
- Tofu
- Unsalted raw nuts and seeds

Note: this is not an exhaustive list.

CARBOHYDRATES

There are two types of carbohydrates: simple and complex. Simple carbohydrates (think white flour and sugar) are also known as sugars. They break down easily and tend to send blood-sugar levels out of control. For the most part, you want to avoid simple carbs, with fruit as the exception. Fruits are simple carbs, but they also contain fiber, which slows down their digestion, as well as vital nutrients and vitamins.

Complex carbohydrates are high in fiber and improve digestion. They provide you with energy, keep you satisfied after meals and stabilize blood-sugar levels. Vegetables, fruits and whole grains are all complex carbs.

STARCHY COMPLEX CARBOHYDRATES

You should eat two to four servings of complex carbohydrates from whole grains or other starchy-carb sources each day.

STARCHY COMPLEX CARBS FROM WHOLE GRAINS

- Amaranth
- Brown Rice
- Buckwheat
- Bulgar
- Cream of Wheat
- Millet
- Oatmeal
- Quinoa*
- Wheat germ
- Whole-grain pasta

Note: *this is not an exhaustive list.*

STARCHY CARBS FROM VEGETABLE SOURCES

These are high-protein complex carbs and may be used as a protein source.

- Bananas
- Carrots
- Chickpeas*
- Beans (kidney, navy, pinto, soy)*
- Sweet potatoes
- Potatoes
- Radishes
- Split peas*
- Lentils*
- Yams

Note: *this is not an exhaustive list.*

depends upon to fight depression. Gasp! Yes, in order to lose weight and keep the body looking fine, you must eat fat. It is a question of what kind of fat and how much.

The best fats are those that are obtained from cold-water fatty fish as well as warm-water lean fish. Cold-water fatty fish include char, salmon, halibut and trout, and warm-water lean fish include such varieties as mahi-mahi, wahoo, snapper, tilapia and grouper among many. Other than fish, healthy fats can also be found in the nuts, seeds and oils of many plants including sunflowers, avocados, olives, peanuts, canola and some vegetables. These healthy fats aid digestion. Their absence would cause digestion to cease and even though you may still be eating plenty, you would starve. Your body cannot run properly without fat.

Factory-produced fats (as opposed to natural healthy fats) are far more dangerous since they carry with them a deadly load of problems, some of which are just beginning to emerge. Trans fats have been linked to cancer, while eating too many omega-6 fats, as many North Americans do, causes inflammation, depression, disease, obesity and heart disease. Trans and industrial fats are highly unstable. If stored or used incorrectly (heated to smoking point or recycled as in French fry vats) they oxidize, unleashing dangerous free radicals. These too are implicated in disease.

"Trans fats have been implicated in causing cancer while eating too many omega-6 fats causes inflammation, depression, disease, obesity and heart disease."

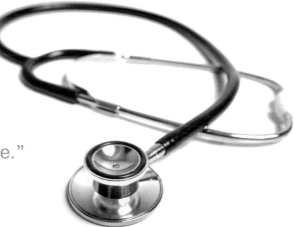

"You are mostly water."

DRINK PLENTY OF WATER!

You may wonder why I have programmed water into every one of the six daily meals in the Eat-Clean lifestyle. For many of us it is difficult, even impossible, to remember to drink enough water. I find that when I make water part of every meal it soon becomes a habit and I never have to worry about getting enough. It is also difficult for many of us to know when we are actually thirsty. The sensation of a dry mouth is not the best indicator of thirst. If your mouth is already dry, it is too late. The elderly have a particularly difficult time maintaining proper hydration because they lose the ability to detect thirst. Programming the drinking of water into your meal times makes it an easy healthy habit you learn to accept sooner.

Water is the very basis of life and composed of two powerhouse atoms – hydrogen and oxygen, and is critical to the Eat-Clean game plan. Both losing and maintaining weight depend on adequate hydration. If you are ignoring your body's need for water, you may be substituting eating for drinking. In other words, you may be confusing your body's hunger for water with hunger for food. This is one of the main reasons that many diets suggest drinking a glass of water before eating – it gives you and your body a chance to decide whether you are actually hungry or in fact just thirsty. Conversely, chronic dehydration has been linked to obesity. The solution? Drink more water.

Roughly 75 percent of your body is water, the bulk of which is stored in the largest organ, the skin. Water is critical for cellular function at every level, from regulating body temperature to keeping joints mobile and maintaining tissue health. Weight loss cannot occur effectively without sufficient water. When you drink cold water your metabolic rate is increased by as much as 30 percent. This happens because your body has to work harder to increase the temperature of the water to match that of your body. Surprisingly, lean muscle tissue is predominantly water. When muscle cells are full of water they help the muscle look toned and increase the body's ability to burn fat. Muscle is metabolically active, which means that it is constantly hungry for fuel, so it is a good idea to pay attention to your thirst. Staying sufficiently hydrated also suppresses the appetite and blunts cravings. Make water your choice for quenching thirst. Try to drink about 10 cups, or a minimum of two to three liters, each day.

> "If you want to be absolutely sure that each meal you eat is going to be Clean, get into the good habit of taking your food with you."

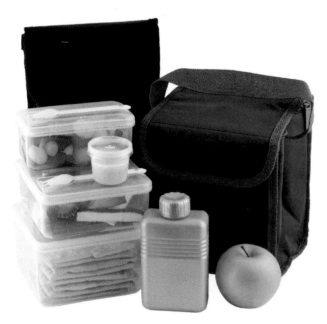

CARRY A COOLER PACKED WITH CLEAN EATS!

It is easy enough to Eat Clean at home since you can stock your pantry, cupboards and refrigerator with wholesome, nutritious foods. However, as soon as you step outside your front door it becomes a far more difficult task. Can you trust what is in that salad you purchased around the corner from your office? How was the soup you ordered at the nearby restaurant prepared? If you want to be absolutely sure from now on that each meal you eat is going to be Clean, get into the good habit of taking your food with you. When you cook Clean fare at home, make extra portions and pack them into smaller containers to take along to work or wherever you may go during your day. An entire chapter in this book deals with strategies that make carrying wholesome foods easier, and don't for a moment assume that you are going to be the only one carrying your lunch to work. Even the famous Dr. Oz, author of the *YOU!* series, carries leftovers to work in his backpack. He munches his meals in hospital stairwells between cardiac surgeries. Now if that busy man can do it, I feel certain you can too!

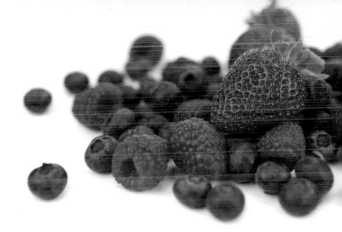

DEPEND ON FRESH FRUITS, VEGETABLES AND WHOLE GRAINS FOR COMPLEX CARBOHYDRATES

Not long ago, carbohydrates nearly did us in! An entire industry sprouted and blossomed overnight in response to other diets that claimed magical weight loss when carbohydrates were removed from the diet. It might make sense to cut carbohydrates completely from the diet. Carbohydrates are not essential because they are not part of cellular structure. In fact, you could manage without them since you can get energy, which carbohydrates provide, from protein and fat alone. But I've tried it, and my experience without these carbon/hydrogen molecules left me a blithering idiot! I could barely dial a number on my phone. The feeling was horrible – I felt robbed of all energy, which is something I normally have in abundance. I was clearly depriving my brain of the fuel it depended upon.

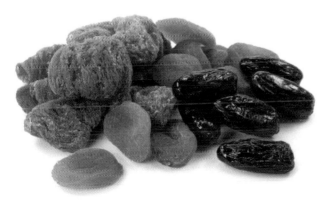

A better approach to consuming carbohydrates is acknowledging that there are two very different kinds of carbohydrates: simple carbohydrates found in sugar and refined foods (bad carbohydrates) and complex carbohydrates found in whole grains (good carbohydrates). Carbohydrates from some fruits and vegetables are simple, but I consider these to be part of the complex group because they occur naturally, and because they contain much needed vitamins, nutrients and enzymes. Once ingested, these energy-giving units behave and are processed very differently from each other. Simple sugars – you might know them as the little guys that sweeten your morning coffee or your breakfast cereal – tear down the body as they are processed. Not only do they remove B vitamins from the body, simple sugars also break down the skeleton by upsetting the delicate calcium-phosphorus balance in bones and teeth. Sugars such as these also wreak havoc on the hormonal chemistry of digestion by causing enormous spikes in blood sugar levels, which insulin must then mop up. However, insulin can do only so much in the face of the vast quantities of sugar that North Americans swill. When insulin cannot keep up with the sheer volume of refined sugar consumed daily by humans, the inevitable result is fat, obesity, diabetes in all its forms, heart disease, stroke and cancer.

On the other side of the spectrum, complex carbohydrates take their time being processed in the belly. As they work their way down the lazy river known as your intestines, a lot happens to help them break down. Complex carbohydrates contain fiber, which takes time to process, and this is the main reason you feel full for a long time after you have eaten a bowl of oatmeal for breakfast. The longer it takes to process a complex carbohydrate, the slower the insulin response, which is a good thing. Another reason complex carbohydrates take longer to digest is that they are complicated molecules that need to be taken apart before the body can assimilate them, again prolonging the blood sugar response. You can see the pattern here: the longer things take to break down in your gut, the slower the insulin response, and the fuller, thinner and happier you are. Yes, it is

true. Maintaining steady blood sugar levels helps prevent weight gain. Additionally, complex carbohydrates contain an array of enzymes, minerals and vitamins essential for optimum health.

STICK TO PROPER PORTION SIZES

Nothing confuses people more than asking them to define the difference between a serving size and a portion size. Maybe you have never thought about it. Are you aware of the difference?

Not long ago, the United States Department of Agriculture (USDA) mandated nutritional and ingredient labeling for all packaged foods. This was the official start of the portion size nightmare. Nutrition labels are now required to list a serving size for every food. If you bother to read the label, this is very helpful information. That being said, nutrition labeling is loaded with tricks. Take that lunch-sized bag of chips for instance. It looks like it ought to be one serving size, but no one considers to check the back of the pack-

"Nutrition labeling is often loaded with tricks. That lunchtime bag of chips you just ate could have contained three servings!"

age to see if it really is only one serving. If you had, you would have discovered a shocking fact — that lunchtime bag of chips contains three servings! Not only that, you just ate the whole thing!

The food guides in North America ("MyPyramid" in the United States and "Canada's Food Guide" in Canada) specify servings — as in, consume five servings of grains each day — but offer no explanation as to what that serving size should be. For your sanity and mine, when you pick up a packaged food item, read the serving size first, then decide what is an appropriate amount of food to eat.

To make the correct decision about how much food is enough or too much for one sitting, I rely on my hands to guide me. I also listen to my stomach. I like to feel full enough to be satisfied, as in not hungry anymore, but not so full that I am uncomfortable. The Okinawa in Japan have a phrase called hara hachi bu, which means you should eat until your stomach is 80 percent full and no more. You can also rely on a method of chewing your food called "Fletcherizing," which is a technique of chewing every mouthful of food slowly and thoroughly, up to 32 times, enough to render the food nearly liquid in your mouth.

"Each morsel you eat, if you'd be wise.

Don't cause your blood pressure e'er to rise

By prizing your menu by its size,"

is a lyric made popular by this method's founder, Horace Fletcher, in the Victorian era. Fletcher's eating technique gives the brain time to pick up signals from the stomach, telling it that you are full. Most of us are already satiated enough when our stomachs are 80 percent full.

"Most of us are already satiated when our stomachs are 80 percent full."

A "HANDY" GUIDE

Using your hands as a guide for portions ensures that you are getting the proper amount of food for your body size. You can see that the portion sizes would not be the same for a burly 6'4" man and a petite 5' woman. Follow the guide below for every meal. If you would like an actual measurement, try using your hands as a guide once or twice, by actually placing the food in your hands. Transfer your handfuls into measuring cups or onto a kitchen scale, and record your findings for future use. You don't need to worry about exact amounts of grams and ounces – just use your hands as a guide. Remember – it's not an exact science!

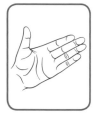

PORTIONS OF PROTEIN

You should be eating six servings of protein each day. A proper portion of meat or other protein is measured by what can fit in the palm of one hand.

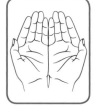

CARBS FROM FRUITS AND VEGETABLES

You should be eating from four to six servings of fresh produce each day. A proper portion of complex carbohydrates from fresh produce is measured by what can fit into two cupped hands.

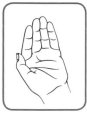

STARCHY COMPLEX CARBOHYDRATES

You should eat two to four servings of complex carbohydrates from whole grains or other starchy-carb sources each day. A proper portion of these complex carbohydrates is measured by what can fit in one cupped hand.

HEALTHY FATS

Gram for gram, about 18 percent of your diet should come from healthy fats from fish, nuts, seeds and healthy oils. Aim to include two or three servings of these foods in your diet each day to ensure you are getting enough healthy fats. A portion of healthy fat is one scant handful of nuts, or one to two tablespoons of healthy oil.

IN SUMMARY

You have now learned that nutrition plays the biggest role in maintaining optimum weight and health. You are also aware that nutrient-dense foods of the highest quality contribute to a lean, robustly functioning metabolism. A minimal 10 percent of your effort should be devoted to exercise and shaping your body into toned muscle. Proper nutrition and exercise work together to yield an improved version of what you may look and feel like now.

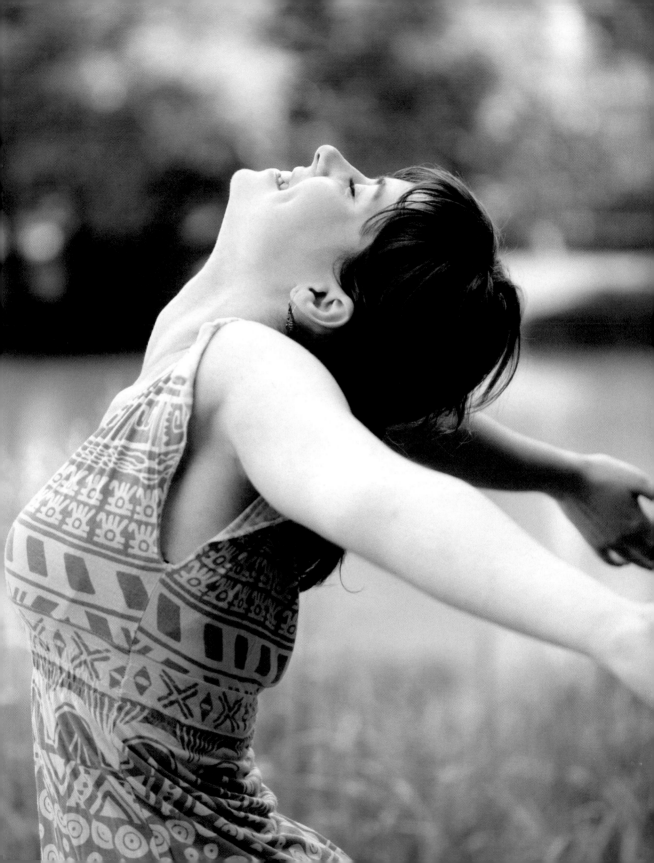

WHAT TO
EXPECT

2

WHAT TO EXPECT FROM EATING CLEAN

What should you expect from Eating Clean? Yet another new diet … why should this one differ from the plethora of diets that seem to emerge every week? The honest answer is that Eating Clean is the simple solution to your overweight dilemma. It is the hit-the-bull's-eye, stay-lean and feel-fantastic remedy to your weight problems. You can expect many positive changes to occur on both the inside and outside of your body right from the start.

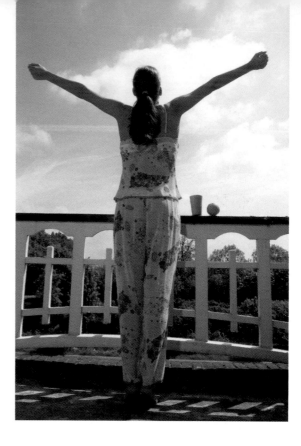

HOW DO YOU FEEL?

When you wake up in the morning, do you leap out of bed with energy, excited for your day to begin? Do you look in the mirror and remark on how clear your skin is? How bright your eyes are? How lean and fit your body looks? How strong and shiny your hair is? When you eat your breakfast, do you think about how every bite you are putting in your mouth contributes to this feeling of health and wellbeing? Do you go through your day with a steady, strong feeling of vitality and end the day with as much energy as when you arose?

Chances are, unless you are already Eating Clean, your day will not start like this. Most people seem to drag themselves out of bed in the morning, groggily stumble into the bathroom, and attempt to avoid the sight of themselves if possible. If they do catch a glimpse of their reflection in the mirror, they are not looking with kindness or pride, but rather with displeasure and disgust. In their mad rush to get ready, most people skip breakfast or hurriedly scarf down a donut or bowl of sugary cereal, and by 10 am they're crashing. Their day is a roller coaster of energy ups and downs, and by evening they are slumped in front of the TV eating potato chips. At bedtime these people lie in bed wondering why their physiques are no longer what they used to be and why weight loss seems like such an impossible task.

ENERGETIC AND FIT

I have good news for you. You *can* be that energetic, fit person, and it really doesn't matter how out of shape you are right now. Your first step is to look in your cupboards and in your refrigerator, throw any "dirty" foods in the garbage and fill up your kitchen with Clean eats. You should start noticing a change in the way you feel almost immediately. I can't repeat this enough: how your body looks and feels is predominantly the result of what you eat. Remember the Body Beautiful/Body Healthy Formula.

Dear Tosca...

TESTIMONIAL

Hi to all,

I thought I might share my success story with *The Eat-Clean Diet* and working out. I have lost a little over 200 lbs now, over a three-year journey. My life has dramatically changed! I had been overweight my entire life, until my wake-up call in 2005. I realized at that time, with profound regret, all of the time and activities I missed with my son because I was morbidly obese.

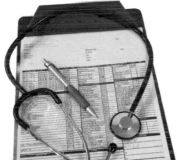

My life is so much better now. I feel very passionate about helping others become healthy, so I now teach classes in my gym – an amazing feat for a former couch potato! At work my patients (I am an RN) are more receptive to my advice because they know I have walked in their shoes. I have promised God that I will use every opportunity I get to encourage people to live healthy lives and avoid all the lifestyle-related illnesses I see in the hospital. The investment in Eating Clean and exercise is most definitely worth it! LIFE IS GOOD!

Terri Stewart

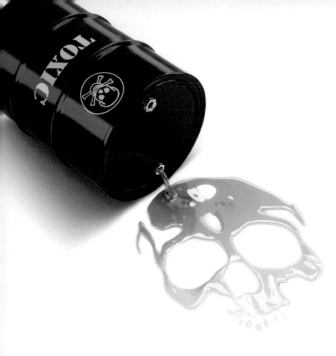

EAT-CLEAN CHANGES

I will get to the fat-loss discussion (which is what likely made you pick up this book), but fat loss, or more specifically, weight control, is only a small part of the numerous positive changes you will see once you start Eating Clean. You've heard the term "you are what you eat." Believe me, even though it's terribly cliché, it's true. If you fill yourself with chemical soup, preservatives, refined sugars and starches, and other trans- and saturated-fat-laden garbage then your whole body will suffer, not just your waistline. When you Eat Clean, the benefits are visible (and perceptible to you on the inside, too) from the top of your head to the tips of your toes.

EYES

Do the whites of your eyes normally have a yellowish tint? Do you ever see streaks of red or a cloudy appearance? Do your eyes appear dull? Within days of beginning to Eat Clean you will start getting compliments that your eyes look bright and alert. You will notice that bags, dark circles and puffiness start to disappear. Your eyes will appear clear and sparkly and the whites will be vivid. Some readers have even reported to me that their eyes feel less dry and irritated thanks to their Eat-Clean regimen. Keeping our diet free from foods that cause inflammation and stress in the body seems to help keep our eyes clear.

"If you fill yourself with chemical soup, preservatives, refined sugars and starches, and other trans- and saturated-fat-laden garbage then your whole body will suffer."

TEETH

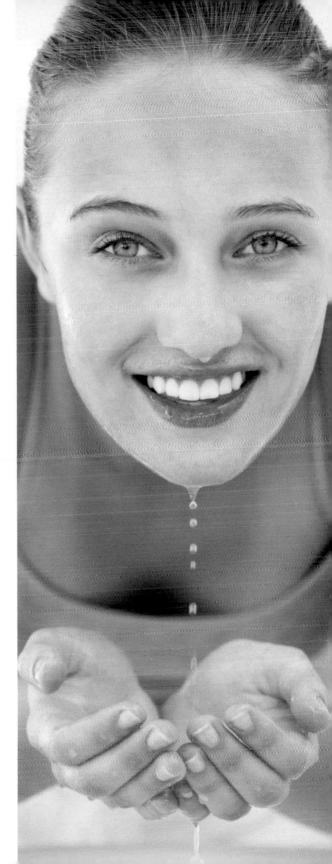

My entire family was happily surprised to discover that our dental health improved when we began to Eat Clean. We hadn't realized what a difference diet made in dental health until our dentist asked us what we'd been doing differently! The truth is, the health of your teeth and gums has more to do with the food you eat than your brushing habits, as archeologists and medical anthropologists have discovered over time. Isolated societies all around the world had good dental health until they were introduced to processed and refined foods, at which point their dental health immediately began to deteriorate. According to Dr. Weston Price DDS, author of *Nutrition and Physical Degeneration*, even without the benefit of toothbrushes and toothpaste, isolate communities who ate abundant plant food, lean protein and no added sugar had no cavities! They did not need braces or orthodontia of any kind because sugar was not part of their diet. No wonder my dentist noticed similar positive changes in my mouth and the mouths of my family.

SKIN

When you begin Eating Clean you will find that your blemishes disappear, while your skin becomes less dry and starts to take on a healthy glow. My skin was never one of my strong points, but since I began Eating Clean, women stop and ask me what my secret to great skin is. They think that I must slather myself with expensive creams and potions. When I am asked, I happily share that my glowing skin comes from what I put *in* my body and not what I put *on* it.

I was recently surprised to read that a celebrity I admire, Angelina Jolie, Eats Clean. When I saw her at the Academy Awards in 2009, she looked so radiant that I wondered to myself whether she was following my eating plan. Her skin looked a lot like mine, which is why I suspected she might be on to what I had discovered by Eating Clean. I realize that she has stellar genetics, but it's nice to know part of her beauty is a result of Eating Clean!

HAIR AND NAILS

Strong, healthy nails and radiant, lustrous hair are two bonus benefits to Eating Clean. Remember that every cell of your body is created from what you put inside it, including the tiniest cells that make up your hair and nails. Have you always had trouble growing nails? Eating Clean is the solution. Does your hair look dull and break easily? Eating Clean will change that. High-quality food, especially protein and essential oils, make for beautiful hair and nails. It's as easy as improving your nutrition intake by Eating Clean.

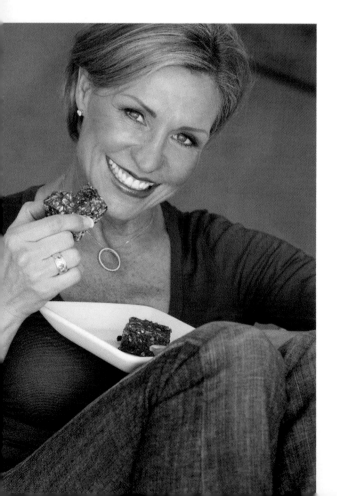

"High-quality food, especially protein and essential oils, make for beautiful hair and nails."

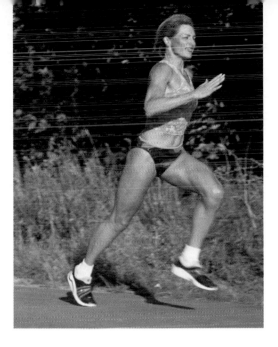

> "An abundance of energy is yours for the taking if you rely on Eating Clean."

CONSTANT ENERGY

For me, constant energy was one of the best results. Before Eating Clean, I would go on sugar highs and then drop down so low I would literally pass out. Your energy swings may not be quite this extreme, but you probably know what I mean by the mid-afternoon slump. That slump, my friend, is caused by unstable blood sugar. One of the many reasons Eating Clean works so well as a fat-loss diet is that it keeps your blood sugar levels stable, which in turn stabilizes energy patterns and prevents cravings.

I love being a totally reenergized person who can not only get up at 6 am and do 45 minutes of cardio-vascular exercise, but carry on to train with weights, look after my family, work a demanding job and still be motivated enough for fun and creative pursuits. I know that I have been able to super-charge my life entirely thanks to Eating Clean.

The regular consumption of small meals (every two-and-a-half to three hours) throughout the day prevents you from feeling sluggish and from overeating. You don't feel like a zombie after a blood-sugar drop either. You feel a steady, solid amount of energy that lasts from the moment you wake up until you get ready for bed.

Have you ever looked at people jogging down the street or at kids running in the park and wished you had their vitality? An abundance of energy is yours for the taking if you rely on Eating Clean. If laziness has been holding you back from your exercise program, reach for your runners hidden at the back of the closet and renew your gym membership right away, because soon you'll have so much steady energy that you'll need a place to burn it off!

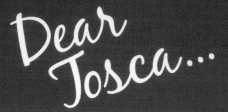

Dear Tosca,

My last few years were terrible health wise. I've been having digestive issues for the past three years. I was finally diagnosed with IBS (Irritable Bowel Syndrome). I was going out of my mind trying to find food to eat without getting the nasty bloating, gas and nausea. As if that wasn't enough, I started having coccyx pain (without falling, I still don't know why). Then came the thorax/back pain. A few months after, the doctor announced that I might have Multiple Sclerosis. All that, and I was having non-stop migraines and headaches! Needless to say, I was about to break down. Instead, I decided to get my life back in control.

I started Eating Clean and joined a gym in September, of 2008. My only goal at that point was to stop feeling sick all of the time. Right away my life changed for the better – no more bloating and plenty of energy!

My weight had been 134 since I was a teenager, and I can't remember weighing any less than that. I do remember weighing 146 at one point. By December, 2008 (three months after I starting Eating Clean), my weight had dropped to 125! I couldn't believe it!

I'd never felt so good, and my confidence increased while my weight decreased!

I started to train more seriously. My goal is now to get my muscles all toned up. I train three to four times a week with weights and cardio, plus yoga and a class at my gym.

Now it is March and I weigh 119 lbs. I still have work to do on my butt, but I'm getting there. My abs are starting to show and I can't wait to have my six-pack. I religiously read my *Oxygen* magazine every month, which keeps me motivated!

I have to say that discovering *The Eat-Clean Diet* has been the best thing to happen to me in a while. Eating Clean has really improved my health, way of life, and made me become a better me. I'm now 30 years old and have never been so healthy!

Josee Perreault

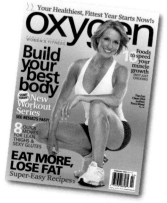

A NATURAL DETOX

I keep hearing about detox drinks, powders, potions and diets, but when you Eat Clean none of this stuff is necessary. Eating Clean is a natural detox, especially when you consume organic foods. Your body does not want to store any garbage in your fat cells, which is where toxins are stored. It wants to be pure and uncontaminated. So when you start Eating Clean, the way nature intended, your body is grateful for the chance to rid itself of unnatural poisons.

If you have been eating or drinking a lot of chemicals, preservatives, caffeine, alcohol and other damaging foods, you might have a couple of tough days before the positive changes arrive. If you feel irritable, tired and headachy, you should be glad! This means your body is getting rid of the toxins you've been pumping into it. The good news is that after your body rids itself of these horrors, you will feel better than you have in many, many years, if ever.

LEAN PHYSIQUE

Here is the part you've been waiting for! Along with your new beautiful skin, shiny, strong hair and nails, bright eyes, gorgeous smile, boundless energy and general feeling of wellbeing, you will lose any excess fat and develop a lean, lithe body. Eating Clean is eating the natural way. By nourishing your body with nutrient-rich foods, you will finally arrive at your physical peak.

People often ask me if they should Eat Clean even though they do not have weight to lose. You need to understand that Eating Clean is not a "diet." It is not only for fat and weight loss. Eating Clean brings you to your optimal weight, no matter what size you start out. So while most people want to lose excess fat, and it helps them do that, Eating Clean also helps underweight people gain, and helps those at their optimal weight stay there but live healthier lives. If you are interested in losing weight, you can

"Eating Clean is a natural detox, especially when you consume organic foods."

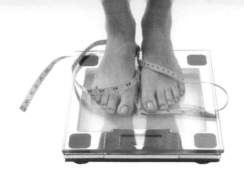

anticipate an average weight loss of three pounds each week, but some people have said that they lost 15 pounds in the first week. Your rate of weight loss will depend on your starting point. If you are obese you will lose weight faster. If you are only five pounds overweight, you may lose three of those pesky pounds in the first week!

You don't have to exercise in order to achieve your optimal weight while Eating Clean, but if you do work out regularly, eating this way will help you create the physique you truly desire. It is a common misconception that if you work out regularly, you will have a lean body, and that is simply not true, especially as we age. Recall the Body Beautiful/Body Healthy Formula. The vast majority – a full 80% – of the way your physique looks and feels comes from what goes into your mouth, so make better food choices and your ideal physique will be yours!

Dear Tosca...

TESTIMONIAL

Dear Tosca,

I just wanted to write you to say thanks so much for helping my family and me make changes!

My teenage daughter has struggled with her weight for years and I have yo-yo'd for the last four years after losing 45 lbs. My daughter has lost 36 lbs to date and I have lost 20 lbs. We both know that this is a lifestyle change, not a diet!

My husband is an OB/GYN and has started telling his patients about your book to help them with their weight struggles – he is a firm believer in it! I sell a line of clothing (at home parties) and I take your book with me to all of them. I have referred so many people (I have lost count!) to buy your book and make a change. Everyone wants to know what I have done, so I share it! I thank God every day for helping us find your book and make a change for better health!

Thank you so much,
Donna Boyd

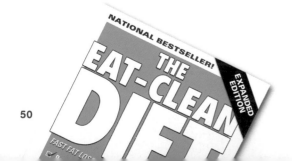

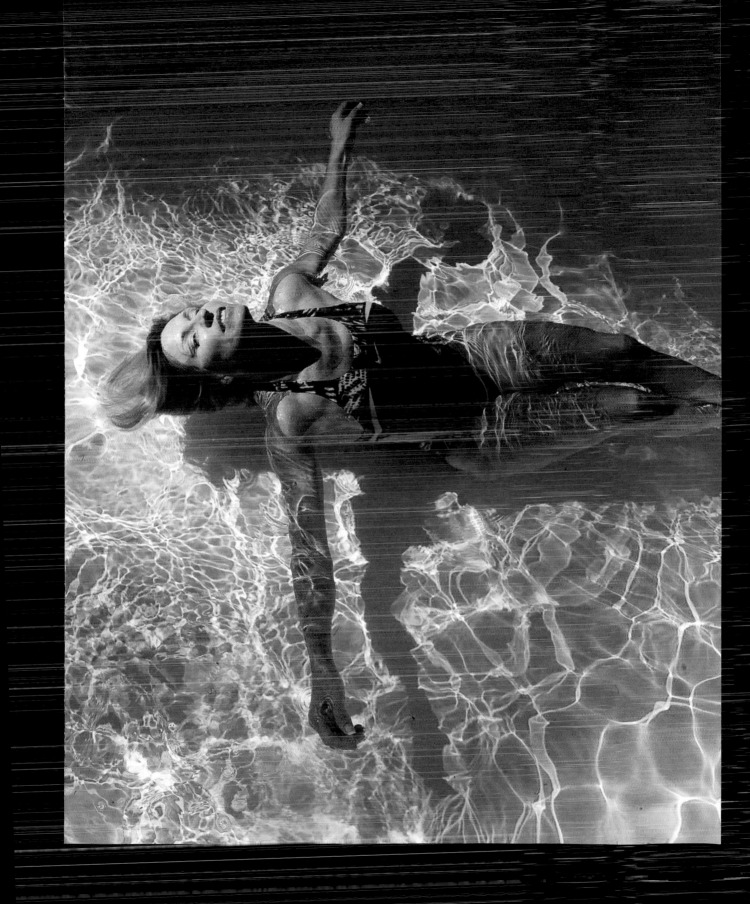

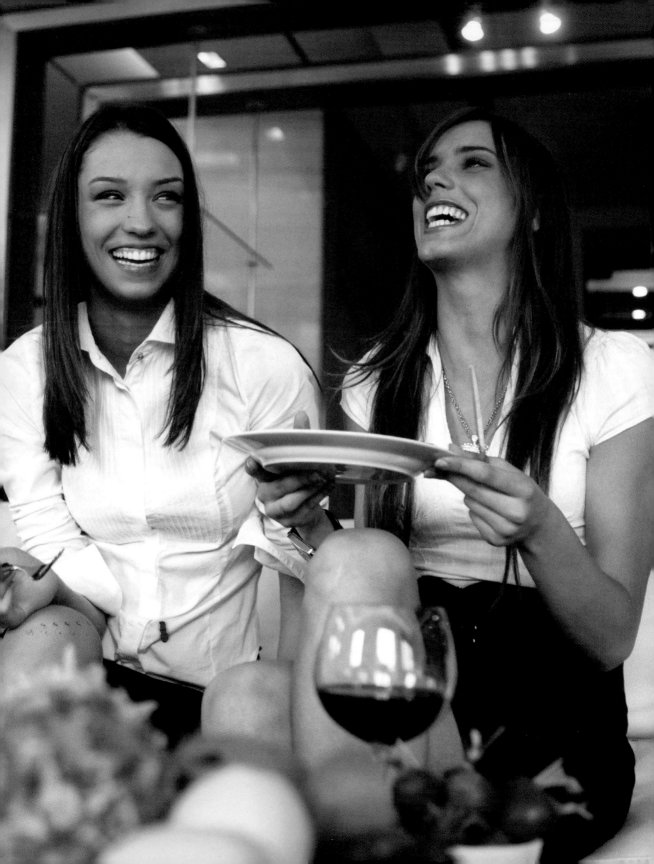

> "We do so many things to damage our metabolism. We skip meals, eat the wrong foods and rely on ridiculous diet trends in an effort to shed weight."

INCREASED METABOLISM

We do so many things to damage our metabolism. We skip meals, eat the wrong foods and rely on ridiculous diet trends in an effort to shed weight. I know plenty of women (and men!) who barely eat a thing and yet cannot lose weight. Why? Because they've been dieting for so long, their poor bodies think they're living in some vast wasteland where food is perennially scarce. I was surprised to discover when I began Eating Clean that I actually ate more than I ever had before and still lost weight. People are shocked at how much food I eat, but I Eat Clean and the food is practically incinerated in my body, because it is so pure and free of chemicals.

When you Eat Clean, your body does not have to create fat cells to store unrecognizable substances. You don't overeat because you consume the ideal amount of food for your body size. Because your body receives quality nourishment every two-and-a-half to three hours, it thinks you've moved from the starving wastelands of Siberia to the opulent farms of Shangri La, and it stops hoarding your fat. How great is that?

GOOD HEALTH

I'm not a doctor and I don't claim to be one, but I have heard from so many people who no longer rely on obesity-related medications, who reduced or eliminated the need for insulin, who have found major health problems improving or disappearing entirely once they started Eating Clean, that I cannot ignore it. I have not performed a scientific study and I'm not going to make any claims here, but based on what thousands of people have told me about their own improved health, I bet that if you bring this book to your doctor, he or she will be very happy you've decided to adopt Eating Clean into your life.

And if you have made such positive health changes, I invite you to send me your doctor's address so he or she can receive a complimentary copy of any one of my books in *The Eat-Clean Diet* series.

The bottom line is that Eating Clean gave me an entirely new life. Before I began this lifestyle, I could never have imagined having the energy I do now. Old friends and family tell me I look better at age 50 than I did at 25. In fact, some say I look better now than I ever did before. Eating Clean is not the only cause of my happiness, but it sure helped turn a miserable, depressed, lethargic, unhealthy middle-aged woman into a healthy, vibrant, radiant, fit and energetic one. I know beyond a shadow of a doubt that it will do the same for you.

MOTIVATION

Ready, set, go! These are the three simple words that have the power to launch a highly trained athlete into top speed in pursuit of athletic records, dominance and personal achievement. When Jamaican sprinting phenomenon Usain Bolt exploded out of the blocks at the 2008 Summer Olympics in Beijing, his motivation was, in his words, "I wanted to be champion and that's what I came out to do." There was no question about his intent or his result. He destroyed existing 100-meter records and the notion that all successful sprinters had to be short and stocky. Bolt, at 6'5", took no notice of that. Motivation to win was all he considered.

Imagine what you could accomplish in your future should you decide to harness the power of motivation! We are not all aspiring Olympians, not by a long shot, but in each of us lies the human desire to live a significant life. It has often been said that with purpose and motivation in hand, all else becomes but a minor obstacle, no matter how daunting the task.

You might consider making changes in your life now, because you are fed up with how you look and feel – this is motivation enough. But what if you are that person who cannot fly on a plane, because he or she is too large to fit in the seat? Perhaps you are the person who cannot tie up his or her shoes, because you can't bend down to do so. Are your hips and knees aching because you have asked your body to support too much weight? Is your health marred by constant illness? Motivation to change may come from any of these factors, which boil down to the glaring fact that you want to enjoy a better quality of life. With nearly 70 percent of North Americans overweight or obese, I would argue that there are many of us who would consider the above reasons as motivation for change.

I once spent too much time lying on a couch with anti-foods, destroying any purpose I might have had in my life. Once I discovered how easily I could change all that, simply by altering what I was shoveling into my mouth, you couldn't stop me from making changes. Motivation poured out of me, helping me regain my health and my physique. I was infused with an intense desire to be better than I had ever been, a passion that continues to burn today. I wanted to run harder, swim faster, lift heavier and write down everything that I had ever stored in my heart – apparently there were many words! I have transformed my life from ordinary, where I did not want to face another day, into extraordinary – blossoming with purpose, where I often feel that there are not enough hours in a day. For me, no day is a monotonous parade of empty hours. Each day brings excitement, possibilities and purpose. This keeps me motivated to do my best.

Try with every cell in your being to live a purposeful life. Sift through your experiences to tease out the notes that sing to you, the memories and people in your life that really matter. Hold them in your heart and make these relationships and moments, along with your personal goals and ambitions, the reasons why you are going to change for good this time. You may wish to simply be able to play with your children and walk down a flight of stairs or you may strive for loftier heights. Without motivating factors nothing will happen – it will only be a wish rather than an actuality. Wishing and hoping accomplishes nothing. They are dead in the water pursuits, unless you act on them and make them your new reality.

Usain Bolt is a prime athletic specimen, who, at 21 years of age, is one of the youngest 100-meter Olympic champions in history. At this early stage of his career, it is safe to assume his best years are yet to come. His motivating force is the urgent drive to test himself – and win. What is your motivating force?

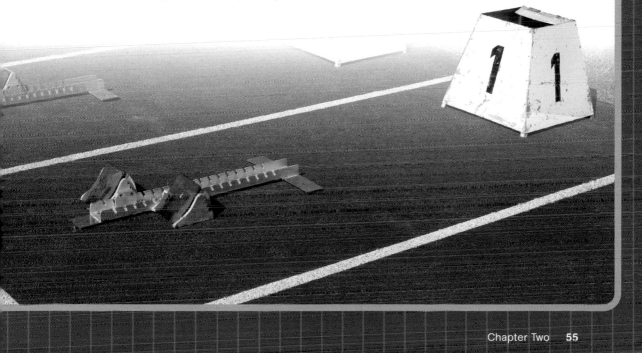

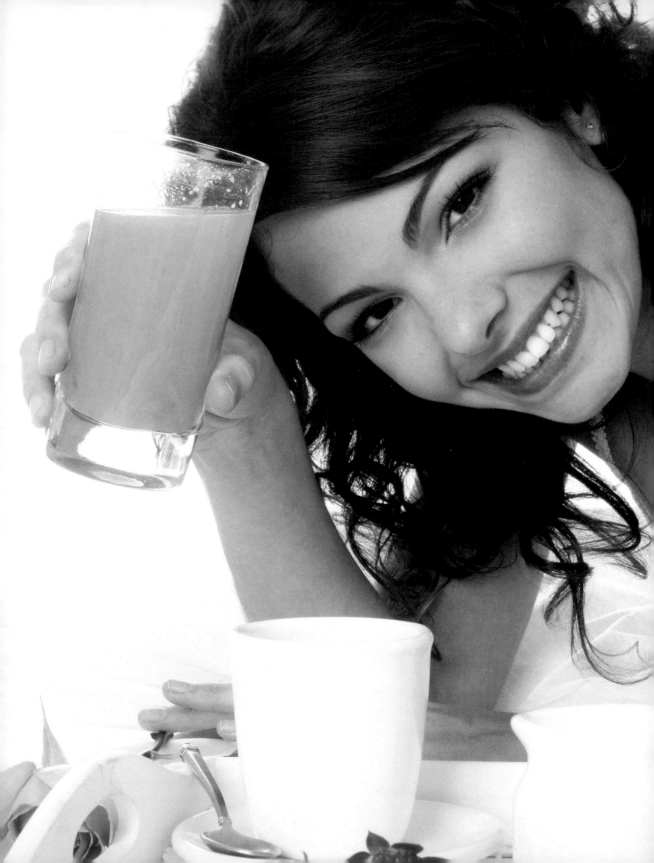

BREAKFAST: AN ENTIRE CHAPTER

3

It is not difficult to work out that breakfast is the most important meal of your day, as I have devoted an entire chapter of this book to it. In my mind, the food I enjoy first thing in the morning sets the tone for both my productivity and eating habits for the rest of the day. I spend time thinking about what kind of nutrients I want to place on my plate and how I can round out the meal with protein. I see every meal, particularly breakfast, as an opportunity to arm my body and consequently my health with disease-fighting, bodybuilding weaponry. This arsenal comes in the form of complex carbohydrates from whole grains, fruits and vegetables accompanied by protein, which I happily consume at breakfast time. I consider myself a mealtime opportunist and I like it!

Since I am the meal planner, chef and bottle washer in my house, I lead the charge for making a healthy breakfast for my entire family. What I eat, they eat. No child of mine is going to leave the house hungry if I can help it. Unfortunately, the same cannot be said for the many children who go to school hungry on a daily basis. When children leave the house without eating breakfast they show up at school hungry and irritable. Starting the day this way interferes with normal brain and physical function. The choice we make to eat breakfast or not has implications for our families and for ourselves throughout the day. The consequences of skipping breakfast include fatigue, the inability to concentrate, irritability, mood and behavioral problems, and poor health to name a few. Hardly a good start to the day!

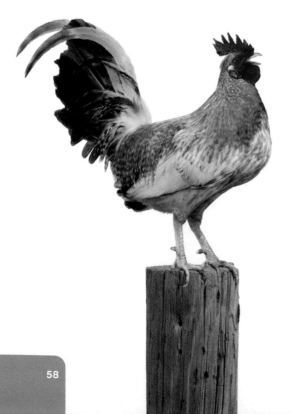

"The choice we make to eat breakfast or not has implications for our families and for ourselves throughout the day."

> "Think of how good you feel once you have enjoyed a bowl of steaming oatmeal topped with fresh fruit and rounded out with scrambled egg whites."

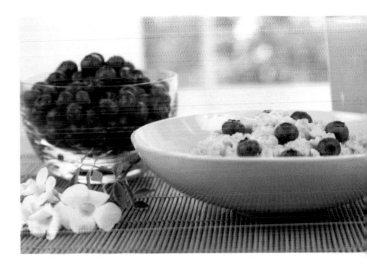

WHAT I KNOW NOW

Before I learned about Eating Clean, I would either skip breakfast in a misguided attempt to reduce my daily calorie intake or I would eat foods saturated in sugar and unhealthy fats. I know many people continue to eat this way. Breakfast is the most skipped meal of any. I was often sick and was, at different times, both too thin and too heavy. From the outside this may have had physical effects, but on the inside losing and gaining the same pounds took its toll on my emotional wellbeing. I was often depressed. I am still stunned to learn how food can affect us positively or negatively in so powerful a manner. In fact, North America is being swept by a wave of depression and other aberrant behaviors, particularly among today's youth. I firmly believe that much of this can be attributed to poor nutrition. Think of how good you feel once you have enjoyed a bowl of steaming oatmeal topped with fresh fruit and rounded out with scrambled egg whites. A breakfast like that can't fail to deliver health and a feeling of general wellness. I know from experience! I live this feeling every day since that is my staple morning meal.

Breakfast is a way of setting the standard for all of your forthcoming meals each day. Once you have upped the ante on this meal you'll hardly want to waste your efforts by gobbling greasy garbage at your next meal. Too many of us squeeze breakfast in by way of a sugary toaster pastry or rush through the drive-thru on the way to work. You can't hope to find quality nutrition in these places and you can't realistically trust the health claims being made about a seemingly sensible yogurt parfait with granola. Read the label for a reality check. (If you can't pronounce it, do you really want to eat it?)

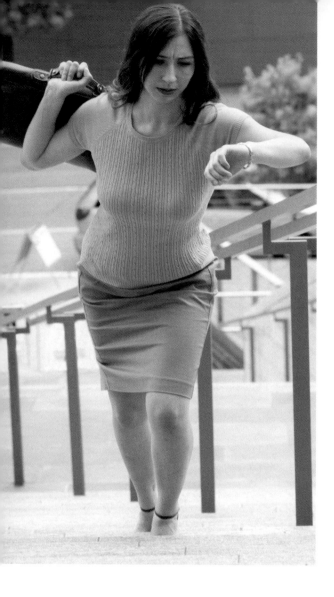

IT'S NOT JUST ABOUT EXCESS WEIGHT

Being overweight is only one negative outcome of overeating. The far more important effect is your deteriorating health and consequently your lost productivity. Skipping breakfast factors heavily into this decline, since it is a missed opportunity, as I like to say, to bolster your body's self-defense mechanisms, particularly in the morning when many of us need to function efficiently at school, home or work. Students who don't have access to a quality morning meal suffer greatly at school. In her article "Overfeeding the Future," Kelly Brownell claims, "It is well documented that poor diet affects cognitive and intellectual performance in undernourished children." The American Dietetic Association would agree, stating that, "Eating breakfast encourages increased concentration and problem-solving skills throughout the day." The cost of poor nutrition, including skipping breakfast, can be measured in millions of dollars. "Researchers estimate obesity-related health care costs in the US alone to be $75 million, with taxpayers financing half of these costs through Medicare and Medicaid," writes Brownell in the same article. If 25 percent of our daily nutrition is attained through breakfast, the enormous expense taxpayers are bearing can be, in large part, attributed to the poor attitude many of us have to this first meal of the day.

"Skipping breakfast factors heavily into your deteriorating health and lost productivity."

THE GROUCHIES SET IN

I have often said that if I am not sufficiently watered and fed, I turn into a bear and an unpleasant one at that. My family members are the same. We know that the Grouchies set in swiftly if we don't eat regularly or start our day with an Eat-Clean breakfast. I can hardly operate my own telephone if I have not had my necessary morning start. Substantiating my own experience, innumerable studies on the subject suggest everyone, from the cradle to walker, benefits from eating breakfast. "Eating breakfast is very important for the brain and the body first thing in the morning," according to Los Angeles registered dietitian Gail Frank, spokesperson for the American Dietetic Association. "Breakfast skippers often feel tired, restless or irritable in the morning." If you are a Breakfast Skipper, you may be one of those irritable people!

FOOD FOR YOUR BRAIN

During sleep your body acquires much-needed rest, allowing it to restore itself in preparation for another day. Unless you are eating throughout the night, this is also a time when your body receives little or no food and water intake. Your entire digestive system uses this chance to clean you up and take a break from processing your food. Your brain goes on idle during this rest time, although I am by no means implying that it is doing nothing! That being said, the brain is not receiving much in the way of its favorite food – glucose – either.

Your morning meal is the perfect time to break the fast your body and brain experienced during the night. Depending on your sleeping and eating habits, this "fast" could last anywhere from six to twelve hours, leaving your brain very hungry – no wonder we wake up a little groggy in the morning! Do not mistake the brain's need for glucose, a simple sugar, as an opportunity to fuel up on white poison. Refined white sugar is most definitely an anti-food and in my opinion, has no place in any diet. Reach for high quality foods such as whole grains, fresh fruits, vegetables and protein instead.

"Refined white sugar is most definitely an anti-food and in my opinion, has no place in any diet."

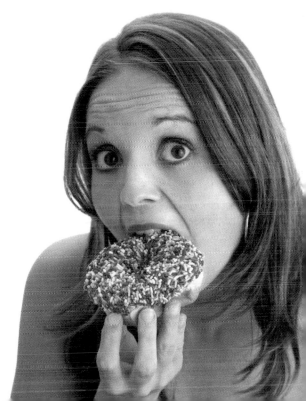

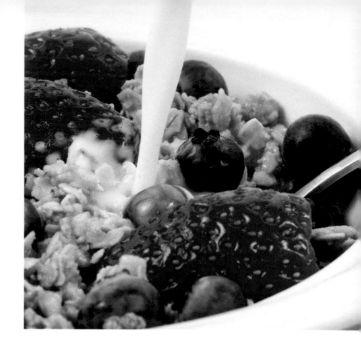

> "Breakfast should provide one quarter of your nutritional requirements each day, even though it is only one of your six daily meals."

EAT MORE – I'LL SAY IT AGAIN

After a good night's rest it is time to break the fast, as the word "breakfast" implies. Even if your brain has not realized how hungry it is, your stomach will really appreciate this meal, and you will no doubt hear and feel what is going on down there. The growling noise that emanates from your tummy is the sound of your stomach walls trying to digest what is not there. Hunger pangs accompany this racket, prompting you to make a beeline for the kitchen. Although I have already suggested that the key to weight loss is not eating less, but rather more of the right kinds of foods, I gamely run the risk of repeating myself to reinforce this principle now. Eating breakfast helps you to both lose and maintain an ideal body weight. This may sound counterintuitive, but study after study has proven it to be true. Simply keeping your stomach moderately full helps curb intense hunger, in the face of which you might be tempted to eat anything in sight without consideration for whether it is nutritious or unhealthy, too much or too little. Additionally, breakfast prevents you from bingeing later in the day when your hunger becomes unbearable should you decide to skip this meal.

Even though breakfast is only one of your six daily meals, it should ideally provide one quarter of your nutritional requirements each day. This is a hefty load of nutrition to be missing out on if you regularly skip breakfast! Those who skip breakfast, because of a lack of time or an attempt to lose weight, miss out on essential nutrients. Studies have shown that people who don't eat breakfast are unlikely to make up for these lost nutrients at other meals. This can have a negative effect on both short and long-term health.

BREAKFAST WITH ME

Forget about rushing out the door to get to work on time. You now know that behavior won't cut it any longer. Instead, come into my kitchen and follow me as I describe my morning breakfast routine. Keep in mind that I too am a busy person with five children, two dogs, a husband, book and magazine deadlines, appearances, travel, a household to manage and an aging parent. Oh, and let's not forget workouts! I don't make excuses about breakfast and I won't let you do it either.

Upon waking, I head into to my kitchen and drink two or three glasses (about one liter) of water. While I am sipping I put on the kettle for coffee or tea. Coffee brewing, I then unload the dishwasher since it appears I am the only person capable of doing so (siigghhh!). I set the table for whoever happens to be joining us for breakfast (anywhere from two to 24 family members and guests), depending on the occasion. If I am really pushed for time, which seems to be a common problem for people in the morning, I simply measure out half a cup of dry oats into a

Dear Tosca...

TESTIMONIAL

Tosca,

I just wanted to thank you for writing *The Eat-Clean Diet*. I am a 43-year-old mother of two who has been into fitness her whole life but, knew nothing about the diet aspect. After having my two kids and buying my first pair of size 11 jeans, I came across your book in the grocery store (as I was going to buy junk food, I might add). I thought I would read it and see what it's all about. It has changed my whole way of eating and thinking.

I just bought my first pair of size 1 jeans! I have NEVER worn size 1! I am now in my mid-40s and I'm in the best shape of my life. Swimsuit season ... watch out!

I am very grateful for your inspiration!

Best,
Vicki Dixon
Columbus, OH

cereal bowl. Then I pour one cup of boiling water over the oats and cover the bowl with a plate so it can "cook," while I prepare the rest of my breakfast and get ready for work. In the meantime, I am also boiling a dozen eggs so I can eat these throughout the day (an excellent protein source). I don't eat all 12 yolks but I will have one or two each day; the rest I feed to my dogs. I can get all of the above done in less than 15 minutes and I honestly do not find this to be a difficult commitment.

On some days I still have time to enjoy a cup of coffee with my husband and answer emails while life chugs along. I haven't shortchanged my health by skipping out on breakfast. Instead, I feel like a healthy, normal person, a feeling I did not often have in those years before Eating Clean.

I expect you will be wondering how I manage to prepare an Eat-Clean breakfast when I am on the road or in the air. You do not have to be at home to Eat Clean. A change in geography does not prevent me from sticking to my Eat-Clean principles – in fact, I have prepared much more on this subject for you in a later chapter. On mornings when I am absent from my kitchen I have developed a plan: I pre-measure baggies of dry oats mixed with unsweetened dried fruits, flaxseed, wheat germ, bee pollen and protein powder. I prepare enough to get me through however many days I will be away from home. I put one in my purse or carry-on and the rest in my suitcase. When it's time to eat I can easily get a cup of hot water from virtually anywhere in an airport or city, mix it with my pre-portioned oatmeal breakfast, and eat. If I am eating my "baggie breakfast" on the plane, I simply request boiling water from the flight attendant and I'm set to jet.

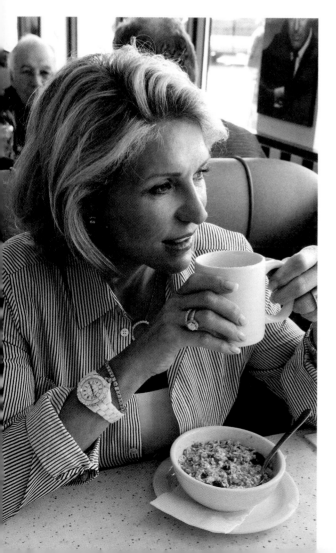

"A change in geography does not prevent me from sticking to my Eat-Clean principles."

COMMON FOODS AND FIBER COUNTS

(The amount of fiber in most packaged foods is found on the nutrition label.)

Fruit	Amount	Total Fiber (g)
Apple, with skin	1 medium	4.0 g
Apricot	3 medium	3.0 g
Apricots, dried	5 halves	1.5 g
Banana	1 medium	3.1 g
Blueberries	1 cup	3.5 g
Cantaloupe, cubed	1 cup	1.4 g
Figs, dried	2 medium	1.6 g
Grapefruit	½ medium	0.7 g
Orange, navel	1 medium	3.1 g
Peach	1 medium	1.5 g
Peaches, dried	3 halves	3.3 g
Pear	1 medium	5.1 g
Plum	1 medium	0.9 g
Raisins	1.5 oz box	1.6 g
Raspberries	1 cup	8.0 g
Strawberries, sliced	1 cup	3.3 g

MORE

COMMON FOODS AND FIBER COUNTS

(The amount of fiber in most packaged foods is found on the nutrition label.)

Vegetables	Amount	Total Fiber (g)
Avocado (fruit)	1 medium	13.5 g
Beet greens	1 cup	3.4 g
Beets, cooked	1 cup	1.4 g
Bok choy, cooked	1 cup	1.7 g
Broccoli, cooked	1 cup	5.2 g
Brussels sprouts	1 cup	3.3 g
Cabbage, cooked	1 cup	2.8 g
Carrot	1 medium	1.7 g
Carrot, cooked	1 cup	4.7 g
Cauliflower, cooked	1 cup	3.3 g
Celery	1 cup	1.5 g
Collard greens	1 cup	4.2 g
Corn, sweet	1 cup	3.7 g
Green beans	1 medium stalk	0.6 g
Kale, cooked	1 cup	2.6 g
Onions, raw	1 cup	1.6 g
Peas, cooked	1 cup	8.8 g
Peppers, sweet	1 cup	1.6 g
Popcorn, air-popped	3 cup	3.5 g
Potato, baked w/skin	1 medium	3.8 g
Spinach, cooked	1 cup	4.3 g
Summer squash, cooked	1 cup	2.4 g
Sweet potato, baked w/skin	1 medium	3.8 g
Swiss chard, cooked	1 cup	3.6 g
Tomato	1 medium	1.5 g
Winter squash, cooked	1 cup	2.0 g
Zucchini, cooked	1 cup	2.4 g

COMMON FOODS AND FIBER COUNTS

(The amount of fiber in most packaged foods is found on the nutrition label.)

Cereal, Grains, Pasta	Amount	Total Fiber (g)
Bran cereal (All-Bran)	½ cup	10.0 g
Bread, whole wheat	1 slice	3.0 g
Oats, rolled dry	1 cup	8.0 g
Pasta, whole wheat, cooked	1 cup	3.9 g
Rice, dry brown	1 cup	6.5 g

Beans, Nuts, Seeds	Amount	Total Fiber (g)
Almonds	1 oz	3.3 g
Black beans, cooked	1 cup	15.0 g
Cashews	1 oz	0.9 g
Flaxseeds	3 Tbsp	8.4 g
Garbanzo beans, cooked	1 cup	12.5 g
Kidney beans, cooked	1 cup	11.3 g
Lentils, cooked	1 cup	15.6 g
Lima beans, cooked	1 cup	13.2 g
Peanuts	1 oz	2.4 g
Pistachio nuts	1 oz	2.9 g
Pumpkin seeds	1 oz	1.1 g
Soybeans, cooked	1 cup	7.6 g
Sunflower seeds	1 oz	3.0 g
Walnuts	1 oz	1.9 g

WHY OATMEAL?

Your grandmother had the right idea when she encouraged you to eat your oats. When cooked into a thick, hot breakfast cereal, this humble grain sticks to your ribs. What does that mean? It means oatmeal is loaded with soluble and insoluble plant fibers. These require a great deal of effort on the part of your digestive system to break down, thus encouraging a prolonged feeling of fullness. These fibers provide bulk, which helps to keep your tummy satisfied for longer. They also help moderate blood sugar levels. Avoiding blood sugar highs and lows is ideal for hormone health, as your pancreas is exhausted from mopping up the deadly white-sugar garbage you have previously been eating. Give it a break!

Oatmeal is so good for you that it was recently given the food version of an Academy Award. Thanks to its high concentration of beneficial plant fibers, oatmeal is one of the first foods ever recognized by the Food and Drug Administration as having a medical benefit to human health. Most North Americans are chronically under-fibered, consuming only a few of the 25 to 30 recommended grams each day. Children need to consume the number of their age plus five grams of fiber every day. North Americans 100 years ago ate 10 times as much fiber as they do today! I wonder if that is why we are so uptight?

I eat oatmeal or a version of oats for breakfast almost every day. If I eat my breakfast at 7 am, and that breakfast contains oatmeal followed by egg whites, I won't be hungry until about 10 am. It is the power of oatmeal at work that keeps me full and free from erratic blood glucose swings. I am no longer the grumpy bear.

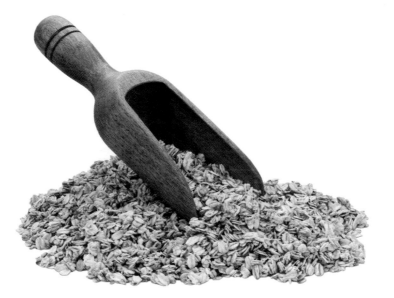

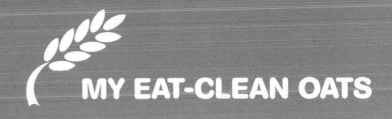

MY EAT-CLEAN OATS

MY EAT-CLEAN OATS AND WHAT I PUT ON THEM

Step 1: Add 1 cup of hot water to ½ cup uncooked oats

Step 2: Place a plate over your bowl to let oats "cook" for about 10 minutes.

When the oats are ready, top with any or all of the following:

* 2 tablespoons coarsely ground flaxseed
* 2 tablespoons wheat germ
* 2 tablespoons bee pollen

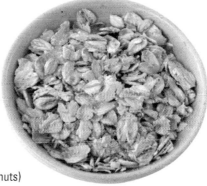

Feel free to add any one of the following:

* ½ cup mixed fresh (or frozen) berries
* ½ cup sliced fresh banana
* ¼ cup unsweetened dried cranberries or raisins
* ½ cup unsweetened applesauce
* 2 tablespoons slivered almonds (or any type of raw unsalted nuts)

You can enhance the flavor of your bowl with any or all of the following:

* Pinch ground cinnamon
* Pinch ground nutmeg
* Pinch ground allspice
* ½ teaspoon vanilla extract

You can vary the moisture content of cooked oats by mixing in any of the following:

* ¼ cup plain fat-free or low-fat yogurt
* ½ cup plain kefir
* ½ cup unsweetened applesauce
* 2 tablespoons apple butter

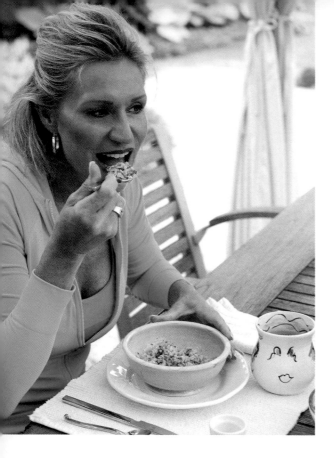

MORE THAN OATS

A bowl of oatmeal alone is not a sufficient breakfast. The Eat-Clean principles recommend consuming complex carbohydrates along with lean protein at every meal to maximize health and weight loss. I also advise that you avoid refined foods, particularly sugars and flours, and steer away from dangerous saturated and trans fats at all costs. There is no point getting your bowl of hot oats right and then messing up with the protein part of breakfast, although I have seen many folks do just that. Greasy bacon, although delicious, should not be a mainstay of your Eat-Clean diet. Yes, that bacon does contain protein, but it is primarily fat.

I prefer to accompany my oats with some form of eggs. I prepare them in many ways, which keeps them interesting day after day. Whether they are scrambled, hard boiled, sunny side up (on a non-stick pan), baked, poached, or in a quiche or frittata, I love them all and enjoy them any way I can. The partnership of complex carbohydrates in oatmeal plus lean protein in egg whites is perfect fuel for a lean body.

I also like to toss a few extras into my oats to give them super nutrition. Everyone who knows me knows that I must eat flaxseed every day. I often opt to put these mighty seeds (coarsely ground) on my oatmeal in the morning (although I have discovered numerous other ways to enjoy them – think salads, smoothies and in baking). Once my oats are cooked I toss two tablespoons of both flaxseed and wheat germ on top. I also add two tablespoons of bee pollen, which I am lucky enough to buy fresh from a local beekeeper in my area. This is followed by half a cup or so of fresh mixed berries. If fresh berries are not available I opt for frozen or use unsweetened applesauce instead. Delicious!

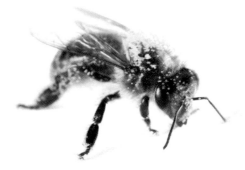

GETTING IT READY FAST

I have heard every excuse in the book for why you think you don't have time to prepare breakfast in the morning. I am not good with tolerating excuses because we are all busy people. We all share the same 24 daily hours to be productive and live our daily lives. I don't want to hear that you don't have time. You must consider what will happen if you don't start now and take the time, which rightfully belongs to you, to put a breakfast meal together and sit down with your gang to eat. Obviously what you have been doing thus far does not seem to be working very

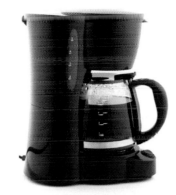

well. If you can get your family to sit down with you, at least for this early morning meal, you will begin to see positive changes from day one.

There are easy ways to minimize breakfast preparations. For example, a little trick I learned from my ex in-laws is to always set the table the night before. It works! Once I see the table ready to go in the morning, I am much less likely to skip out on the meal. It is also a time saver. Here are a few more time-saving tips:

☀ I try to **set the coffee machine on automatic if I know I will be rushed in the morning.** It's much easier to wake up when you can smell fresh coffee brewing! With all of the technology we are privy to, there is no reason why we can't pull off breakfast.

☀ Another thing I like to do is **soak my grains overnight, especially harder grains such as Irish oats.** It takes less than five seconds to douse the grains with water in a bowl and cover them. Not only does this cut down on cooking time, but it also releases more nutrients from the grains.

☀ I often **prepare a bowl of mixed berries big enough to get my family through at least three days of breakfasts.** That is about how long the berries will last before they all get eaten up or go bad. Leftover berries should be stored in the fridge.

☀ You can follow my travel tip and pre-measure and **mix your dry oats and toppings the night before so they are ready to go in the morning.** I always stash an extra "baggie breakfast" at the office in case I am caught short. It has saved my bacon more than once!

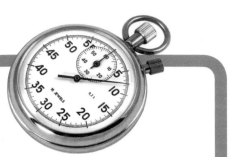

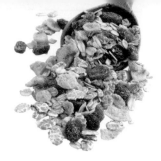

QUICK EAT-CLEAN BREAKFAST OPTIONS

- ☀ Drinkable fat-free or low-fat yogurt mixed with muesli or granola
- ☀ Kefir mixed with muesli or granola
- ☀ Ezekiel bread spread with hummus, topped with hardboiled egg whites
- ☀ Protein smoothie made with fat-free or low-fat cottage cheese, yogurt or kefir, 1 banana, ¼ cup uncooked oatmeal or 1 whole-grain breakfast wheat biscuit, 1 tablespoon natural nut butter, 1 tablespoon ground flaxseed, and soy, rice, almond or skim milk
- ☀ 2 whole-grain breakfast wheat biscuits spread with natural nut butter, topped with sliced banana, sprinkled ground flaxseed and a splash of soy, rice, almond or skim milk
- ☀ Bowl of Ezekiel cereal with fat-free or low-fat milk and fresh berries
- ☀ Scrambled egg whites with tomato and spinach on toasted Ezekiel or other whole-grain bread or wrap

If you do not enjoy oatmeal, consider cold breakfast cereals with high nutritive value such as granola, muesli and whole-grain breakfast wheat biscuits. These cereals are easy to pour into a bowl, douse with your favorite milk (cow, sheep, goat, rice, almond, soy) and top with the same wonderful additions I throw on my oatmeal. For an interesting flavor kick, try pouring your hot skinny latte onto a couple of whole-grain breakfast wheat biscuits. It's delicious and portable.

I like to make egg frittatas, since they are an easy one-dish egg meal. Here's how: preheat your oven to 350°F. Crack your eggs into a bowl, mixing approximately eight whites with two yolks. Meanwhile, have an ovenproof (no plastic bits) skillet ready and heat up a tablespoon of olive oil. Chop up some various vegetables and don't ignore the already cooked ones from last night's supper. I love spinach leaves, onion, garlic, broccoli and tomatoes in my frittata, but any vegetable will work. Sauté the vegetables until they become soft, then pour the egg white mixture over top. Season the dish with salt and pepper and cook until almost set. Then pop it into a hot oven to finish cooking. In 10 to 15 minutes, or when the dish is baked, remove it from the oven and cut into wedges. Serve hot. Make enough for leftovers because this dish is delicious cold too.

Ultimate Smoothie, see recipe p.293

A WORD ABOUT EZEKIEL AND OTHER SPROUTED-GRAIN PRODUCTS

Breads and other cereal products made with sprouted grains are recommended in the Eat-Clean lifestyle, but what are they? An explosion of live grain products has become available in response to the movement that supports a more conscious way of eating. Sprouted grains of any kind are beneficial to the diet since the sprouting process releases more nutrients. Traditionally, all grains and seeds were sprouted, which yielded as much as 10 to 20 times more nutrients than are found in processed seeds. A further benefit of consuming sprouted grains, seeds, nuts and their products, is that they foster the growth of good bacteria in your gut, which in turn helps to keep your colon clean. It doesn't hurt that sprouted grains also contain plentiful concentrations of antioxidants, potent anti-cancer agents.

In general, sprouts and sprouted-grain products are more readily digested than your typical store-bought loaf of whole-grain bread. In addition, their nutritional profile is high in fiber, protein, vitamins and minerals. It is the cooked form of wheat that causes mucus congestion, allergic reactions, constipation and bowel irritability. When wheat is sprouted the starch is converted to simple sugars and this has no negative effects on the digestive tract.*

Ezekiel bread is but one of many sprouted-grain products available today. The recipe was inspired by the verse in the Holy Scripture that guides Ezekiel to prepare for his journey in the desert. **Ezekiel 4:9** reads, "Take also unto thee Wheat, and Barley, and beans, and lentils, and millet, and Spelt, and put them in one vessel, and make bread of it ..." The combination of sprouted grains and legumes used to make Ezekiel (whether made by you or by a company) yields a complete protein that is almost comparable to the protein found in eggs, which are the gold standard for protein. In your Eat-Clean lifestyle, you may want to consider choosing products made from sprouted grains, particularly if bread is part of your meal.

*Those with gluten intolerances should check with their doctor before trying any new products.

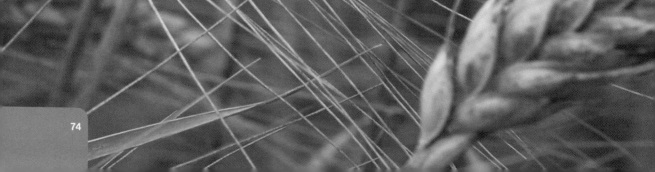

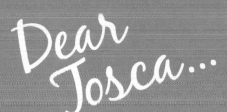

Dear Tosca,

I just wanted to say thank you. Even though I've never met you, you have changed my life.

For more years than I care to count, I have been overweight and unhappy, and not even aware that I was poisoning myself with unhealthy foods. I was literally being poisoned. I was dealing with unexplained panic attacks, poor sleep and depression. I have read so many books with guaranteed cures and watched countless infomercials on pills and machines, but it was your book that got into my heart and soul. Your words somehow sunk in and I decided to put my fate in your hands.

I look back now 26 weeks later and am happy to tears. I have lost 50 lbs (down from 204 to 154) and I have lost a total of 28". I have found my smile and my confidence – two things I feared I would never see again. Tosca, thank you for being who you are and for helping those who are willing to listen. Whether you know it or not, you pushed me through my workouts, and you made me get up at 5 am every morning no matter how tired I was. I am so thankful every day that I am here and that I have found healthy eating and fitness (both of which I now couldn't live without). I have even been asked by my co-workers and a neighbor to help put them on track to a healthier lifestyle.

Thank you for helping me get my life back.

With deepest admiration and thanks,
MaryBeth Dilauro

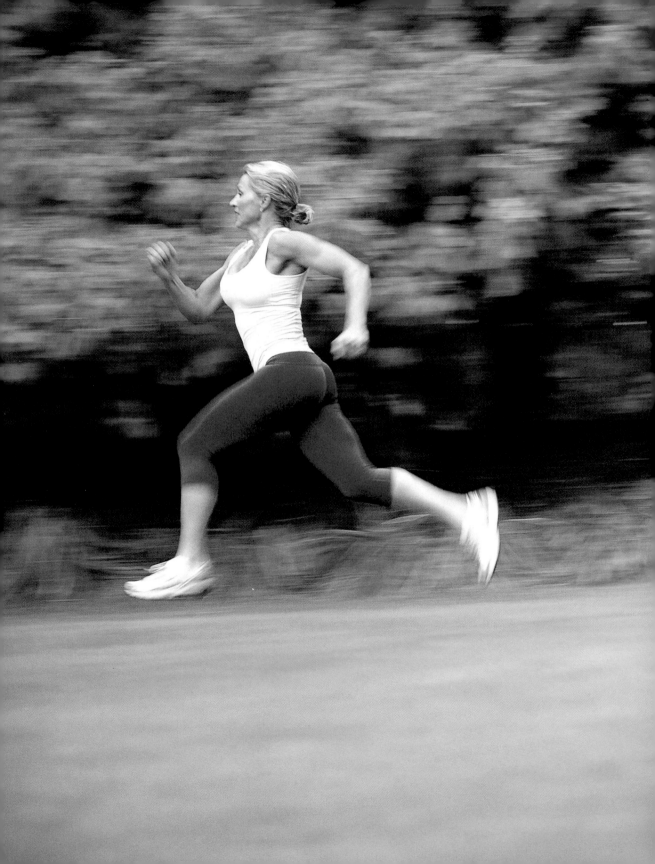

THE BASICS OF METABOLISM

4

"My son is a bottomless pit, but can eat anything he wants" or, "Everything I eat goes right to my hips." Sound familiar? Some people have a fast metabolism, making it easier for them to lose weight and, in certain cases, difficult to gain. These people seem to be able to eat anything in sight and never gain a pound – and yes, that might make you mad! Other people have difficulty dropping pounds. The needle on the scale never seems to budge. The whole business seems unfair, doesn't it? Fortunately, your metabolism can be altered such that you can speed it up (that's a good thing) or slow it down (not such a good thing). Eating Clean is one way to accomplish this change for the better and it is a *very* good thing.

WHAT IS METABOLISM?

Metabolism is a steady process that begins when you are born and ends when you die. It's a balancing act of two different activities that occur in the body – the building up and breaking down of energy stores and body tissues. To put it in simple terms, your metabolism is what breaks down the energy you get from food and turns it into fuel for regular body functions including breathing, staying warm, basic body movements such as moving our arms and legs and, of course, working out.

The speed of your metabolism, which is called your metabolic rate, establishes how much food you need to consume to maintain a stable weight. If you find yourself gaining weight, you are consuming more energy than your metabolism can process and you begin to store the unused fuel as fat. This is your body's natural response to excess. In times of famine, this response holds onto your fat as a protective reserve of energy in order to guarantee your survival.

Your basal metabolic rate, or BMR, is the rate at which your body uses energy at rest. Your BMR and metabolism depend on a variety of factors such as your height, weight, muscle mass and activity level. A muscular person who runs marathons will have a much faster metabolism than a couch potato who remains horizontal for most of the day.

"A muscular person who runs marathons will have a much faster metabolism than a couch potato who remains horizontal for most of the day."

FOR BETTER OR WORSE

The state of your metabolism depends not only on how you treat your body right now, but also on the relationship you've had with it in the past. If you've followed a consistent weight-training program for any period of time, you will likely have an efficient, fat-burning metabolism. It's like money in the bank earning interest. Your metabolism works for you all the time even when you aren't working out and, surprisingly, even when you're sleeping. On the other hand, if you have dieted for years, gaining and losing the same weight over and over again, it's more likely that you have interfered with your metabolism, meaning that you burn fuel from food energy at a slow rate, making it more difficult to lose weight.

I was firmly in that sluggish, interfered-with category until I discovered Eating Clean through the tutelage of Robert Kennedy. I struggled every time I wanted to shed pounds, ultimately gaining and losing the same few until today.

Yo-yo dieting confuses your body. Cleverly designed to withstand feast or famine, your metabolism is trained to take it easy or work overtime, depending on available food sources. When food is scarce or when you skip meals, your metabolism slows down in response to your reduced caloric intake. Your body is protecting itself by avoiding starvation – making it less prone to shed excess fat in case you need to use it for future fuel. That also means

"Metabolism is the steady process of building up and breaking down energy stores and body tissues."

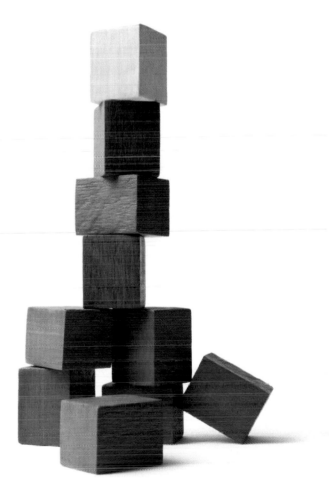

METABOLIC PROBLEMS

A very small percentage of the population can blame an extremely slow (or fast) metabolism on medical problems. Two common problems, both controllable by medication, are:

1 **HYPERTHYROIDISM** ~ caused by an overactive thyroid gland. The thyroid releases too much of the hormone thyroxine, which increases a person's BMR. Symptoms include weight loss, increased heart rate and blood pressure, neck swelling (from an enlarged thyroid, or goiter) and protruding eyes.

2 **HYPOTHYROIDISM** ~ caused by an absent or underactive thyroid gland. In children this condition can result in stunted physical and mental growth. Symptoms include severe fatigue, a slow heart rate, weight gain and constipation.

when you go on a diet and begin to lose weight, your body revolts, making it harder for you to reach your weight-loss goals.

Eliminating specific food groups from your diet also bewilders your body. When you remove certain foods from your diet, such as carbohydrates or fats, your body reacts in a negative way. You may lose weight, even a substantial amount, but it won't last. When you stop eating entire food groups, your body is missing out on essential nutrients. Then, as you reintroduce those foods back into your diet, your body clings to the long-lost nutrients, causing rapid weight gain.

STEP ON THE GAS

Fortunately, there are things you can do to speed up your metabolism. It can be retrained to function efficiently after long periods of dieting. Your BMR is not a fixed number. Whether you have 10 or 100 pounds to lose, you can speed up the rate at which your body burns energy with regular resistance training. One pound of muscle burns approximately 25 times more calories than a pound of fat. If you are not overweight, there is more muscle tissue in your body than any other type of tissue. Muscle tissue demands the most energy, thus it is your muscle tissue that determines the rate at which your body burns energy. By building a layer of muscle tissue through training with weights, you will increase your metabolic rate.

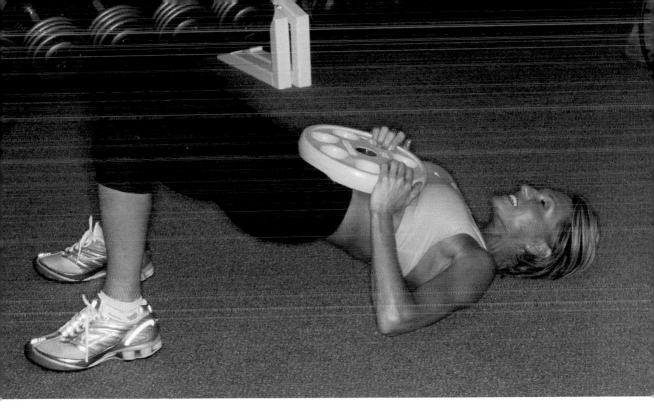

WEIGHT TRAINING

A number of things happen immediately inside your body in response to increased physical activity. As soon as you begin moving your muscles, your fat cells become smaller in a process called lipolysis. Exercise and weight training quickens and encourages muscle growth. Remember that the more muscle you have, the faster your metabolic rate, so you want to build as much muscle as possible. I'm not talking about becoming the next Arnold Schwarzenegger – even if women spend hours in the gym every day, they cannot build huge manly muscles without the help of steroids. It's more than likely that the slender, toned bodies you envy were created through exercise and lifting weights.

Weight training not only stimulates your muscles while you are working out, but for hours afterwards. Exercise triggers the release of testosterone into your body, a reaction that works to destroy fat. To make the most of your lifting sessions, be sure to train the large muscle groups such as the quads, glutes, chest and back. Training these areas (especially quads and glutes) starts up the vehicle that drives your body to increase its metabolism and burn more calories. Squats, leg presses and lunges are effective exercises that work the large muscle groups. When you perform exercises that work major body parts, hundreds of your muscles contract at once, increasing your metabolic rate by as much as 2,000 percent! Your body uses all of the calories you eat for fuel and draws on its fat stores for energy.

BURN IT OFF

Intense activity is another key factor in maintaining a fast metabolism. When you are lifting weights, hiking up a mountain, performing push-ups or running on the treadmill, really focus on maintaining intensity in your workouts. In other words, put your mind into the muscle. You can build more muscle and burn more energy by concentrating on the task at hand instead of staring into space. If you are daydreaming about what's on TV tonight while working your biceps, reading a novel on the treadmill or worrying about financial problems between sit ups, you aren't making the most effective use of your time and you won't achieve the results you desire. When you grab the weights, mentally be there when you lift them and think about your muscle when you bring them down again – this maximizes your results.

Your aerobic workouts don't need to last forever to deliver results. You can speed up your metabolism in the shortest amount of time through high intensity interval training (HIIT). HIIT is especially handy if you are pressed for time and need to train with weights and then do a cardio workout during one trip to the gym. Interval training involves performing any cardiovascular exercise at a high exertion for a short period of time and then dropping the level of intensity, to recover, for the same period of time. For example, you might run as fast as you can for two minutes, then pull it back to a slow jog for another two minutes. These short, volatile sessions fire up a sluggish metabolism by surprising your muscles. Studies have shown that people who incorporate high-intensity interval training into their workouts lose twice as much weight as those who don't. I remember a radio interview with Dr. Mehmet Oz, who said that he loves to do intervals or sprints to keep himself in top shape because that is the time when the body works at its maximum, releasing hormones to help bring about healthy changes in the body. I always picture him doing his sprints as I am running mine.

TIP!

If you want to rocket your metabolism into the stratosphere, split your workout into two daily sessions. Do your cardio in the morning and lifting in the evening, or switch it around. Your metabolism will be on fire all day long!

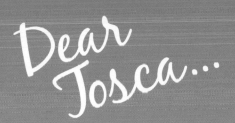

TESTIMONIAL

Dear Tosca,

I wanted to tell you a little bit about my journey, since you had so much to do with it. I am a 37-year-old mother of two with a wonderful husband who has always been into fitness, but I just couldn't seem to get as enthusiastic as he was. I worked out, but never saw the results I thought I should. I discovered *The Eat-Clean Diet* last April and was immediately inspired by you to change my eating habits. Since that time I have been completely amazed at the transformation in both my body and my life. I have much more energy and look better now than I did in my twenties.

The biggest accomplishment, however, is the effect this has had on my family. My husband began Eating Clean and he looks like an underwear model. Yay! My children love the recipes and so do their friends. They don't even know how good they are for them.

Recently, my 12-year-old daughter was getting an academic award at her middle school, so I went to watch the ceremony. During it, they also awarded her a certificate for being the "Most Health Conscious." I almost cried! ☺ I think I was more proud of that than the good grades. She has recently begun cooking with me and asked if she could have *The Eat-Clean Diet Cookbook* as her first recipe book.

Thank you so much for helping me to be such a great, healthy example for my children. Your influence has made our lives much better.

Sincerely,

Holly Williams

Summerville, SC

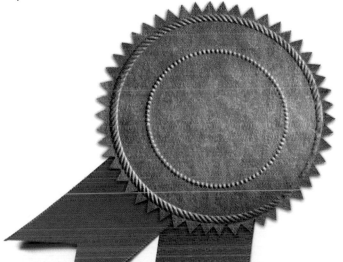

83

FOOD IS FUEL – BUT WHAT KIND?

The food we eat also works to either stimulate or slam the brakes on our metabolism. To maintain a healthy weight you must nourish your body with high-quality food at regular intervals. When you wait too long between meals or skip one entirely, you trigger a starvation response in your metabolism, which causes it to slow down. Eating small meals every three hours ensures that your metabolism will stay hyped all day long.

Eating Clean supports a healthy metabolism. Increasing the frequency of your meals, as well as eating the superior food combo of lean protein and complex carbohydrates at each meal, prolongs digestion and encourages your blood sugar to remain stable between meals. If you feel tired or lethargic throughout the day, especially mid-morning or mid-afternoon, it's usually a direct result of unstable blood glucose and insulin levels. When you Eat Clean you slow the release of sugar into your bloodstream, causing your blood and insulin levels to stabilize, and giving you energy that lasts all day long.

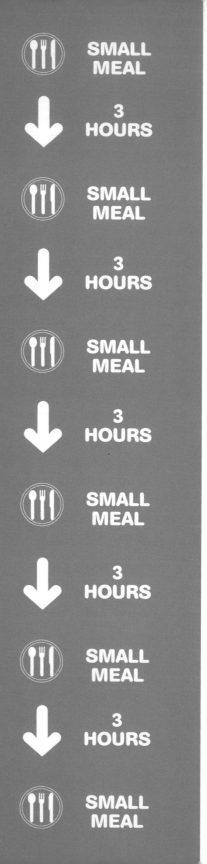

PRO-DUCTIVE PRO-TEIN

Eating protein causes your metabolism to speed up as a direct result of the numerous chemical reactions required to digest protein. This number is far higher than those needed to digest other macronutrients. This is called the "dynamic action of protein." The amino acids (building blocks) in protein stimulate cellular activity, thereby increasing your BMR. Eating carbohydrates alone increases your BMR only slightly for a short period of time. This is why you feel tired after a big meal loaded with carbohydrates. Eating a meal that combines lean protein with complex carbohydrates causes your BMR to begin to rise within one hour. This increase lasts from three to twelve hours – that's a long time! What I have come to appreciate about Eating Clean is that I no longer struggle with the afternoon crash that virtually knocked me out in the past. Today, thanks to that high-octane fuel combo of lean protein and complex carbohydrates I eat at every one of my six daily meals, I have energy to spare. I can't imagine my life any other way.

"Combining lean protein with complex carbohydrates causes your BMR to rise and can help eliminate that afternoon crash."

SAY NO TO SIMPLE CARBS

If you want to eat for peak metabolism, you've got to remove all simple carbohydrates from your diet, especially those that are chemically charged and refined. Get up right now and look through your cupboards and cabinets. Cookies, gummi bears, crackers and potato chips must all end up in your garbage can. Foods with added sugars, or made with processed white grains and flours, have a high Glycemic Index, and cause a spike in insulin levels, which in turn makes your metabolism slow down. Throw out the white rice, bread and pasta and rely on the complex carbohydrates found in whole grains, and fresh fruits and vegetables for energy. There is no question. Eating nutrient-dense foods makes an enormous and notable difference both in your health and your physique.

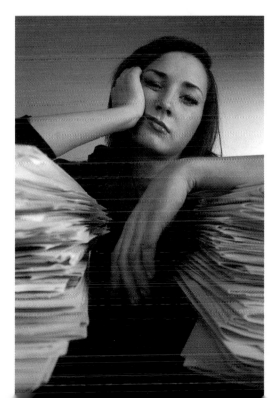

WHAT TO EAT TO SPEED UP YOUR METABOLISM

Eat your body on fire by depending on the following five foods (and liquids) each day:

① WATER

Keep your water bottle in sight at all times. Drinking water (otherwise known as the miracle liquid) keeps your body lean by helping nutrients flow through it, and by washing away waste and free radicals. A recent study in Germany suggests that 90 minutes after drinking it, cold water will boost your metabolism by 24 percent over your average BMR. Sounds like a pretty good reason to keep the Brita filter full!

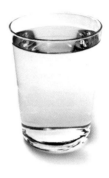

② LEAN PROTEINS

Eating protein raises your metabolism. Remember the dynamic action of protein I mentioned earlier? Lean protein found in poultry, fish, bison and egg whites keeps you feeling satisfied while helping your body burn through energy faster, resulting in a higher calorie burn. There is also less of a chance that protein will be stored in your body as excess fat, so make sure to eat a portion with every meal.

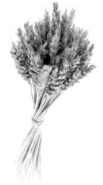

③ FIBER

Fiber is nothing short of fiberrific! Complex carbohydrates such as oatmeal, wheat germ, bran and flaxseed are a great source of fibrous energy. They provide steady, long-lasting energy without the crashes that can accompany simple carbohydrates. Fiber also keeps you feeling satiated between meals. The best time of day to eat oatmeal is in the morning. You need the energy from these complex carbohydrates to efficiently run your brain and body throughout the day.

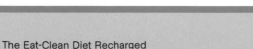

④ BLACK COFFEE OR GREEN TEA

Even though some nutritionists may turn their noses up at coffee, a lot of people (including me) refuse to give up their daily dose of java. Recent research suggests that drinking a cup of black coffee raises your metabolism, increases your concentration and improves heart health. Drinking green tea packs an even more powerful punch. Its high antioxidant content raises your metabolism better than coffee.

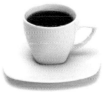

⑤ SPICES

Spices that contain the chemical capsaicin, such as jalapeno, habanero and cayenne, have thermogenic properties that speed up your heart and heat up your body. Your body has to burn calories to cool itself down. A recent study from Laval University in Quebec suggested that men who sipped coffee alongside spicy foods were able to burn up to 1,000 more calories per day than a group who ate bland foods.

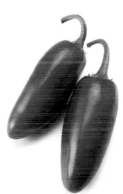

"To maintain a healthy weight you must nourish your body with high-quality food at regular intervals."

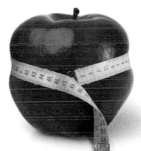

5 MORE!

Keep your metabolism moving by incorporating these foods into your diet:

⑥ HEALTHY FATS

It sounds like an oxymoron, but there are fats that help you burn fat. Monosaturated fats (found in olive oil, canola oil, cashews, hazelnuts, peanuts and chicken fat) help reduce cholesterol, triglycerides and blood pressure, and work to control diabetes. Polyunsaturated fats (omega-3 fats found in canola oil, walnuts, flaxseeds, hempseeds, salmon, mackerel, trout, tuna, sardines and herring) reduce triglycerides, inflammations and tumor growth. They also improve immune function and protect against sudden death from heart disease. Fats isn't always a four-letter word!

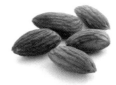

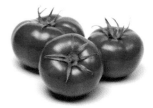

⑦ TOMATOES

Tomatoes taste great and are very healthful. Along with Vitamin C, tomatoes contain citric, malic and oxalic acids that accelerate your metabolism. These natural acids flush more water through your kidneys and prompt them to filter out large amounts of fatty deposits, which you then eliminate from your system. Tomatoes are also rich in lycopene, a cancer-fighting antioxidant that works to stimulate your body's metabolic rate by up to one third.

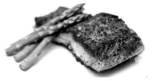

⑧ LOW-FAT PLAIN YOGURT

Yogurt contains healthy fats, some protein and many probiotic cultures that are vital for a healthy digestive tract. Probiotics are dietary supplements that contain beneficial bacteria or yeasts that play a role in your metabolism. A recent study at the Imperial College in London found that foods containing probiotics, such as yogurt, could have a significant effect on metabolism.

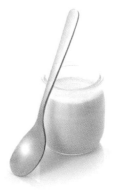

⑨ GARLIC AND ONIONS

Bad for your breath but good for your metabolism! Garlic is a natural diuretic. Garlic contains mustard oil, which act like a cleanser in your body. This oil encourages muscular contractions that loosen fat and help to wash it out. It also breaks down clumps of fat in your body. Onions, like garlic, also contain minerals and oils that break down fatty deposits in your body and speed up your metabolism.

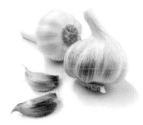

⑩ GREENS

It may not be easy being green, but it sure is easy to eat greens, especially when you think of the magical things they do for your body.

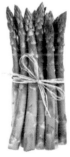

Asparagus contains the chemical asparagines, an alkaloid that stimulates the kidneys, improves the circulatory process and breaks down fat. Asparagus also contains a chemical that helps to remove waste from the body by breaking up the oxalic acid – this acid tends to glue fat to cells, so by breaking the acid up, it helps to reduce fat levels.

Cabbage, a natural diuretic, is especially beneficial if you have a potbelly or spare tire around your waist. Cabbage contains sulfur and iodine, which helps to cleanse the mucous membrane of your stomach and intestines, breaking up the fat in and around that area.

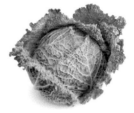

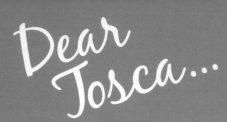

Dear Tosca...

Tosca,

I love your books and have all of them. I use them every day as a resource. I have been Eating Clean for about a year now, but really hardcore for the past four months or so. I had never worked out in my life until the past year where I have done cardio four or five days a week and lifted with a personal trainer two times weekly. I love it! I am 49 and look better than ever.

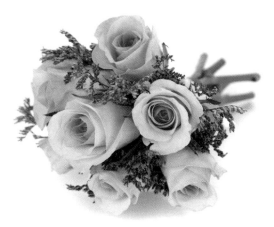

I recently got to show off at my 24-year-old daughter's wedding. I definitely did not wear a typical, matronly mother-of-the-bride dress, but one that was sleeveless and backless. I received many com-

pliments. My daughter was so proud of me that she asked the photographer to take a picture of me in a double biceps pose surrounded by the groom's men! Thanks for the inspiration, Tosca!

Sharon Harr
Ann Arbor, MI

P.S. My husband, who runs marathons and is in great shape, has dropped his cholesterol over 45 points since I changed our diet. All the running did nothing, but Eating Clean did!

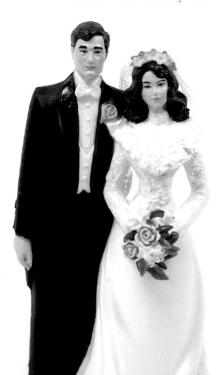

MENOPAUSE AND YOUR METABOLISM

With every advancing year metabolism declines – the rate is about 10 percent for every decade. Studies have shown that over the age of 30, the average person will gain about a pound of fat and lose half a pound of muscle each year if they continue to eat a constant number of calories. Fortunately, this is not a fate you're forced to accept.

Women – listen up! Menopause (also called change of life) is the time in a woman's life when she ceases to ovulate and her period stops entirely. The average age of menopause is 51, but it can happen much earlier or later.

It is common for women to experience rapid weight gain during menopause. In fact, most women will gain 10 to 15 pounds. This weight tends to accumulate gradually around the abdomen, creating an "apple" shape. During menopause, women undergo hormone fluctuations that directly impact appetite, metabolism and fat storage, making weight loss more difficult but not impossible.

To combat menopausal weight gain, follow the Eat-Clean Principles (eating small meals every three hours, combining lean proteins with complex carbohydrates at every meal, and adding regular exercise and resistance training to your routine). Go to bed early, drink enough water and try to avoid stress – the result will be a healthy, lean physique for years to come.

WHAT YOU CAN DO TO AVOID MIDLIFE WEIGHT GAIN

- Eat breakfast
- Exercise regularly (cardiovascular activity and weight training)
- Eat enough protein
- Get a good night's sleep
- Avoid alcohol
- Drink lots of water
- Try to reduce or limit stress

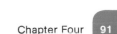

When you admire the beauty of a blooming flower or a babbling brook you are looking at the magic of water. It is a powerful force that maintains life in the most crucial way. This clear liquid, composed of oxygen and hydrogen molecules, infuses the body and all living things with hydration and is a substance humans cannot survive without.

Simple water is often overlooked for fancier beverages, but these imposters can never do what clean, fresh water does. Water is the main component of the blood that courses through our veins and the fluids that bathe our brain, cells, muscles, joints and organs. The human body is nearly 70 percent water and can survive without food for weeks but only a few days without water.

Studies show that most of us don't consume sufficient water, despite the ubiquitous water bottle. Soft drinks, coffee, teas and juices seem much more appealing to our taste buds and our purchasing habits prove we prefer them, but water is actually what we need. Best of all, water is Clean!

WHERE IS WATER USED?

The better question is: where is water *not* used?

The composition of water, two hydrogen molecules combined with one oxygen molecule (H_2O), makes it a universal solvent, meaning that it can dissolve virtually everything! Aside from the countless tasks water handles in nature, it also serves our bodily functions in innumerable ways.

Water is the main facilitator of digestion. It acts as a solvent for the foods we eat, so every nutrient in each mouthful of food is made available to the human body. Water also helps deliver nutrients to our tissues, and facilitates the removal of toxins and waste from the body. Our cells are bathed in a material called extracellular fluid, which makes up one third of the amount of water in the entire human body. Cells are filled with intracellular fluid, which makes up the remaining two thirds. As you can see, the human body is very watery! These fluids act to protect our organs, lubricate our joints, float our brains, bathe our tissues and protect a growing fetus in the womb. Can you imagine how our body would shut down without constant hydration?

Water is also crucial for maintaining a constant body temperature. The body doesn't want to overheat or become too cold. You are probably familiar with sweat and the perspiration process, which is necessary even if it is a little smelly! When we get too hot, we sweat as a means of releasing heat from our system. Can you guess the main component of sweat? That's right, it's water!

Water is necessary for proper bodily function. Without it we'd dry up and ... well, you get the picture.

> "Water is the main component of digestion."

DEHYDRATION

The body uses water in so many ways that it is easy to see how we might get dehydrated if we don't keep our water consumption constant. The role of water in digestion and sweating, among other things, means it is quickly used up. If we don't replenish our water levels throughout the day it is easy to become dehydrated. One dictionary defines dehydration as "deprivation of vitality," so you can see how crucial it is for the body to stay hydrated. Water is vital!

20 WAYS WE DEHYDRATE

1. **Breathing:** We depend on water to keep our lungs moist, but we also release moist air with each exhale.
2. **Stress**
3. **Digestion**
4. **Sweating**
5. **Pregnancy**
6. **Aging:** The thirst reflex is blunted with age, leading to less water consumption.
7. **Growing**
8. **Obesity:** More water is needed to run a larger body.
9. **Diets high in processed foods** that contain chemicals, sugars, salts, alcohol and caffeine.
10. **Consuming toxins** including contaminated foods, alcohol and drugs.
11. **Diarrhea**
12. **Vomiting**
13. **Fever**
14. **Chronic illness**
15. **Sun exposure**
16. **Exercise**
17. **Not drinking enough water**
18. **Decreased mineral levels:** They act to maintain water balance.
19. **Medications**
20. **Burns**

"Be more concerned about dehydration."

You probably have found yourself dehydrated without even knowing it. The symptoms of early dehydration are very subtle and include:

- headaches
- mood swings
- lethargy
- confusion
- dry lips
- constipation

These symptoms are similar to those felt during the slump experienced by many people during the mid-afternoon. You may not have realized that you were simply experiencing thirst. When I start to feel this way, I reach for a drink of water before trying anything else because most of the time I have simply allowed myself to become too thirsty. When I struggled with yo-yo dieting I would pick up a candy bar or have something sweet as my first line of defense, attempting to conquer the afternoon blahs with sugar. Now I would much rather suck on my water bottle, knowing my body is actually craving moisture. Decreasing your total body water by only one percent can decrease your ability to work effectively by 10 percent. Think about it. A decrease of three percent means your ability to function is reduced by 30 percent! That's a lot and certainly not good for your productivity.

If dehydration is taken too far it can lead to serious issues. Symptoms of late dehydration include dark yellow urine, hallucinations and general achiness. Within a few hours you could stop making urine altogether, at which point your kidneys will begin to shut down. This is severe and needs to be treated with a visit to the emergency room. Other effects of severe dehydration include:

- heat injury
- swelling of the brain
- seizures
- hypovolemic shock
- constipation
- kidney stones
- urinary tract infections
- increased risk of developing certain types of cancers
- coma
- death

Overdosing on water is difficult to do if you have healthy kidneys. However, it is possible. I recently saw on the news that a woman who challenged herself to drink an incredibly large amount of water had a negative reaction and died. This is not the desired effect of keeping the body adequately hydrated.

Be more concerned about preventing dehydration. Learn to recognize the first signs of thirst, with a headache, sluggishness and a lack of concentration as a warning that you need water now!

HOW MUCH IS ENOUGH?

The question of how much water a person should drink each day has been raging for ages. Some people suggest that one liter is sufficient, while others maintain that seven liters is adequate, hence the confusion. I like to stick to between two and three liters of water each day, depending on how active I have been. My body usually tells me when it needs more. More accurately, when I'm thirsty, I notice that I start to lick my lips a lot and become tired and foggy in the head. That is when I listen up and start drinking!

HERE'S A FUN ACTIVITY:

Take your weight in pounds and divide it in half. This is how many ounces of water you should consume each day at the bare minimum. So if you weigh 140 pounds, you should be drinking at least 70 ounces (about nine cups) of water each day, plus more if you exercise, travel on a plane or consume alcohol.

I've also heard that for every 50 pounds of body weight, one liter of water should be consumed. 150 pounds = three liters of water.

TIP!

Drink a glass of water when you are having a craving to determine if you are thirsty before heading to the food cupboards. It won't hurt and it will keep you well hydrated at the very least, if not leaner.

It's crystal clear (just like water!) that there are plenty of theories out there about how much water you need to drink and perhaps not enough answers. Most importantly, you need to listen to your body when it tells you that you are thirsty. The thirst function can be weak and is often disguised as hunger. You should practice listening to your body to find out what it needs. Better yet, incorporate water into each one of your six daily meals. If you study the menu plans in this book and others I've created In *The Eat-Clean Diet* series, you will notice that I have programmed water consumption into the plans. I have done this because I find so many people cannot discipline themselves to consume sufficient water. Once it becomes part of your Eat-Clean habits, keeping yourself hydrated is no longer a problem.

The theory is: you need to do something 10 times and then it becomes a habit.

If you Eat Clean and maintain a balanced diet of fruits, vegetables, lean protein and whole grains you will easily obtain about 20 percent of your recommended daily water intake from food. The remaining 80 percent is attainable from the fluids you drink. Now you just have to make sure you choose the right fluids.

DECIPHERING THE GOOD FROM THE BAD

Just as there are Clean foods and dirty foods, there are also Clean drinks and dirty drinks (and I'm not talking about a dirty martini). As you may have guessed, plain water is your best bet. It is pure and simple, and gives you everything you need.

"You need to listen to your body when it tells you that you are thirsty."

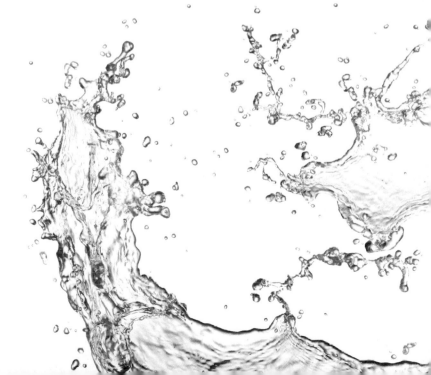

Coffee and teas are also sources of fluid. Unfortunately, these beverages usually contain a hefty dose of caffeine. Caffeine is a diuretic, which means that it makes you have to urinate, so it nulls water's hydrating effects. I am definitely not one to skip out on my coffee in the morning, so I stick to one cup when I rise and balance it out by drinking plenty of water throughout the day. Caffeine-free herbal teas are also an excellent option. These are especially comforting in the late afternoon or in the evening to calm you after a busy day. I actually have an entire drawer in my kitchen at home dedicated to my herbal tea collection — that's how much tea I drink!

Fruit juices and soft drinks are over-consumed and unnecessary beverages in my opinion. Most of these are loaded with sugars, toxins and empty calories. For example, consider the average 10-ounce bottle of orange juice. It contains two or more servings — at least the juice from three or more oranges. That is more than enough fruit and fruit sugar than anyone needs to consume in one sitting, and it comes without the fibrous goodness of the fruit skins and pulp to boot. Consuming enormous amounts of sugar in the form of fruit juices puts a strain on your pancreas and kidneys as these organs struggle to mop up the offending sugars. I would encourage you to stay away from fruit juices and carbonated beverages.

Sports drinks are abnormally high in sugar although the packaging tries to convince you they are healthy. You must scrutinize the ingredients label to be sure!

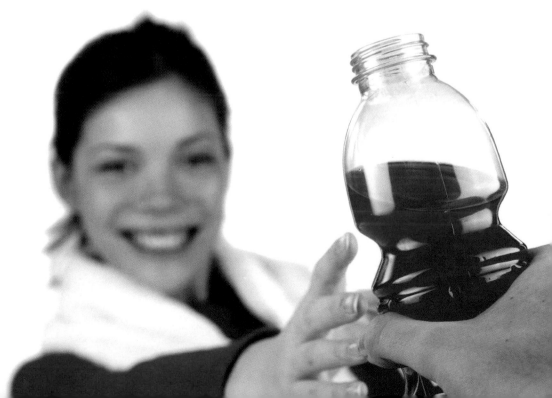

The sugar in these drinks is disguised as high fructose corn syrup (HFCS) and other sugar alternatives. Sports drinks have been touted for their hydrating effects, but they aren't really necessary unless you are exercising for an extended period of time, like when running a marathon.

I'm sure you already know that alcohol is not a great option for maintaining your hydration. For those of you who do enjoy the occasional drink, you might be familiar with the need to urinate soon after having a cocktail or glass of wine. This is because, like caffeine, alcohol has a diuretic effect. I am not one to avoid a glass of wine or light beer once in a while, but you need to balance out your water levels in order to stay hydrated. I am two-fisted drinker. I keep a glass of wine in one hand and a glass of water in the other. You could also try alternating one glass of water for every glass of wine. You'll likely avoid a nasty headache, too.

> "Sports drinks are abnormally high in sugar although the packaging tries to convince you they are healthy."

GETTING ENOUGH AND TAKING IT WITH YOU

Drinking enough water can be a daunting task, especially if you are new to the game, but once you pick up the habit you will find yourself craving water (believe it or not). Eventually you will stop running for the bathroom, too.

On your new Eat-Clean regime, you are encouraged to have water with each of your six daily meals. I like to start the day with a tall glass of water before any food hits my stomach. This encourages a lovely morning bowel once-over and helps to revitalize your cells.

You may know that I bring a cooler of Clean foods with me wherever I go. I also take my water. It's important to have it at my fingertips, so I always carry a one-liter stainless steel bottle. It helps me keep track of how much water I've had throughout the day. It also means I never have to go without. You don't have an excuse for picking up a soda when you have water by your side at all times.

Make sure you have water with you during your workouts, too. This is an important time to rehydrate, since you are losing so much water by sweating.

Get into the habit. Water is the way to go!

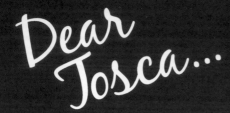

In August of 2008, a very dear friend introduced me to Tosca Reno's *Eat-Clean Diet*. At first I was not interested in a "fad diet" and had a difficult time grasping the idea of NOT counting calories and simply watching my portion sizes and intake of certain foods to ensure a balanced, nutritious diet. I thought that I knew what I was doing and if I wanted, I could drop the weight. Then the realization that my friend had lost all of her "baby weight" and then some by Eating Clean and working out hit me. If she could do it with a new baby and a full time job – why couldn't I? She seemed so excited and motivated about the plan that it was contagious! I started to ask questions about what it meant to Eat Clean.

A month later, my friend convinced me to purchase Tosca's *Eat-Clean Diet Cookbook* – just to try it. I was instantly hooked! Tosca's way of simply explaining the way our bodies require nutrition made much more sense than anything else that I had read. It was a no-nonsense approach to eating. Soon thereafter, I purchased Tosca's *Eat-Clean Diet* book and read it cover to cover in a matter of days. I cleaned out my cupboards and we started from scratch. At first my husband didn't understand, but blindly trusted that what I was doing would make me happy. He was such a good sport. Now, he is just as into Clean Eating as I am and has leaned out and bulked up in the process. He jokes that he has lost "sympathy weight."

In the first month of Eating Clean I lost 8 pounds! I was following the open Cooler 3 plan and wasn't really working out. In November, I decided to take my workouts seriously. I followed Tosca's advice and started weight training – that is when the transformation really began.

I managed to follow the Eat-Clean Principles and lose a decent amount of weight through Thanksgiving, the loss of a very close uncle, a vacation to Mexico at the beginning of December, three Christmas celebrations, New Year's Eve and five birthday celebrations. When we travel to relatives's homes I pack my cooler for the weekend. I resist temptations as much as possible and treat myself instead of holding myself back – and at all times I try to make smart, Clean decisions about what I eat.

I am amazed at the changes that have occurred in the shape and form of my body from Eating Clean and being dedicated to my workouts. I look at myself in the mirror and sometimes do not recognize the person staring back at me. My friends that have not seen me lately tell me that I do not look like myself – that I look like a new person!

Maria Peters

WHAT IS BPA?

As we begin to realize how much garbage is dumped on the land, water and air we exist in, we have started to make great strides to "green" our environment. It's also important to green our bodies. In the past few years, one significant change has been the shift from using plastic water bottles to ones made out of glass or stainless steel. Have you ever wondered why?

Most plastic water bottles contain a chemical called bisphenol A (BPA). This nasty chemical acts as a hormone disruptor, which can ultimately harm both male and female reproductive organs, among other things. BPA leaches into your water under a number of conditions, including leaving your water bottle sitting in your car, in your purse or briefcase, or on your desk. The best way to avoid BPA is to put your plastic bottles to rest in the recycling bin and avoid purchasing plastic bottles of water in the future. Instead, purchase a refillable water filter for your refrigerator or your faucet and fill up reusable stainless steel or glass bottles. Wash them regularly with warm water and soap to avoid bacterial development.

By choosing a reusable bottle, you will not only be reducing the amount of toxic waste that gets into your body, but also decreasing the amount of environmental waste that ends up in our landfills. That means you are taking two steps to reducing your carbon footprint. Good for you!

"By choosing a reusable bottle, you will not only be reducing the amount of toxic waste that gets into your body, but also decreasing the amount of waste that ends up in landfills."

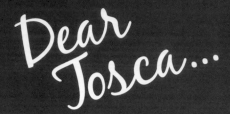

TESTIMONIAL

I started my weight loss journey four years ago at 230 pounds. I had to put my size 22 pants on when they were a little damp so they would stretch. As a single mother of two, I realized something had to change, and it had to be me. I started reading books and websites, and fought hard not to fall victim to gimmicks and promises. Finding the truth in a quick-fix, fast-paced society was very hard. I initially stuck to portion control and just the basic baked or grilled anything. I went up and down in weight trying to find the best plan for myself. I could never commit to exercise. I had just become so lazy, but I had always been. Never in my 24 years had I been small. I have been the "fat girl" all my life.

I sit here writing you today in my size 4/5s weighing in at 120 pounds!!!!! I made it to my goal. It was the best choice I ever made for myself, by far! I am moving forward to the new slamming me and I am not looking back. My couch will miss me! I just wanted to thank you for the knowledge and inner strength that you have provided for me.

I also found out two weeks ago that my husband is Type 1 Diabetic. I have him following *The Eat-Clean Diet*, which he is actually enjoying. In two weeks, by Eating Clean and using his insulin, his sugar dropped from 450 to 130-150. It's amazing and he says he feels much better.

Keeping it tight,
Miranda Henderson

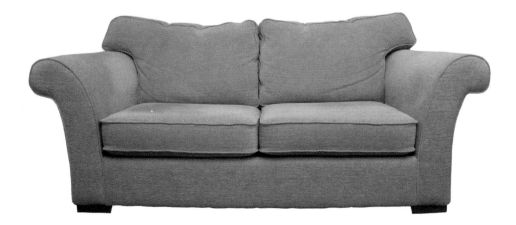

FANCY WATER

The latest craze is deluxe water. Every marketing agency has jumped onto the fancy water bandwagon. From fizzy to fruity to vitamin-enhanced, this new fancy water can be found everywhere, but is it necessary? If flavored water is something that helps you get your liquids down, I highly recommend it. But before chugging away, be smart and read the nutrition label. Flavored waters should not contain artificial flavors and colors. Furthermore, they should not be loaded with sugars and salts. Watch out for artificial sugars, such as aspartame and sucralose. These are found in flavor crystals, which should be avoided at all costs. These can often make you thirstier. Take a long, hard look at the ingredients label before buying fruity or flavored water. Better yet, make your own with fresh fruit.

HAPPILY HYDRATED

Along with your Clean eats and liquid treats you are in for a big surprise. Within no time your body will be thanking you for giving it the gift of hydration. Watch your skin start to glow, your bowels start to move and your head start to clear. Another exciting benefit from drinking water is that keeping yourself adequately hydrated will boost your metabolism by as much as three percent. What an incredibly simple way to lose weight! Feeling better?

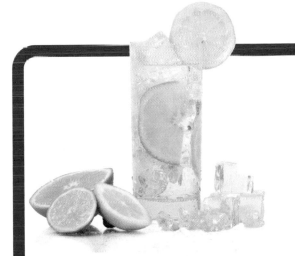

MAKING WATER BETTER

Let's face it: there are some days when we just want a little something more. You can have your water and drink it too (enjoy it), with the right combination of extra ingredients. Adding these little splashes of flavor will perk up your water and keep you sipping all day long:

- Slices of lemon or lime (my personal favorite)
- Slices of cucumbers and oranges
- A splash of unsweetened fruit juice (orange, cranberry, pomegranate, apple)
- Caffeine-free herbal tea bags
- Flower essences
- Peppermint leaves
- Mineral water (use sporadically, as the phosphorus present in the bubbles can leach important minerals from your bones)

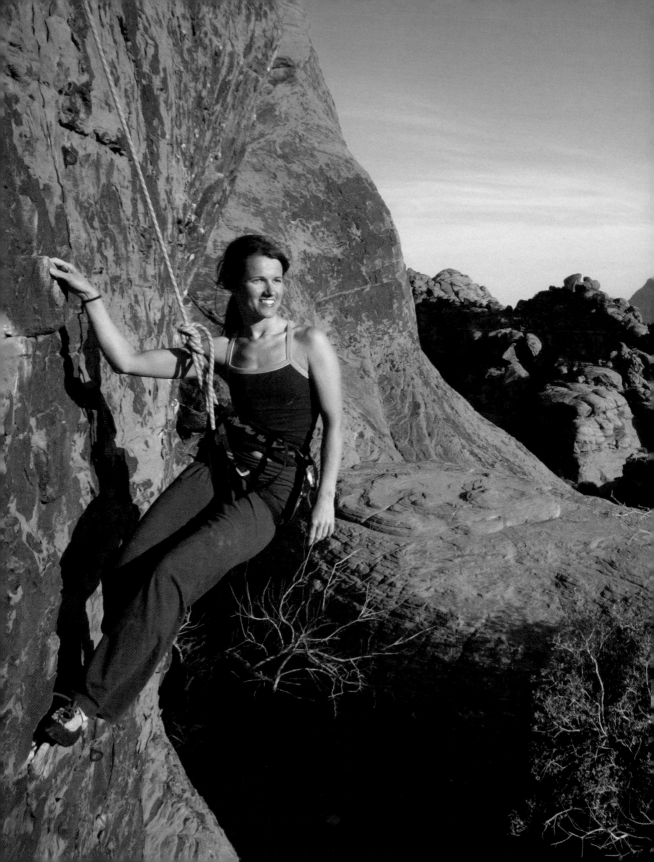

RECLAIMING YOUR LIFE

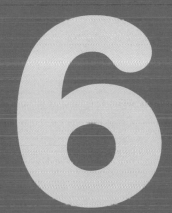

Think back to when you were a kid. What were your dreams? Is your life now as you pictured it then? Chances are it's not. I know when I was chasing through my teens I had no clear vision of what my life would be like, although I did have a recurring dream that I was on stage. My visions for my life became even blurrier once I focused on raising my children. My 30s were clouded with "must dos" and I lost sight of any aspirations I once had.

We can't go back in time and change our decisions, just as we can't magically make ourselves great actors or singers, but we always have the opportunity to find a path that brings us back to the essential us – the person we know we truly could be. It takes a mix of fearlessness and, as I like to say, "the courage to plug your nose and jump off the cliff into the great unknown."

Just before my transformation at the age of 40, I no longer recognized myself. I had once been a happy, fun-loving, active girl filled with dreams and potential. I ran or cycled everywhere and I was always positive and upbeat. Something changed. As the decades progressed I became miserable, middle aged, over-weight, unhealthy and crying into stacks of laundry. I was unhappy in my marriage and more importantly, unhappy with myself. What had happened to me? The person I once was had disappeared!

THE AHA! DAY

I consider the day I decided to change my life to be my true rebirth. Not only did I escape the miserable life I was living, but I also unearthed the person I had always wanted to be. Now, 10 years later, I'm still that new person – the real me. I wake up in the morning full of energy, ready to take on whatever the day brings. Each day is a new day of promise.

This is possible for you too! There is no reason for you to remain in the state you're in. Why would anyone want to stay lonely, forgotten, unhappy and increasingly addicted to food? Over and over again, people tell me they can't do it. It's too late. I've heard this from men and women in their 40s, 50s and 60s, but I've also heard it from people in their early 20s. Yes, really! Logically, you must know deep inside that you can make change regardless of how old you are. Just because you haven't done it yet doesn't mean you can't or never will. I firmly believe that there is no "best before" date on health and fitness. Anyone who is 40, 50, 60 or beyond does not have to accept slippers, curlers and crutches as the natural fate of their increasing age. I can't wait for you to discover your true potential.

"I can't wait for you to discover your true potential."

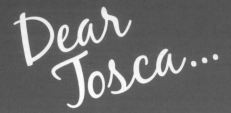
In 1998 I became a registered dietitian. Eat Clean is the advice we (dietitians) tell to those with diabetes and other diseases. However, as I was always carrying extra weight (at that time 20 lbs), I never felt very motivated to be teaching others.

After I got married and had some trouble with pregnancies I reached an all time high of 220 lbs at the height of 5'6". I decided to go to therapy to look at what I thought were weight issues and over that year lost 20 lbs by walking and very likely 'letting go' of past issues. After taking some drastic measures, I was able to shed a lot of weight. My body was defi-

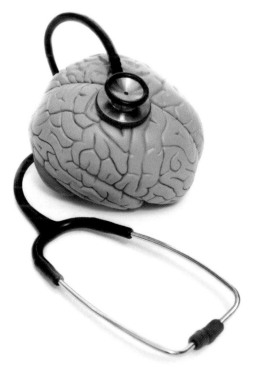

nitely smaller, but I was soft and out of shape. It was like the biggest clunk over the head, asking me, "So, when are you actually going to treat your body well enough that you NEVER have to go through such extreme measures again!?"

I found *Clean Eating* magazine and through that YOU. You, the way you write, your story, your passion, your articulate way of writing 'clicked' me on to the Eat-Clean lifestyle. My body has been changing so drastically! I feel grateful for my entire journey, as I've been struggling with my weight since the age of 9. My choice – the ONLY choice for me – is Eating Clean.

Thank you from the bottom of my heart for making the knowledge I already possessed a true internal realization. It never ceases to amaze me that the vibration and energy of one individual can permeate to another that she has never even met!

With much gratitude,
Arlene Moshe
Thornhill, Ontario

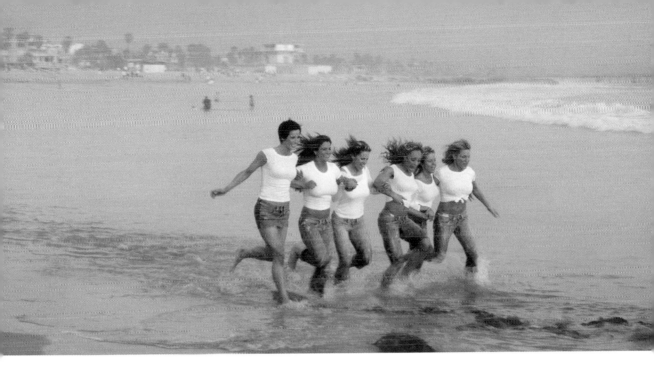

OTHERS BEFORE ME

Grandma Moses began a successful art career in her 70s. Her breathtaking images have moved us all. Laura Ingalls Wilder, author of the classic *Little House on the Prairie* series (which later became a popular TV show), did not begin writing until her 60s. Julia Childs parlayed her love of cooking into a cultural phenomenon in her 50s. The Dutch Olympian, Fanny Blankers-Koen, won four gold medals at the 1948 Summer Olympics, breaking both track and world records, all at the age of 30 and as a mother of two! These are examples of women who did not regard age as a reason to stop living, but instead got fully energized about life, precisely when others were putting up their feet to rest on the couch.

I did the same. My friends say I always do things backwards. It was not until I faced the age of 40 that I began to pursue a career in fitness and swimsuit modeling, bodybuilding and motivational speaking. This at a time when most of the other models were barely 21! It was also at this time I finally found the courage to begin another youthful passion of mine, writing. Once I started I couldn't stop, although I felt like I had run out of words with every book I finished. Not so! There are numerous projects on the table and I am more excited about each one.

A short time ago I received a letter from a woman in her 70s. She decided it was time to lose the 75 extra pounds she had been carrying around with her for most of her life, and she did so. She started attending fitness classes. Eventually the health club she attended asked whether she might like to teach a class. At the age of 75 she got her fitness certificate and is now an aerobics instructor. Wahoo for her!

One of my favorite stories is about Andora Quinby. After giving birth to eight children and having served as a physicist in WWII, Andora became an aquatics instructor at the age of 46. At 75, she earned her master's degree in Human Services Management. At 78, she was introduced to weightlifting and now at 89 (at least 90 by the time you read this), she is a world-champion weightlifter. Andora still teaches aqua-fit classes once a week, where she sometimes scoffs at the young 60-somethings who say they're getting too old for this.

> "Taking good care of yourself, and looking and feeling your best is the only way to live!"

Ask yourself if anything is holding you back. Is it fear of the unknown? Are you comfortable where you are? Is your mindset programmed to believe that you will fail anyway, so why bother trying? I know how you feel because I felt that way too before I resurrected myself. Thoughts like these are normal and even the most successful among us encounter them, but to retain them in your mind prevents you from being the "best you" possible. It's a self-limiting, cruel way of thinking because it robs you of the richness to be found in living a full, happy, purposeful life – the only kind of life worth living.

FEAR OF THE UNKNOWN

Imagine if you never did anything you hadn't done before, just because you didn't know what the outcome would be. You might still be an infant unable to walk, talk or eat. You wouldn't have played in puddles. You wouldn't have gone to school. You wouldn't have traveled. You wouldn't have sung, danced, kissed or have gotten married. Life begins with the unknown and if we're lucky, we continue to experience the unknown throughout our lives.

It's reasonable to fear the unknown if the unknown is entering a dark cave at night or driving down a dark country road not knowing where you are going. That's sensible and is an instinctual, built-in response designed to keep us safe. The fear of losing excess weight, however, is not sensible. Fat gained from uncontrolled eating is not who you are; it is simply an outer coating. As weight is lost and a leaner physique emerges, you simply unveil your inner self – the person you were always meant to be. Your brain, your soul and your heart have not changed, although your heart will be in better shape, your brain will think how wise you are to make such positive changes and your soul will rejoice at your newfound happiness!

If I could grant any wish for you in this life, I would wish for you to discover what I have found to be true, that taking good care of yourself, and looking and feeling your best is the only way to live!

COMFORT ZONE

You may not like what you see in the mirror but your reflection is familiar. It's your old, comfortable self. It turns out that the average person spends at least 45 minutes each day getting ready for work or his or her other daily activities. A good portion of that time is spent in front of the looking glass, and we continue to check ourselves out in front of the mirror around five times each day. We are so very familiar with ourselves, many of us are a little tuned out to the reality of our own appearance.

I see my daughters constantly standing in front of the mirror and I have observed a pattern. First they stand facing the mirror full on. They suck in the tummy and then, preferring the side view because you can look thinner this way, they turn sideways and really suck in the waist. At this point some kind of decision is made regarding how they feel about themselves and their appearance that day. I do the same thing. I think we all do, but that sideways view can be a little misleading.

We may look thinner sideways than from the front, but that really doesn't tell the whole truthful story. To effectively manage your weight and make changes, you must step out of your comfort zone, which means you must break the old constructs of how you view yourself. Stepping out of your comfort zone requires bravery and a heck of a lot of discipline, attributes you may have left in a younger, more hopeful version of yourself. It is far more comfortable for you to remain sitting on the couch, remote control in hand. But staying ensconced on the couch is a bad habit that leaves you inactive and wondering if and when things will ever change.

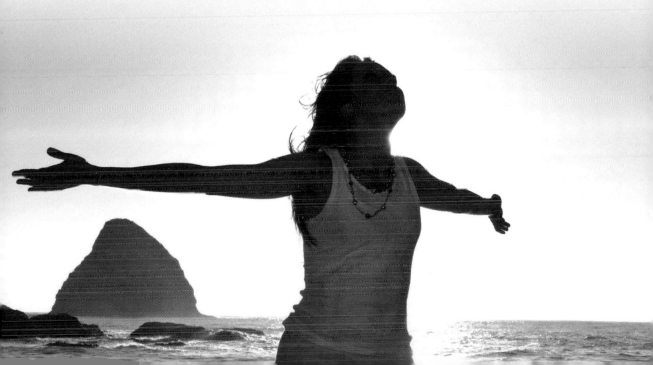

"If you want to reclaim your life and if you want to be the leaner version of yourself that is currently hidden from view beneath an insulating layer of fat, then you're going to have to break out of your comfort zone. You cannot change anything by sticking to your current habits."

Habits tend to become routine activities in our lives, and they have either positive or negative consequences. Brushing your teeth is a good habit. Parking yourself on the couch at every opportunity is a bad habit. Eating sugarcoated cereal for breakfast is an unhealthy habit, but you were used to eating it every morning. Switching to a bowl of oatmeal with some scrambled egg whites would bring you out of your comfort zone. By changing your breakfast, you could start to rebuild and reenergize yourself, but which is stronger, your desire for a new you or that familiar bad habit?

Pulling yourself off of the couch is darn hard work and it's something that feels awful the first time you do it. It's difficult because you are leaving your comfort zone, but the payoff is huge if you can make the change. You may be in the habit of going to the coffee shop for a cream- and sugar-filled coffee and jelly donut to pick yourself up mid-morning. (I recognize this routine; I did it myself every day before my Reno-vation!)

The woman who works behind the counter expects you every day. In fact, when she sees you coming, she gets your coffee and donut ready without even asking. That makes you feel special because someone knows exactly what you like. It's comfortable. If you don't show up for your morning fix, "Donut Lady" will think something is wrong. Here's a habit you will need to change if you want to see something different in the mirror.

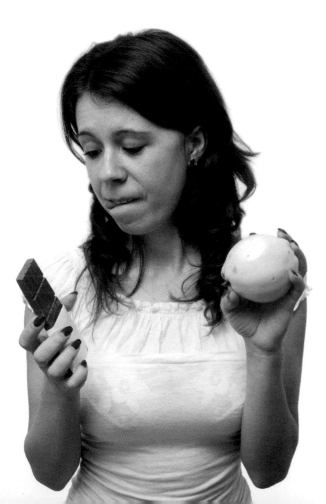

> "Taking small steps to become this new vivid you will change you for the better!"

Your evenings are spent sprawled out in baggy sweatpants on the couch, watching TV and munching on nacho chips with your spouse. It's comfortable. It's your routine. The opposite of your routine would be to go for a workout after dinner, come home, shower and get into bed early. Whoa! That would be way too uncomfortable for you! I have heard both men and women say they don't work out because they don't like to get sticky and sweaty from training. I must be an odd duck then because I love it! A little bit of hardworking sweat never put me off anything.

If you want to reclaim your life and if you want to be the leaner version of yourself that is currently hidden from view beneath an insulating layer of fat, then you're going to have to break out of your comfort zone. You cannot change anything by stick-ing to your current habits. I think the movie starring Jack Nicholson, *As Good as it Gets*, says it all. Jack plays a character with obsessive-compulsive disorder (OCD), and is literally paralyzed with fear about germs. As the movie progresses, Jack's character takes risks that little by little, expose him to the messiness that is life, until he eventually finds love and a whole new meaning to life, living fully and vibrantly.

Taking small steps to become this new vivid you will change you for the better. Before long, a healthy, luminous, beautiful Eat-Clean lifestyle will become your new comfort zone. You will get so exhilarated by the positive transformations you have made by Eating Clean, you will never want to give it up! I make that a promise.

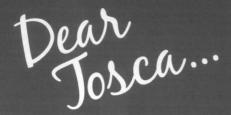

TESTIMONIAL

I had always been the big girl or the skinny girl ... never in between. I'm in my 20s so I don't have too many years under my belt, but I have lost 40+ lbs THREE TIMES in my life. People would ask why I had gained weight again, and I told them that I was the size I was meant to be, because I working out four times a week with no results. I woke up one day and felt like an idiot. I could barely fit into regular-sized clothes. I drank too much, had stomach problems and stopped working because I had no energy. I was 5'9", 180 lbs and had no muscle.

I finally decided to order *The Eat-Clean Diet* from *Oxygen* magazine. I read it, and after the first chapter I called off all of my appointments. I read the entire thing in a day. I get it! I get why I have to eat often, what protein does and why sugar is bad. Everything clicked! I started right then and there by cutting out all of the sugar in my diet. I quit the sugar in my coffee, and stopped eating cookies and ice cream.

The weight began falling off of my body. I lost 3 – 4 lbs per week for the first few weeks, and then I started to follow the program in the back of *The Eat-Clean Diet* and kept losing and losing. The only exercise I did was walking my dogs. I lost 25 lbs in six weeks before I hit my first plateau. I bought a gym pass, cleaned up my diet, ate more veggies and lost 10 more lbs.

I get up at 4 or 5 am and go to bed at 11 at night and feel amazing! I work out every day, work long hours, prepare my food, take care of my house, three animals, my beautiful boyfriend and our property, and I have so much energy! My stomach problems are gone. I don't crash at 3 pm EVER. I love eating and still get to do just that - six times a day. I run faster, I look firmer, my skin is healthier and I have more confidence.

Eating Clean truly is 80 percent of the battle. If you want to change your life but not the way you eat; you're wasting your time. This is not a diet, it's a lifestyle, and I know that I won't gain back the fat because I live Clean. Woohoo!

Jenna Begin

ATTENTION IS SCARY

Many overweight people tell me they use their excess fat to insulate themselves from others, and this was certainly the case for me. There are many reasons for protecting oneself this way. For some, the fatty layer is a form of protection against abuse, shyness and unhappiness. For others, it's more of an awareness of the affliction they suffer with, being overweight, and a sense that they are different from most other people in the world.

This is flawed thinking because ultimately, excess fat is already a common problem, and is the source of much heartache and even disease in many cases. There is still a very real stigma against overweight people, even though the vast majority of us do carry excess poundage. In my experience, I have found that the greatest degree of depression arises from lowered self-esteem and unhappiness, both of which describe how an overweight person feels about their looks. My heart aches for you.

If you have demons that make you want to hide from the world under a layer of fat or in another destructive way, then you'll have to learn to deal with those issues in a different way. Hiding or avoiding your situation does not yield positive change; it simply prolongs your prison sentence inside an unhappy, unhealthy body. Only you can free yourself! Bob Marley once said, "Emancipate yourself from mental slavery," and while he was not referring to the

"I have found that the greatest degree of depression arises from lowered self-esteem and unhappiness associated with being overweight."

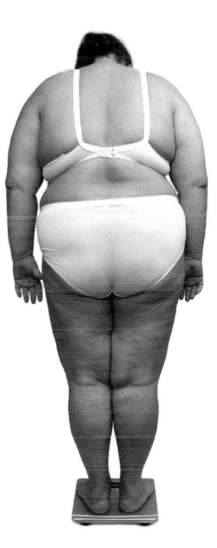

"The way people perceive you depends on the way you present yourself."

subject of weight, his command is relevant to any person allowing him or herself to remain in a personal prison against his or her true will.

If you are uncomfortable with sexual attention, do not fear. Although your new, leaner self will, without a doubt, make you feel more attractive, you don't have to attract sexual attention unless you want it. The way people perceive you depends on the way you present yourself. At her heaviest, Anna Nicole Smith was an estimated 100 pounds overweight, and she still had plenty of men lusting after her. Conversely, the most in-shape wallflower will still go unnoticed. Being large doesn't take the attention off of you, and likewise, being lean doesn't put the attention on.

It's a matter of how you carry yourself and how you show yourself to the world. Marilyn Monroe was famous among friends for being able to disappear into a crowd. One of the biggest celebrities in history, Marilyn could walk down a street and have no one notice her. This was because she knew how to "turn it off." She made her posture more average, drew her face inward and after a few minutes of being "off" she could "turn it back on." She held herself more confidently, walked with more purpose and she would shine from her eyes, truly giving herself to the world. People would notice her again and she controlled it. You can do this too, if you wish. Although, you might find that once you start looking great you will want *more* attention, not *less!*

FAILURE IS MY LIFE!

You may think "failure" is your middle name. You have tried to achieve again and again, and failure is always the end result. The average number of times a smoker attempts quitting before he or she stops for good is 14 times. If that smoker said after the 13th try, "What's the point? I'll never succeed," then he or she would be right. Those who say, "This time I will succeed!" do succeed. Thomas Edison, an inventor who only had a few weeks of formal schooling, attempted to create the electric incandescent lightbulb over 10,000 times! 10,000?! One of the things he said regarding his efforts was, "I had to succeed because I was I running out of ways to fail, I had to keep going!" I love this philosophy!

The truth is that the more you do something, the better you get at it. Practice really does make perfect. An excellent illustration of this point is the fact that you are reading this book, right now, instead of one that claims you can lose ten or more pounds in a few days. After countless attempts to lose unwanted pounds, you know fad diets simply don't work. None of your previous weight-loss efforts have yielded long-term results. If you were to be totally honest with yourself, you might even say you are even heavier now, from repeated diet misfires, than you were before you tried losing weight!

With my book in your hands, as you read on, you are beginning to understand that to lose your excess weight you can't cut out food groups, and that good health depends on consuming fresh, nutrient-dense foods while avoiding anti-foods.

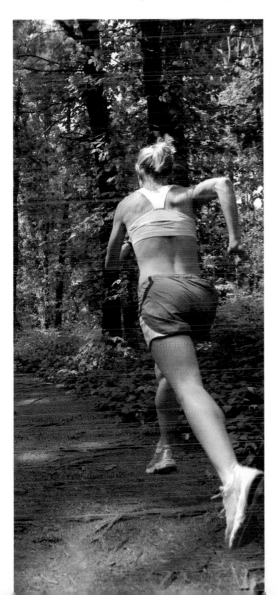

> "Those who say, 'This time I will succeed!' do succeed."

Becoming familiar with your weaknesses is part of successfully living the Eat-Clean lifestyle, and if you are determined to lose weight and live a healthier life, you have to know how to work around them. There are chapters in this book that will give you strategies for Eating Clean during times when temptation is at its highest. Many of you will need an Eat-Clean plan for celebrations and parties. A lot of people cannot stay on course without planning their meals in advance, especially if they are eating outside of the home. Temptations also exist at home. You know if you keep goodies in your cupboards they'll be calling to you till you give in. Why keep them around in the first place? Your new life begins right now.

Losing weight is not a mad dash to the finish line. You know that even if it takes a little longer to lose weight by Eating Clean, the weight loss will be permanent. One year, five years, 10, 20, 30 years from now, you will still be lean, healthy, vibrant and wonderful instead of bemoaning the fact that you've once again put on another 10 pounds on top of what you weighed before. If you're young and haven't wasted years trying fad diet after fad diet, then good for you! You're smarter than I was!

It doesn't matter that up until this point you have not achieved your weight-loss goals. What's past is past and you can do nothing to change your history, but you can absolutely change your future. From this point on choose the direct, home-run path that will get you to your goals.

Try this visualization exercise: picture two paths. At the end of one path is a bleak, miserable, polluted, gray city, populated with sick, unhappy people. At the end of the other path is a beautiful village by the sea, with fresh air, happy people and a general feeling of wellbeing. The path to the beautiful village might have steep hills or rocky terrain and the path to the polluted city might be easier. However, if you found yourself accidentally walking on the path that leads to the miserable gray city, would you simply stay on that path until its inevitable outcome? Or would you switch over to the other path, even if getting there might be less comfortable?

If you are choosing to Eat Clean, you are making the choice to walk on the path to the beautiful seaside village. If you continue to eat junk food and not look after yourself, you are choosing to walk on the path to the miserable, polluted city. Make the right choice and make it every day. If you find you've slipped and gotten sidetracked, don't fret and give up. Cross over to the other path. Continue to do this day by day and you will soon wake up and realize that Eating Clean is not really a diet at all. It is a lifestyle that has allowed you to reclaim your life. What a wonderful life it is!

"At the end of the other path is a beautiful village by the sea, with fresh air, happy people, and a general feeling of wellbeing."

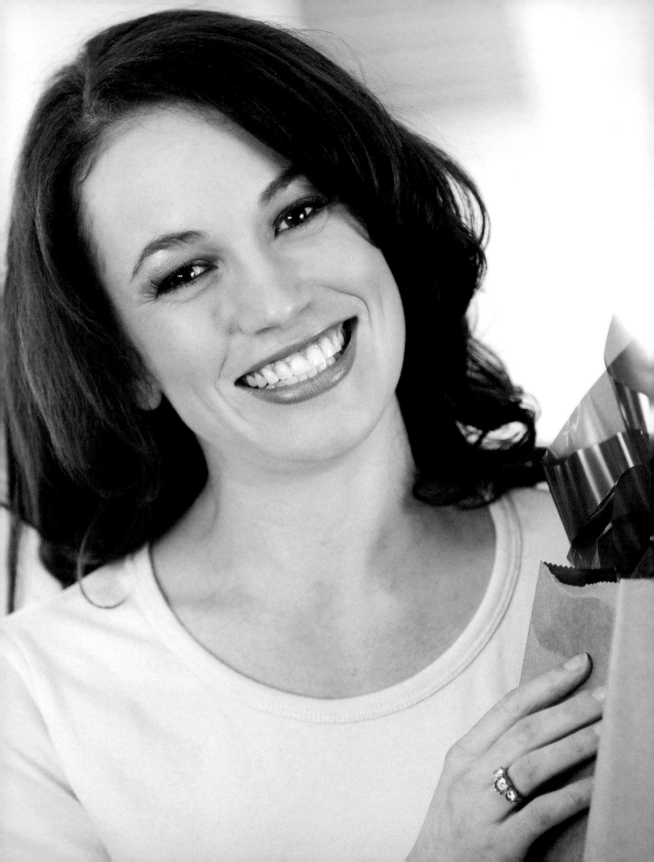

SHOPPING CLEAN

7

FINDING THE FOOD THAT BUILDS A LEAN, FAT-BURNING PHYSIQUE

You're well on your way to Eating Clean, congratulations! You're already picturing a new, slimmer version of yourself, with better health and increased energy. You've thrown out the junk in your cupboards and beer in your fridge. Family-sized bags of potato chips are now in the garbage and liters of soda have been dumped down the drain. Your poor eating habits are a thing of the past. You're ready… and a little bit hungry – so now what? When your pantry is bare, it's time to go shopping!

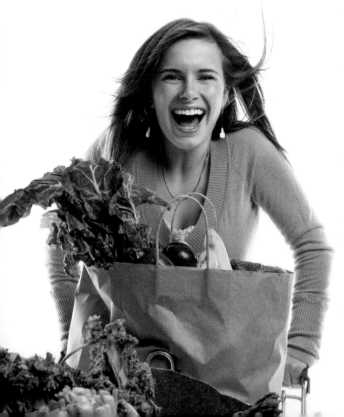

This may seem like a daunting task at first. Where do I shop for Clean foods? What foods should I buy? How can I avoid the temptation of the cookie aisle? How much is Eating Clean going to cost me? If you find yourself asking some (or all) of these questions, don't worry, you are not alone. When I started Eating Clean, shopping was an intimidating experience. I worried I wasn't going to make the right food choices. It's so easy to focus on what you can't eat anymore, instead of all of the wonderful, fresh, natural foods you **can** have in abundance. My fear didn't last long. I am very much an all-or-nothing girl, so for me it was as straightforward as telling myself to jump in and go, which I did, naturally!

NO MORE QUESTIONS!

You'll soon realize that Eating Clean takes the guesswork out of shopping. Going to the grocery store can be a pleasant experience and quite possibly an adventure when you know what to buy and where to look for it. It's exciting when you are on the lookout for that next unusual food item that fits the Eat-Clean lifestyle. Yes, I admit I get excited when I find dinosaur kale or star fruit in the produce aisle. When I line up at the cash register I feel proud that my grocery cart is overflowing with healthy, nourishing foods that will sustain my family. I know you will soon be proud to feel the same way.

BEFORE YOU BEGIN

Plan ahead! Whether you are shopping for your-self or your entire family, it's a good idea to think about the food you're going to need for the upcoming week. My family ranges in size from five to ten people, depending on who is home that week, so I need to be really organized to avoid an empty fridge!

Start by planning a menu. Even if you eat most of your meals alone, this is a definite must. Take stock of the foods you already have in your fridge and pantry, and combine these with the foods you plan to buy to create enough Eat-Clean meals for the entire week. There will be foods you need to buy once a week, such as dairy products and fresh produce, and those you need to buy less often, such as canned goods. Keep an eye on the items in your pantry and restock as needed – you never know when you are going to need that can of chickpeas. I gain more confidence with my cooking when I know my pantry is well stocked with basic items that can yield a meal with little or no trouble. Our grocery list will help you create a similar pantry (see Chapter 14 for grocery lists).

Make a shopping list and stick to it! Not only will you be more efficient with your precious time and hard-earned dollars, but you will find it much easier to avoid tempting foods. The cookie aisle still calls my name from time to time, but I know that if something is not on my shopping list, it's not going in my cart. This is a good rule to stick to but allowances can be

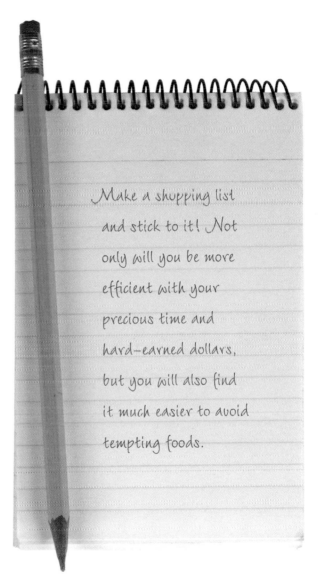

Make a shopping list and stick to it! Not only will you be more efficient with your precious time and hard-earned dollars, but you will also find it much easier to avoid tempting foods.

made on occasion. I'm talking about those deep red strawberries that are too plump and juicy to pass up, not the Pop Tarts on sale at the end of Aisle Four!

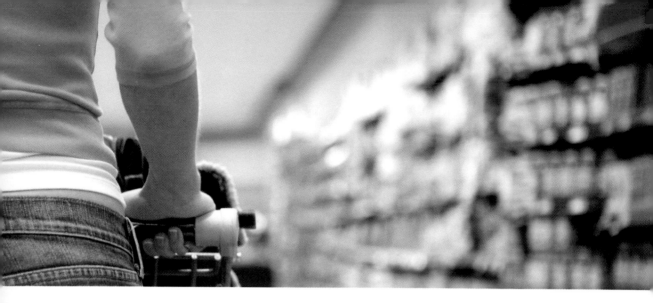

If you are shopping for your entire family, it may make sense to shop alone. It may be easy to deny yourself the junk you used to eat, but I can tell you from experience it's much harder to resist those cute little faces begging you for just one treat. Until those chubby little fingers are grabbing for bananas and carrot sticks, it's best to shop solo. There will also be more room in your cart for must-have Clean eats – it's amazing how quickly the grocery cart fills up. Soon enough your family will also be interested in the Clean shopping experience and you can make going for groceries an event. My children don't mind coming with me, especially if we are going to a farmer's market or Whole Foods. They enjoy selecting good foods too.

One last thing before we begin — eat something before you go. Studies have shown we have a hard time sticking to our shopping lists when we are hungry. Not only will you buy too much food when shopping on an empty stomach, but you'll also make choices you wouldn't ordinarily make. Sounds like a recipe for an Eat-Clean disaster!

THE GROCERY STORE

The grocery store can seem like an overwhelming place. It's like a casino. It's huge, there are no windows, no clocks and temptation is everywhere! Now that you know how to Eat Clean, you don't want to compromise your goals for achieving a lean, healthy body by gambling away your health on anti-foods. Did you know that grocery stores are designed to draw you in? Think about it. In every grocery store you've ever been to, when the front doors swing open you are immediately confronted with the sight of colorful, shiny ripe fruits and vegetables, and the overpowering (albeit delightful) scent of freshly baked breads and other goods. It's heavenly, and storeowners want you to be sorely tempted by these delicious aromas – that is part of their game to get **you** to spend your money in **their** store.

One of the best things about standard grocery stores is that they have everything you need in one place. From whole-grain breads to fresh produce, low-fat milk and eggs to lean meats, it's all there for you. Personally, I don't always do all my shopping at the grocery store (as you'll see later on in this chapter) but it does have everything you need to Eat Clean. How convenient!

Have you ever heard the term, "Shop the Perimeter?" This means to stick to the outer walls of the grocery store, avoiding the aisles in the middle. Of course it's unrealistic to assume that you'll never go down any of the aisles, but for the most part, shopping the perimeter is a helpful tip for any Clean Eater. Think about it – all of the freshest foods such as fruits, vegetables and freshly baked breads (sometimes made right in the store!) are kept close to the outer walls of the store. Foods that need to be chilled, including meats, eggs, yogurts and milk will also be found on the outer aisles of most grocery stores.

Make a plan upon entering the grocery store to shop the perimeter first and then work your way through the center aisles. By that time your cart will already be filled to the brim with fresh, healthy foods so you won't have much room for packaged goods. Look at your list and load up on fruits, vegetables, lean meats, fresh whole grains and whole-grain products. Include breads and wraps, low-fat milk and yogurt, and milk alternatives such as soy, almond and rice milk.

Keep focused when browsing the center aisles. Food choices tower over you on each side. Shelves are stocked from head to toe with no room between products. Cans of sardines are literally packed like a can of sardines! You can see now why I advise you not to go grocery shopping on an empty stomach. Hunger pangs plus endless food options right at your fingertips does not equal sensible shopping. It's not necessary to browse every single aisle of the store, either. There are some aisles that I choose to avoid completely. Can you guess which these might be? If your answer was the junk food or soda aisle, you're right.

Start with the frozen food section. Here it's easy to decipher between Clean foods and anti-foods. Anything advertised as a one-step, heat-and-serve, or ready-to-go meal in a box is most likely not what you want to be feeding your family. Learn to read nutrition labels. Look at the ingredient list. If you can't pronounce some of the words or if they look like they belong in a science laboratory, put the product back on the shelf. Skip the frozen pizzas, lunch-sized meals and canned sugary drinks. Try unsweetened frozen fruits. They can be a huge money saver in the winter when fresh varieties are out of season. Frozen vegetables are perfect in a pinch, as long as the vegetables are the only ingredients listed on the package.

DECIPHERING NUTRITION LABELS

They may look like a foreign language, but nutrition labels are here to help – not confuse – you. Learning how to read them is easy, as long as you know what you are looking for. It is also a good idea not to believe everything you read once in the grocery store. Many Big Food Companies "trick" the unsuspecting consumer by making all sorts of ridiculous claims about food. Beware the glitzy packaging and outlandish claims!

Nutriton Facts
Per 1 cup (54 g) serving

Amount	% Daily Value
Calories	200
Fat 2 g	3 %
Saturated 0.4 g	2 %
+Trans 0 g	
Cholesterol 0 mg	
Sodium 115 mg	5 %
Carbohydrate 41 g	14 %
Fibre 4 g	17 %
Sugars 15 g	
Vitamin A	8 %
Vitamin C	15 %
Iron	50 %
Niacin	10 %
Zinc	10 %

(1) Serving information is listed at the top of the nutrition label and is important, because the information on the rest of the label is based on one portion of the package only. You'd be surprised that some products (one bottle of juice or one cookie) often contain more than one serving. Now that you know, you'll never be fooled again! Be mindful of what constitutes a serving. The number of servings in the entire package is also listed here.

(2) Below the serving information is the amount of calories, fat(s), sodium, carbohydrates, sugar, protein and fiber in the product. This is where it can get confusing, so I'll try to make it as simple as possible. Saturated fats, trans fats, added sugars and sodium are things we want to avoid. (These are generally absent from Clean foods anyway.) We want to consume healthy fats and foods with high amounts of protein and fiber, because these are the foods that will keep our blood sugar stable, stomachs satisfied and our health optimal. The percentages to the right of this information are based on a 2,000-calorie a day diet. Since Eating Clean does not include calorie counting, this is not something you need to be overly concerned about.

(3) Further down is the part that shows you how much of the recommended amount of certain vitamins and minerals are in the food. Your goal is to reach 100 percent for each vitamin and mineral every day.

The canned foods aisle can be a Clean Eater's dream. Look for low-sodium versions of your favorites. Canned tomatoes, tomato paste, canned beans (white beans, chickpeas, lentils, kidney beans, mixed beans), peas and corn, tuna and salmon packed in water, and low-fat soups are excellent options to have waiting in the pantry. A well-stocked pantry can be lifesaving when it comes to mealtimes.

When shopping for grains, always choose whole grains. Oatmeal (not the instant kind), wheat germ, Cream of Wheat, bulgur, millet and quinoa can be found in the cereal, grains or baking aisle, depending on your store. If your grocery store has a section for organic products, some foods may be located there as well.

It's also necessary to venture down the baking aisle. Here (along with the Devil's Food Cake and chocolate chip cookies) you'll find whole-grain flours, baking supplies including vanilla, baking soda and baking powder, high-quality oils, seeds and nuts, and a variety of spices. Using various spices is a key element to Eating Clean. You can cut out the fat and chemicals while keeping the taste and flavors of your favorite foods. Like spicy food? No problem, just add a little Cajun seasoning. Prefer the tastes of India? Try curry powder or a five-spice blend. One of my favorites is garam masala.

"The canned foods aisle can be a Clean Eater's dream. Look for low-sodium versions of your favorites."

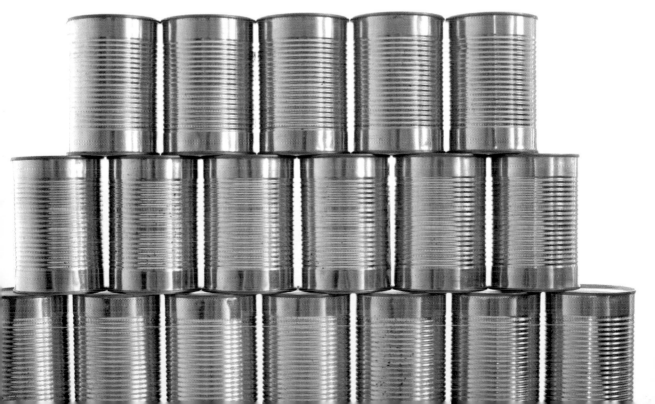

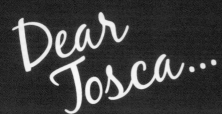

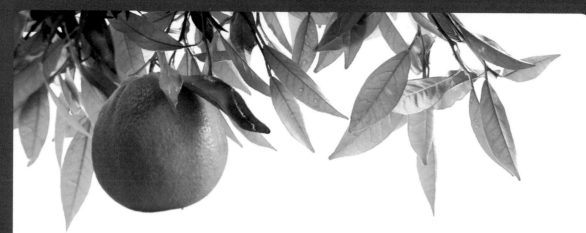

I am 23 years old and I have had a battle with my weight and food for most of my life. I was an overweight child until I was diagnosed and treated for having an underactive thyroid.

My family would tell me to lose weight. They cared, but it hit me hard and I developed a negative mindset towards my physical appearance. When I lost the weight I looked great, but in my mind I was still too heavy, so I wanted to lose more and more and more without caring what it would do to my body. I tried starving myself, skipping meals, eating only very low-calorie foods, Weight Watchers, The Atkins Diet, The South Beach Diet, diet pills, etc.

Like a drug addict, I never thought that I would be able to go a week without bingeing, but Eating Clean has really taught me a healthy way to live and made me a better me. I don't even remember the last time I even had an urge to binge. I am a better daughter, girlfriend, teacher, student, and every role that I play – I'm better at it. I can think clearly now. I was constantly wondering: is that too many calories? Do I have control? When can I have a brownie? I constantly nagged myself about my weight and food choices. It truly came to a point where I could not enjoy life. I now know that I was a slave to food.

When I Eat Clean, I breathe a sigh of relief, because I get to enjoy the true tastes, the smells, and the textures of REAL FOOD. I am not sitting with a box of processed, manmade food. I am fueling my body with something the Earth produced. I would recommend this way of life to anyone and I hope that more people catch on to Eating Clean.

Mary Milhalchik

OTHER PLACES TO SHOP

If you are lucky enough to live in a big city or close to a metropolitan area, you likely have a few more shopping options than just a grocery store when it comes to searching for Clean food – and I'm not talking about the 24-hour convenience store around the corner. Although it might take a few different trips to get everything you need, shopping at several different places can be beneficial for numerous reasons.

Shopping around allows you to be choosier in terms of the foods you are putting in your body. Visiting several stores means you can choose the brands you know and trust. It also means you can aim to purchase foods in their most natural state, guaranteeing they will be tastier, more nutritious and the healthiest for you and your loved ones. For example, doesn't it make more sense to buy your summer vegetables directly from the farmer who grows them locally, as opposed to a grocery store that ships them in from across the country, allowing them to ripen on the truck? In my mind this makes sense on many levels, particularly from a carbon footprint point of view. It also improves the local economy. Following are some of the alternative places I like to shop:

THE SPECIALTY GROCERY STORE

The kind of grocery store often referred to as a natural or organic foods market is a great place to start shopping because it caters to people who are looking for healthier, more natural options – people like you! The downside is that these stores can be more expensive. The upsides, however, are plenty! Organic stores often have several options of harder-to-find products, such as kefir, low-fat natural cottage cheese, strained natural yogurt, spelt, buckwheat and rice pastas, Ezekiel breads and whole grains. The produce at specialty stores is incredibly fresh and sometimes entirely organic. Specialty stores often work together with local farmers and charities creating initiatives that help local communities and planet Earth in general. When we make food choices we are essentially voting with our dollars, and those dollars end up supporting either big food companies, who don't care about anything but making a profit (there are exceptions), or the local organic farmer who has your health and your planet in mind. So don't underestimate the importance of making good food/Eat-Clean food choices. Your dollars add up collectively to make a big difference.

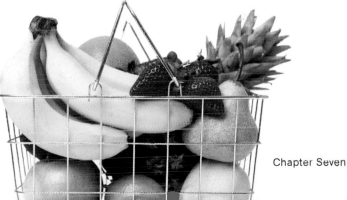

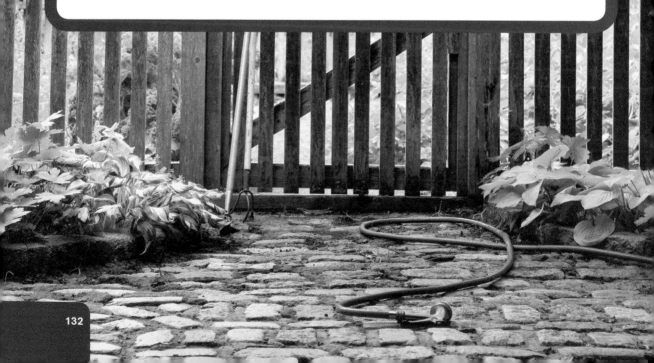

SHOULD I OR SHOULDN'T I SHOP ORGANIC?

We've all seen organic fruits and vegetables in the grocery store, sitting there, looking holier than thou with their claims of health and expensive price tags. Are they really that much better for you than regular produce? This question is becoming more and more important, especially in light of the fact that not all organic companies have the best in mind for you either. You, the Eat-Clean consumer, need to be on the alert, even in the Organic Section of town.

There are a few good reasons to shop organic. First, shopping organic supports small local farmers, who are paid a fairer price for their organic produce. Organic fruits and vegetables are also better for you. Studies have shown that chemicals and residual pesticides linger on fruits and vegetables even after they've been washed. Organic farmers work hard for their organic certification – it takes three years to achieve this – and so supporting the efforts of these farmers also supports the greater cause of keeping our planet clean and green.

In a perfect world we would all shop organic. Actually, if we lived in a perfect world, we wouldn't need to use any chemicals or pesticides to begin with! Since we don't, we can shop smart by choosing to buy organic versions of the produce most heavily affected by pesticides and regular versions of the produce that is not.

THE 12 FRUIT AND VEGETABLES MOST CONTAMINATED BY PESTICIDES ARE:

1	Apples	7	Peaches
2	Bell peppers	8	Pears
3	Celery	9	Potatoes
4	Cherries	10	Raspberries
5	Imported grapes	11	Spinach
6	Nectarines	12	Strawberries

THE TOP 12 FRUITS AND VEGETABLES (A LOT OF THESE HAVE THICK, PROTECTIVE SKINS) LEAST CONTAMINATED BY PESTICIDES ARE:

1	Asparagus	7	Kiwis
2	Avocados	8	Mangoes
3	Bananas	9	Onions
4	Broccoli	10	Papaya
5	Cauliflower	11	Pineapples
6	Corn	12	Sweet peas

> "If you haven't been to your local bulk store in a while, it's time to take a second look."

THE HEALTH FOOD STORE

The health food store is a smaller version of the natural food store, with more emphasis on nutritional supplements and wellbeing. Here you can find whole grains, small quantities of fresh fruits and vegetables, vitamins and supplements, and some less common items like seaweed, miso, tempeh and kombu. Health food stores are often independently owned and the owner (or shopkeeper) is knowledgeable about the products sold there. The health food store is a great place to find daily vitamins, bee pollen, flaxseed, wheat germ and protein powders. If you are looking for more natural protein sources, this is the place to go. Health food stores carry many different protein powders, including options for vegans, such as hemp and soy.

My favorite health food store also carries grass- and grain-fed meats and poultry, wild fish, and eggs from free-range hens, along with numerous exotic oils, vinegars and spices that make my Eat-Clean food preparation far more interesting.

THE BULK FOOD STORE

If you can avoid the giant bins of sour gummies and chocolate chips, the bulk food store is an amazing place to load up on Clean foods. The best part is the savings! By buying bulk, you are avoiding brand packaging, which can save you a lot of money in the long run. Again, buying foods with less packaging is a Green initiative, which you are voting for with your all-important dollars. If you haven't been to your local bulk store in a while, it's time to take a second look. Bulk food stores often carry a vast selection of natural products, including spelt, kamut, wheat and gluten-free flours, raw unsalted nuts of all varieties, herbal teas, coffee and flaxseed (ground and whole). Most bulk stores even carry natural nut butters – some you can even grind yourself. If that's not the freshest option out there, I don't know what is!

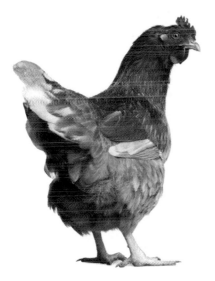

MEAT, PROTEIN AND MORE

You don't have to buy your meat in the grocery store. In today's age of convenience, we rarely think of visiting our local butcher or farmer to purchase meat. However, it can be done and it's easier than you think! Buying meat from local farmers is not only cheaper than purchasing regular grocery store meats, it's also healthier. You can choose to purchase animals that have been allowed to roam freely and fed natural foods and grass. The flavor of these meats is also superior to anything you'd find in a grocery store. The treatment of these animals is far more humane than what goes on in concentrated feed lots (CFLs) all across North America.

If your only option is the grocery store, you can save money by buying your meat in bulk, sometimes referred to as the "family pack." Most meat, including boneless, skinless chicken breasts, freezes very well. I keep stacks of chicken breasts in my freezer at all times — I stock up when they are on sale.

Although I emphasize the importance of consuming protein at every meal, this is by no means a command to eat animal protein at each of these meals. In fact, I prefer to switch out meats as much as I can, in order to introduce other alternative protein-based foods into my diet. I do this not only because it is healthier, but also because eating more plants is cheaper and more environmentally friendly than consuming only animal protein. In the eye-opening book, *Food Matters*, author Mark Bittman writes, "According to one estimate a typical steer consumes the equivalent of 135 gallons of gasoline in a lifetime … try to imagine each cow on the planet consuming almost 700 barrels of crude oil." He lands at this hefty oil consumption number by virtue of the petroleum based "fertilizers, land use, pesticides, machinery, transport, drugs, water and so on …"

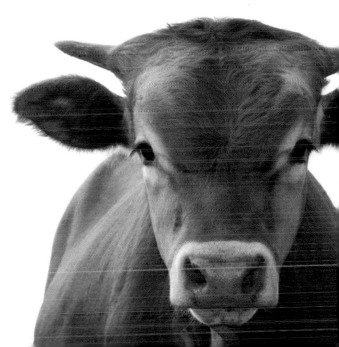

FRUITS AND VEGETABLES

Shopping at your local farmers market is one of the smartest decisions you'll ever make. Not only is the produce cheaper and often organic, it's grown locally, which means it's as fresh and nutritionally charged as it can be. Food offered at the market is usually picked from the field at its peak. At farmers markets you can talk to the people who actually have a hand in growing, looking after and picking your produce. They are proud of their crops and for good reason! I have also found many hidden gems at my local farmers market; heirloom tomatoes, apples and other fruits are true and rare finds for me.

If you live out in the country, you may be lucky enough to find farmers selling their produce right at the end of their drive. There is nothing quite like fresh tomatoes and Indian summer's corn on the cob. Mmmmmmmm!

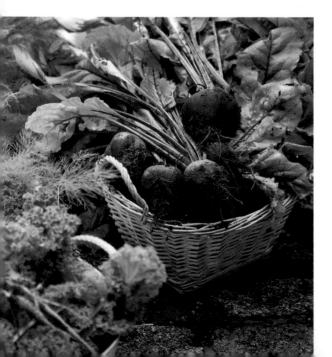

If you live in a big city, you can look into joining a food service program. For a small monthly fee, a big box of fresh, local in-season fruits and vegetables will be delivered right to your door. It doesn't get much more convenient than that! A lot of big cities host in-town farmers markets in parking lots on the weekends. Look into it – you may be surprised at what's already going on in your city.

GROW YOUR OWN

For those of you with a green thumb, a little spare time and some land, create a garden in your backyard. Grow your own pumpkins, tomatoes, zucchini squash and herbs. Gardening can be a relaxing pastime and you can rest assured that your produce won't carry any residual chemicals or pesticides if you make the choice to grow your vegetables organically. I learned to plant plenty of garlic, alyssum and marigolds amongst my plants to stave off pests naturally. Best of all, you can brag about it to your friends over a freshly cooked homemade dinner, made quite literally with the fruit of your labor! The bigger reward is the valuable lesson you will be teaching your children. We need to set the example of how to be good stewards of the land. As I write this book my own little garden is sprouting blue potatoes, shallots, garlic, romaine, Bibb and butter lettuce, arugula, kale, tomatoes, peas, beans, peppers, fennel, squash, cucumbers, squash, carrots and radishes. Every day is a surprise when I step into my little patch of heaven!

"Every day is a surprise when I step into my little patch of heaven!"

CLEAN EATING IS GREEN EATING!

THE GREEN MOVEMENT

It's hard to miss the Green and Blue Movements happening across our earth and oceans. The time has come to accept responsibility, not only for our wasteful consumerism, but also for cleaning up the mess we made. As I write this, plastic shopping bags are being banned in many states and provinces in North America, replaced with reusable shopping bags. Europeans have been bringing their own bags to the market for decades already. Just making this simple change keeps several billion plastic bags out of our landfills. Earth Day and Earth Hour are events in which the global community can participate and make a small but significant contribution to the clean up and green up of our planet. But I bet you didn't know this: If you Eat Clean, you also Eat Green.

CLEAN EATING IS RESPONSIBLE EATING

By making more informed food choices you are doing your part to improve not only your own health, but also that of the planet. The foods we eat every day have an enormous impact on the world in which we live. This impact has been given a name – the carbon footprint – and is a way of measuring how much carbon human beings generate. Carbon exists in all living things in various forms including gas, minerals and rocks. It moves between the atmosphere and the ocean via the Carbon Cycle, following nature's course, and there is a fixed amount of carbon in the world. The system goes out of kilter through irresponsible human activities including the burning of coal and oil for energy as well as the use of petroleum-based fertilizers for farming.

Your carbon footprint can be measured in many ways, but for you and me on a practical level it makes a greater sense to consider the foods you are eating, where they came from and how they became "food." Stopping to think about blueberries shipped from Chile in the winter makes you wonder about the land the berries were harvested from, the way it was farmed, the plane that carried those berries to your grocer and the packaging for those little gems. Most packaging is made with petroleum products. The day is gone when we can blindly eat and not consider what we are eating.

Here's where Eating Clean can help. By reviewing your diet and making Eat-Clean choices you are essentially voting with your dollars to select foods that have a responsible provenance (along with improving your health). The berries you eat could come from the local farmer who lives not 10 minutes from your home. The beef you eat could be grass fed, so it did not require enormous doses of antibiotics, fertilizer and petroleum to get it onto your plate. Your eggs could come from the chicken farmer down the street.

Along with the positive changes you will make on your body when reaching for Clean foods, you will also make changes that will clean up our water, air and soil. Purchase food from local growers, especially when foods are in season. When you do this you not only get the freshest foods possible at their nutritional peak, but you also lessen your carbon footprint by reaching for a berry grown in local soil rather than one grown in and flown to you from Argentina. Have you ever noticed how little packaging there is with produce and whole foods? By eating more whole foods and plants and rejecting processed foods, you are eliminating excess packaging, which helps to keep garbage out of landfills.

I feel as if I am doing my part for the environment by following a Clean lifestyle. Going Green is just one more reason to Eat Clean.

"This impact has been given a name – the carbon footprint – and is a way of measuring how much carbon human beings generate."

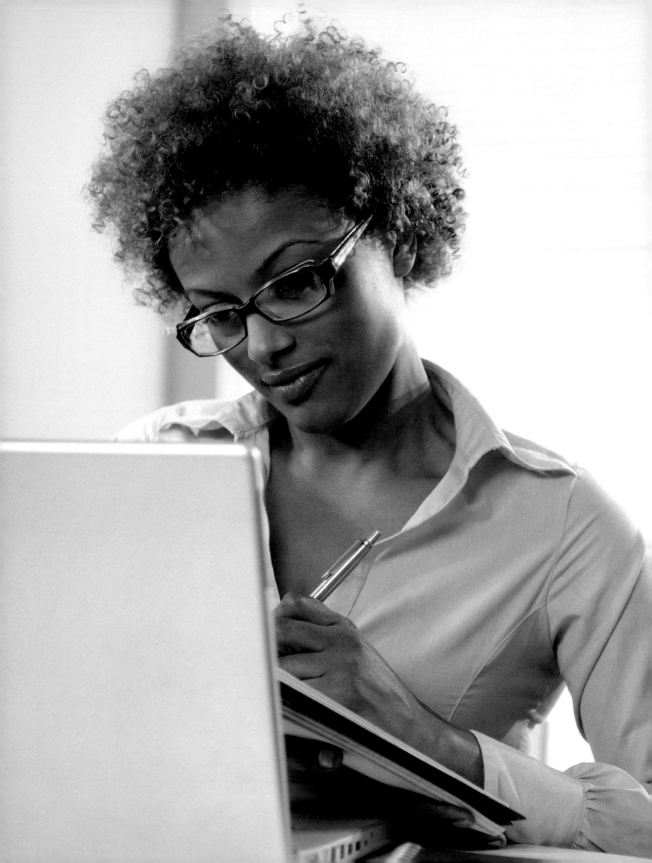

EATING CLEAN
ON THE GO

8

There's no point in denying it; life is simply not what it used to be! A few decades ago your parents and mine lived a different life. Chances are you walked or biked to and from school and possibly even went home for lunch. Today, few households manage to survive without two incomes. This reality has brought about frantic mornings and hurried dinners, along with such lunchtime nutritional disasters as Lunchables.

WHERE DOES THE TIME GO?

Most of us have at least an idea of what we should be eating, but life can get in the way of our best intentions. You start the week by saying that you'll make sure you and your family eat proper meals. The next thing you know, you're skipping your own breakfast, pouring sweetened cereal into a bowl for the kids and throwing a few bucks at them to buy a hot dog or slice of pizza from the school cafeteria as you rush out the door.

Dinner is no better. Your children probably get home before you do, and have already rummaged through the cupboards to fill their tummies by the time you open the door. You are too tired to even think about preparing vegetables or lean, unadulterated meat, so you throw some chicken fingers and frozen

> "Most of us have at least an idea what we should be eating, but life can get in the way of our best intentions."

fries into the oven because it's quick, easy and the kids will eat it. Meanwhile, you devoured donuts in the morning, grabbed a mayo-laden sandwich for lunch and are now so hungry that you're nibbling on cheese and crackers while you wait for the chicken fingers to finish cooking.

IS TOO MUCH EXPECTED OF US?

I understand what this kitchen crunch feels like because I have lived it too. After arriving home after a long day's grind, I remember dreading the walk from the front door to the kitchen because I knew I would be expected to make magic happen with my pots and pans. The pressure can be intense to "whip up a meal," especially when your gang is demanding to know when dinner is going to be ready. This book will help you make those snap decisions about food and what to eat, using healthier foods and food-preparation options.

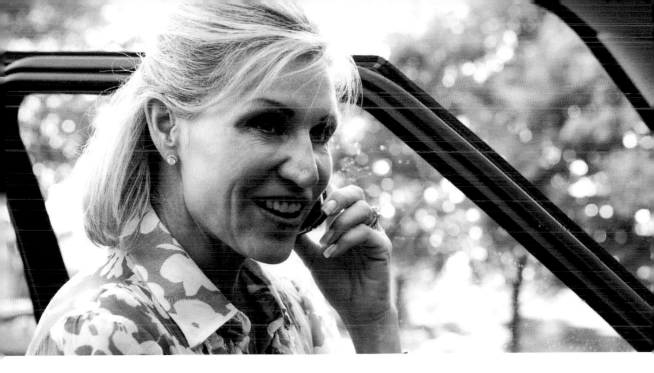

You obviously don't want your eating lifestyle to continue the way it is going now, so your new game plan is here, in the pages of this book. You and your family will begin to eat foods that not only nourish, but also rebuild your health and wellness. Wouldn't it be wonderful if you could get through the day bursting with energy and feeling in control of your decisions about food, instead of feeling like you are crashing by mid-afternoon and lost when it comes to what's for dinner?

You want to get home and spend family time with your kids instead of being grumpy and miserable. You want to go to sleep easily, thinking what a great day you just had, instead of lying awake wishing you could change. Living life to your fullest is one of the best gifts you can give yourself and your family, and yet it's so easily taken for granted.

CHANGE IS POSSIBLE

Change can happen. I know it can because I made many of these changes myself. My kids ate healthy foods, but they ate a lot of junk too, as a result of Mommy's ignorance. I lived on coffee with cream and sugar, and then skipped meals in an attempt to lose weight, which is why I would sometimes pass out from low blood sugar. Once, famously, I fainted right in the grocery store.

Learning how to Eat Clean has not only changed the way my body looks, it also changed the way I feel. No longer do I lie awake all night or wake up so tired that I might as well have not have gone to bed at all. The old exhausted me would drink an entire pot of coffee in the morning to try and wake myself up. Eating Clean brought my energy to levels higher than I ever could have imagined. Eating more food didn't make me sluggish. In fact, quite the opposite. I am filled with so much energy that making extra food and working out regularly are no trouble at all.

Getting started on this or any new lifestyle plan is often the biggest stumbling block. Right now changing feels like moving a mountain of rocks. Sitting where you are right now, you don't have the extra energy because you're not Eating Clean yet. It's like trying to get a job with no experience – no one will hire you without experience, but you can't get experience because no one will hire you. Now, here is your opportunity to get all of the answers and experience you need. In this chapter, I'm going to give you so many ideas for making fast, easy Clean food that you'll have no excuse not to start Eating Clean this very second!

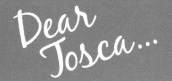

TESTIMONIAL

I'm 44 and have been working out in the gym for three years consistently, after quitting smoking. My goal had always been to lose 10 - 12 lbs, but I weighed the same, week after week, with absolutely no change on the scale. I ran, I walked and I strength trained. I read everything I could get my hands on. But still, the scale had never changed until I found *Oxygen* magazine, then you, and then *The Eat-Clean Diet*!

This is a true testimonial, Tosca – I hit a nine-lb weight loss this morning after only eight weeks of Eating Clean! I haven't seen this number on the scale in at least 10 years! The weight has been coming off steadily; a few pounds each week. I'm still doing the same gym routine – still running and walking - but the difference now is how I eat and the pounds are coming off!

Thanks again,
Kathy Temple
Ithaca, NY

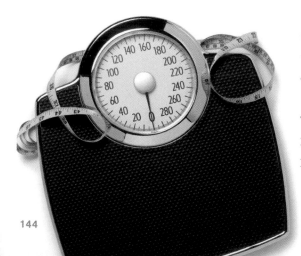

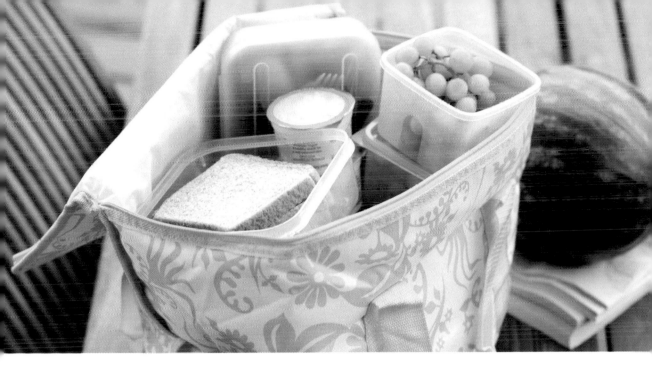

TAKE IT WITH YOU

If you don't pack a cooler each day filled with the foods you need to get you through, you'll have a tough time following and achieving success with the Eat-Clean lifestyle. If you can't pack a cooler, at the very least pack a few foods that will keep in your purse or briefcase, so you won't crash from hunger midday.

If you were going camping for an entire week, you would make sure to pack enough food to last until the end of your trip, right? If you went sailing for two days, you would make sure you had enough food for two days. Why is it then, when you go to work and leave home for eight hours, you don't plan ahead? Do you think you don't need to eat for those eight hours? Maybe you think that eight hours is not a long enough time to be concerned with. Your quick solution to eat-ing away from home probably includes fast food, take-out, eat-it-in-a-hurry, slapped together meals. Yet, according to the Eat-Clean Principles, you should be eating three meals in those eight hours. What will you eat if you haven't packed any food?

LOOK OUT FOR NUMBER ONE – YOU!

Your ancestors had to have their food planned out a full six months in advance. They had to survive the winter and spring before food started growing again. If they didn't plan this correctly, their family might starve. Since you're alive and reading this, it means your ancestors succeeded, year after year. They survived through the harshest conditions, and yet you say that you can't plan meals for you and your family for just one day? I don't think you give yourself enough credit!

If you remember nothing else from this chapter, remember this! Just like the grocery store with its tempting smells, the fast food places you drive by on your way to work, the coffee truck, snack shops and hot dog stands all exist only to take your money. That's it! They do not have your best interest, and certainly not your best health, in mind. They create food that will tempt the largest group of people and that they can make the most profit from. That means refined and processed foods with a lot of extra salt, sugar and fats (likely trans fat), none of which is Eat-Clean food.

If you truly want to make the change to a healthy, Clean way of life, you will have to get in the habit of taking your food with you. If you make and pack your own meals, you know exactly what is in them. You don't have to question the nutritional content or wonder if it's Clean food or anti-food. Packing your own food means worrying less – we could all use a lot less stress in our lives! Also, remember that you need to eat every two-and-a-half to three hours! You can't leave that to chance.

Dear Tosca...

TESTIMONIAL

I don't know what else to say other than THANK YOU! I was introduced to your books just last Sunday by one of the instructors at Gold's Gym where I work out in Charleston, SC. I have been struggling to lose the 10–15 pounds that I've been dragging around for the past couple of years. I fell prey to yo-yo diets. In January I decided that enough was enough and that I was going to eat properly (so I thought) and

exercise. The exercise came back naturally, but those nagging 15 pounds were still attached to my rear end! So, after buying your book (I read it twice from cover to cover!) and Eating Clean for only one week, I can honestly tell you that I feel amazing! There are no words to describe the difference between how I feel today and how I felt just a week and a half ago. My husband loves it, too!

Nicole Alexander
Charleston, South Carolina

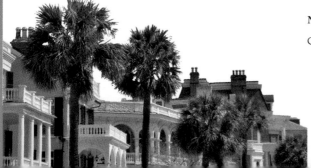

YOUR COOLER

These days we're lucky. The companies that manufacture coolers have listened to us Clean Eaters! Just a few years ago, we had a very hard time even finding coolers adequate to carry throughout the day. Now we can choose a cooler in every size and color. They come in styles that look good at a picnic or with a business suit. I've even seen coolers that look like beautiful handbags! I can understand why you wouldn't want to bring a hard plastic lunchbox to work, but what's your excuse when your cooler is a "cool" fashion accessory?

Now that you have your cooler (or a few!), what else do you need to think about? First, you need some reusable containers to seal your food in. I'm trying to avoid plastic in an effort to reduce unnecessary waste in landfills, exposure to toxins emitted from plastics and my carbon footprint. It is not an easy thing to do, although many companies are recognizing the significance of using responsible materials in their products and packaging. I have purchased Pyrex glass containers with tight-fitting lids, available in numerous sizes and perfect for packing lunch. Whether you choose containers made of glass or plastic, you will need ones that seal well.

Next, you will want to pick up some foil, plastic wrap or parchment paper and paper lunch bags. You will also need to remember to bring along some cutlery. Interesting bamboo utensils are now available. They are sustainable and environmentally friendly. I like to avoid plastic utensils when possible — I just feel so guilty tossing these things into the garbage after one use! If most of your cooler-packed meals will be

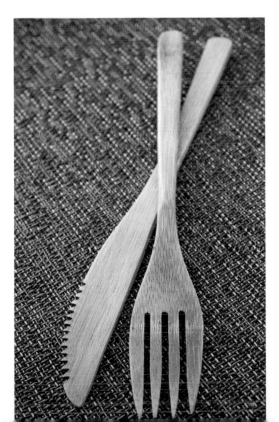

"Bamboo utensils are sustainable and environmentally friendly."

LEAN PROTEIN/ COMPLEX CARBOHYDRATE COMBINATIONS

- ⮑ Hummus and crudités
- ⮑ Apple or banana with natural nut butter or raw unsalted nuts
- ⮑ Grilled chicken breast with fresh vegetables in a whole-grain wrap
- ⮑ Beef stew containing vegetables and potatoes
- ⮑ Fat-free or low-fat cottage cheese with flaxseed, raw unsalted almonds and chopped fresh fruit
- ⮑ Chunk tuna (packed in water) mixed with salsa and served over salad greens
- ⮑ Protein shake made with natural protein powder, fresh or frozen fruit, skim milk and nonfat plain yogurt
- ⮑ Brown rice pilaf with flaked salmon and vegetables
- ⮑ Beef curry with rice
- ⮑ Salad with chickpeas
- ⮑ Whole-grain pasta with homemade meatballs and tomato sauce
- ⮑ Boiled egg whites in a wrap with hummus and baby spinach
- ⮑ Ezekiel wrap with nut butter and banana

eaten at work, keep some extra cutlery there. Even the most organized of us forget sometimes. It's also a good idea to pick up a few re-freezable ice packs. You don't want your food spoiling and the ice packs will keep your food chilled just enough.

WHAT TO PUT INSIDE

Now that you're ready to start packing your cooler, what will you put inside? First, figure out how many of your daily meals will take place away from home. For most people on Monday to Friday (or whatever days you work), this will be three meals. You'll have breakfast at home, and then you'll eat your midmorning meal, your lunch and your mid-afternoon meal out of your cooler. You midmorning and mid-afternoon meals are smaller and won't take much prep time. Your third meal is lunch and it will require a bit more effort to get it organized, but is still very doable. According to the Eat-Clean Principles (see page 21), you will need to pack three meals that contain both lean protein and complex carbohydrates.

Don't forget your water bottle! You'll also need to make sure to drink enough water with your meals or throughout the day. As I suggested earlier, I'm trying to avoid plastic and so I use stainless steel bottles, but that choice is up to you. Just be sure to consume a bare minimum of two liters of water each day, preferably three, especially if you exercise.

PLANNED LEFTOVERS

One of the most common excuses people use to avoid following a healthy eating plan of any kind is not having enough time to prepare meals. When you are hungry and have nothing to eat and you are not in your own kitchen, what do you do? Too many people choose to head to McDonald's, Taco Bell or even the corner store for a candy bar. These are not good options, but you are still hungry! So, what is the answer?

Having a plan of action to handle hungry times is essential to weight-loss and weight-management success. Planned Leftovers is the strategy you need. Having leftovers already prepared and taking them along in your cooler guarantees that you will have Clean foods on hand. This is your game plan for surviving hunger on a busy day. When you have Clean Planned Leftovers in your cooler, you have no excuse to turn to fast food – think of it as weight-loss insurance. Your cooler and your planned leftovers both work equally hard to keep you trim and healthy.

There is no worse feeling than being trapped at the office or on the road with nothing to eat but burgers, doughnuts and sodas. Extra food prepared with care the night before saves your bacon and your hard-earned cash, which is why I recommend cooking more food than you need, every time. Cooking more food at one time requires less effort and energy than cooking on multiple occasions, so you might even

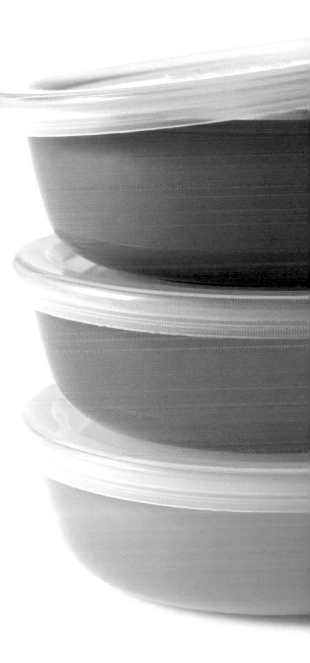

say you are doing your part for the economy and the environment by making Planned Leftovers. Grilling up eight chicken breasts takes the same amount of time as grilling four. Making a big pot of brown rice takes just about as long as making a small pot. Boiling a dozen eggs takes the same amount of time as boiling three. It only makes sense to cook extra at each meal! You can freeze the leftovers or use them for tomorrow's lunch.

As for vegetables, which should make up the bulk of your Eat-Clean fare, it is sheer genius to wash and prepare a bulk portion every time. After stocking up on produce, wash your carrots, celery, peppers, cucumbers, broccoli and more right away. Cut up your vegetables immediately so they are ready to eat raw or steamed – what a time saver! I bank on cooked leftover vegetables on nights where the traffic on the drive home robs me of valuable time. Another great timesaving tip is to soak your beans or legumes the night before. In the morning, toss them in a slow cooker with vegetables, meat (if you are so inclined) and broth. This takes virtually no time and the flavor can be varied depending on what is in your pantry or refrigerator at the time.

The general approach to cooking and Eating Clean is to be prepared by making and eating more of the most nutrient-dense foods available. Forget about fast food from the drive thru – you will have instant food the next day, and possibly the day after that too, and it will be Clean food that both nourishes and slims your body.

When we Eat Clean – the way we should eat in order to keep our bodies functioning the best they can – we will be eating 2,190 meals a year. That's a lot of meals, so we'd better figure out how to do it right. Why leave it (and along with "it," our health, our bodies and our happiness) to chance, especially when all it takes is a little foresight to succeed? You've made the decision to Clean up your life, now don't throw it all away just because you didn't plan ahead! For me, planning ahead, just like saving money, gives me confidence. When I am prepared I feel better able to take what life may throw at me. I don't want to be caught short. Being prepared with food is just one more way to keep my life in line.

"Vegetables, which should make up the bulk of your Eat-Clean fare, should be cut up immediately so they are ready to eat raw or steamed – what a time saver!"

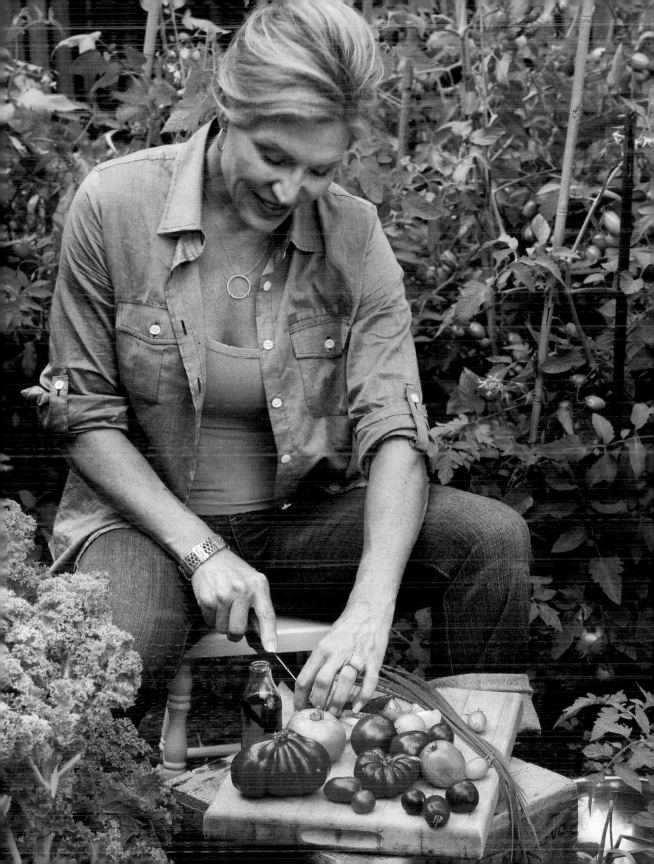

PLANNED LEFTOVERS AND THEIR NEXT DAY INCARNATIONS

Dinner	Next-Day Meal
Salmon fillet with brown rice and sautéed spinach	Green salad with cold brown rice and flaked salmon fillet
Grilled chicken skewers with ½ baked sweet potato and grilled asparagus	Ezekiel wrap spread with tzatziki sauce and filled with greens and grilled chicken

A FULL PANTRY

Along with keeping Planned Leftovers in your fridge, there are a number of items you should keep in your pantry at all times to make quick, Clean meals when time seems to evaporate. Among my favorites are frozen vegetables, particularly spinach, edamame, peas, frozen berries, oatmeal (of course!), canned chickpeas and other dried lentils and beans, rice in every color imaginable (except white), canned low-sodium broth, canned tomatoes and whole-grain pasta. I also make sure to have a good selection of spices on hand to electrify meals.

I almost always have leftover cooked brown rice in the fridge, along with hardboiled eggs, grilled chicken breasts and a few bulbs of roasted garlic. I used to fear the kitchen as a place where I would discover only failure – failure as a cook and as a mother. Now I rule with a wooden spoon. I love to play with foods and ingredients. Sometimes I make a mess and sometimes I make a meal worthy of a high-class restaurant, but most of the time I make homemade food bursting with nutrition and love.

With just this small group of foods you can cook an endless array of meals. Thinking about it makes my mouth salivate with anticipation! The combinations are endless: pasta with black beans, spinach and roasted garlic chicken soup with rice, rice pilaf with eggs and chickpeas. Not only that, you can have dinner ready for the whole family in less time than it takes to drive to McDonald's, and for less money too!

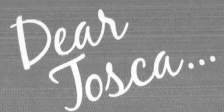

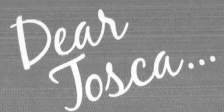

TESTIMONIAL

I'm a 33-year-old mother of three, wife and full-time teacher who has been Eating Clean for a little over a month now. My oldest child is nine years old, and I have been very busy for the last 10 or so years … so busy that I completely let myself go and made myself believe that I really didn't have time to care about my looks (or my health).

A little over a month ago, my dad had some heart-related health scares, and it really opened my eyes to my unhealthy lifestyle. I had convinced myself that putting my children first meant feeding them whatever they wanted and not taking care of myself. Dad's heart issues made me realize that I truly needed to make some major changes in my life.

A friend of mine recommended *The Eat-Clean Diet* to me. She is 48 years old and looks fantastic, so I willingly took her advice and read the book. It made perfect sense! I was surprised at how easy it was to incorporate Clean foods into my diet, replacing the junk I had previously been feeding myself and my family.

To make a long story short, a month ago I weighed 242 pounds (at 5'9"). I have currently lost 22 pounds (and 2 clothing sizes!) and have more energy than I ever remember having before. I started by drinking lots of water and changing my diet to eating Clean foods only. That worked well so I started walking and running, and decided to purchase weights to use a few times a week.

I am so excited about my new lifestyle. People are noticing my changing body and actually asking ME how to lose weight! All of their compliments just make me even more motivated. I'm excited about the results and am looking forward to losing a lot more weight and reshaping my body.

I truly want to thank you, Ms. Reno. Reading your book is one of the best things I have ever done in my life. You offer such a true-to-life story of yourself, and clearly you know what you're doing! I appreciate you so much.

Sincerely,
Jennifer King
Marshfield, MO

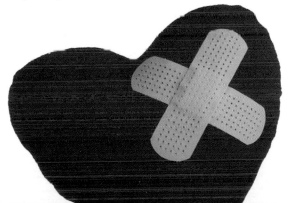

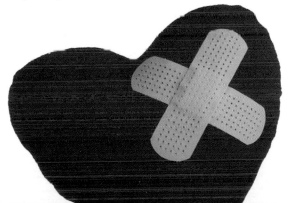

153

FAST FOOD:
THE WORST CHOICE, THE BEST CHOICE AND HOME ALTERNATIVES

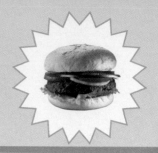

MCDONALD'S

WORST

McDonald's Big Mac, Large Fries and Large Coke

Total Calories	1410	Trans Fat	1 g
Total Fat	56 g	Sodium	1460 mg
Saturated Fat	13 g		

WORST

McDonald's 6-piece McNuggets with Barbeque Sauce, Large Fries and Large Fruitopia Strawberry Passion Awareness Drink

Total Calories	1270	Trans Fat	0.5 g
Total Fat	48 g	Sodium	1430 mg
Saturated Fat	7 g		

BEST

McDonald's Garden Fresh Salad with Warm Crispy Chicken and Reneé's Balsamic Vinaigrette and water

Total Calories	390	Trans Fat	0.2 g
Total Fat	22 g	Sodium	1250 mg
Saturated Fat	4.5 g		

BEST

McDonald's Chicken Fajita, Apple Slices (without the carmel dipping sauce) and water

Total Calories	240	Trans Fat	0.1 g
Total Fat	6 g	Sodium	570 mg
Saturated Fat	2.5 g		

ALT

Smoked salmon bagel (sliced smoked salmon, capers, low-fat cream cheese, on half of an Ezekiel bagel) and water

Total Calories	380	Trans Fat	0 g
Total Fat	8 g	Sodium	1120 mg
Saturated Fat	2.7 g		

ALT

Hardboiled egg whites with sliced cucumber and tomatoes on rice cracker, and a handful of grapes with water

Total Calories	240	Trans Fat	0 g
Total Fat	6 g	Sodium	240 mg
Saturated Fat	2.5 g		

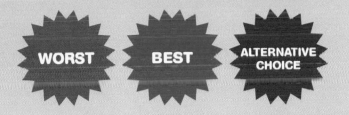

BURGER KING

WORST

Burger King Whopper Sandwich with Cheese, Large Onion Rings and Large Sprite

Total Calories	1460	Trans Fat	1.6 g
Total Fat	67 g	Sodium	2120 mg
Saturated Fat	19.5 g		

BEST

Burger King Flame-Broiled Hamburger, BK Side Salad (with no croutons or dressing) and water

Total Calories	330	Trans Fat	0.5 g
Total Fat	12.3 g	Sodium	535 mg
Saturated Fat	4.6 g		

ALT

Roast chicken wrap (4 oz. roasted chicken, lettuce, tomato, cucumber, hummus in a whole-wheat wrap), handful mixed berries and water

Total Calories	254	Trans Fat	0.1 g
Total Fat	7 g	Sodium	273 mg
Saturated Fat	1.6 g		

TACO BELL

WORST

Taco Bell Burrito Supreme, Nacho Supreme and Large Coke

Total Calories	1130	Trans Fat	2.5 g
Total Fat	67 g	Sodium	2000 mg
Saturated Fat	13 g		

BEST

Taco Bell Fresco Chicken Burrito and water

Total Calories	350	Trans Fat	0.1 g
Total Fat	9 g	Sodium	1390 mg
Saturated Fat	2 g		

ALT

Tuna salad (salad greens, tomatoes, cucumber, 5 oz. tuna canned in water, 2 Tbsp balsamic vinegar, 1 Tbsp olive oil), handful of grapes and water

Total Calories	338	Trans Fat	0 g
Total Fat	14.5 g	Sodium	399 mg
Saturated Fat	0.3 g		

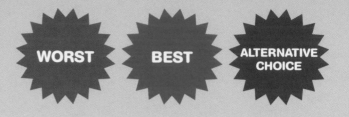

WENDY'S

SUBWAY

WORST

Wendy's Double Jr. Bacon Deluxe, Large Fries and Small Strawberry Frosty Shake

Total Calories	1320	Trans Fat	1.5 g
Total Fat	57 g	Sodium	1520 mg
Saturated Fat	21 g		

WORST

Subway 6" Tuna Sandwich, Chocolate Chip Cookie and Large Coke

Total Calories	1060	Trans Fat	0.6 g
Total Fat	40 g	Sodium	1095 mg
Saturated Fat	12 g		

BEST

Wendy's Homestyle Chicken Go Wrap, Plain Baked Potato and water

Total Calories	580	Trans Fat	0 g
Total Fat	15 g	Sodium	825 mg
Saturated Fat	4.5 g		

BEST

Subway 6" Turkey Breast and Ham Sub, 1 (or more) package Apple Slices and water

Total Calories	325	Trans Fat	0 g
Total Fat	3 g	Sodium	500 mg
Saturated Fat	1 g		

ALT

Greek roasted chicken salad (4 oz. roasted chicken, tomato, cucumber, onion, low-fat feta, lemon juice, 1 Tbsp olive oil), Wheat Thins crackers and water

Total Calories	395	Trans Fat	0 g
Total Fat	23.5 g	Sodium	597 mg
Saturated Fat	1.9 g		

ALT

Turkey Sandwich (4 oz. turkey breast, lettuce, tomato, Dijon mustard on Ezekiel bun), 8 baby carrots and water

Total Calories	266	Trans Fat	0 g
Total Fat	2 g	Sodium	566 mg
Saturated Fat	0.1 g		

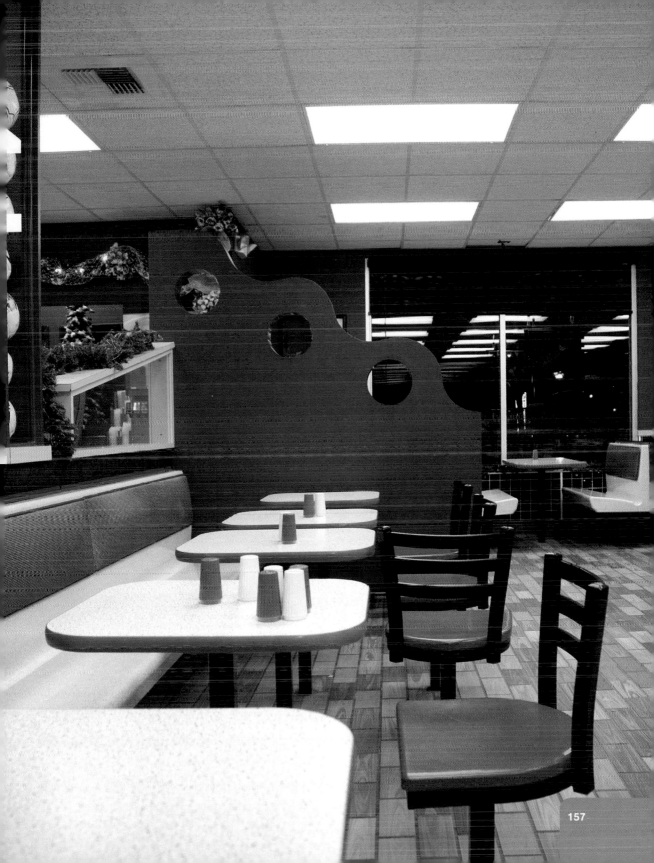

RESTAURANT GAME PLAN

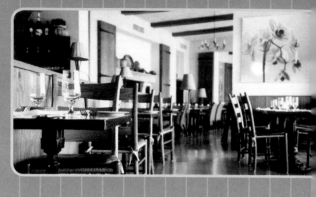

Eating out is part of the North American way of life, not only for families and friends, but also for many of us who travel as part of our job requirements. I face this difficulty often since I am on the road about 50 percent of the time. Ordering at a restaurant can be riddled with difficulty, so it is essential to have an Eat-Clean Game Plan. You can find more on this topic in the next chapter, but I've included this handy guide for quick and easy reference.

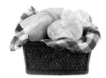

ORDERING STRATEGIES MADE SIMPLE:

Forget about the breadbasket. Having it on the table (especially when you are hungry!) just tempts you to eat it. Opt for nothing or crudités and/or olives instead.

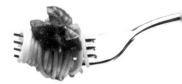

Order the leanest cuts of meat, especially if you are considering red meats. Beef or bison tenderloin is leaner than a T-bone steak or prime rib. Chicken and turkey breast are leaner still. Don't be afraid to choose exotic red meats such as bison, elk or venison. These are usually grass fed and allowed to range, which improves their nutritional profile substantially.

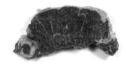

Order pasta (whole wheat if possible) with a red, tomato-based sauce, rather than a white sauce, which is normally made with fatty butter and cream.

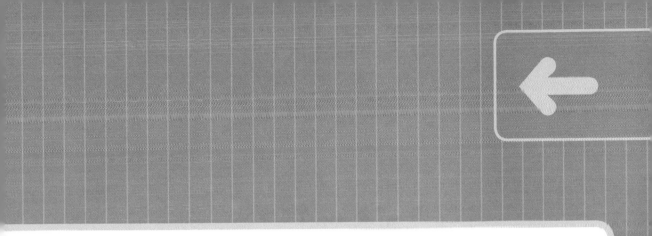

Try to visualize your entrée on the plate and manage your ordering so that you have about 1/3 protein and 2/3 complex carbohydrates. Of those complex carbohydrates, be sure to place the emphasis on vegetables. Use the hand serving guidelines to help estimate proper portion sizes.

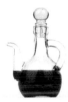

When ordering an appetizer, always opt for a salad with dressing on the side. If the dressing is white, it is usually heavy cream or fat based. Switch it up for citrus or vinegar and oil-based dressings instead.

Decide if this is a celebratory occasion. If it is, then order dessert to share, rather than indulge in an enormous slab of decadence. It's very likely that the dessert will be so rich you wouldn't be able to finish it on your own anyway.

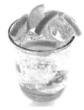

Opt for sparkling or flat water with a squeeze of lime or lemon, rather than a cocktail. Most cocktails contain loads of sugar thanks to both the juices and the alcohol. Avoiding sugar is one of the surest ways to stay on target with your dietary goals

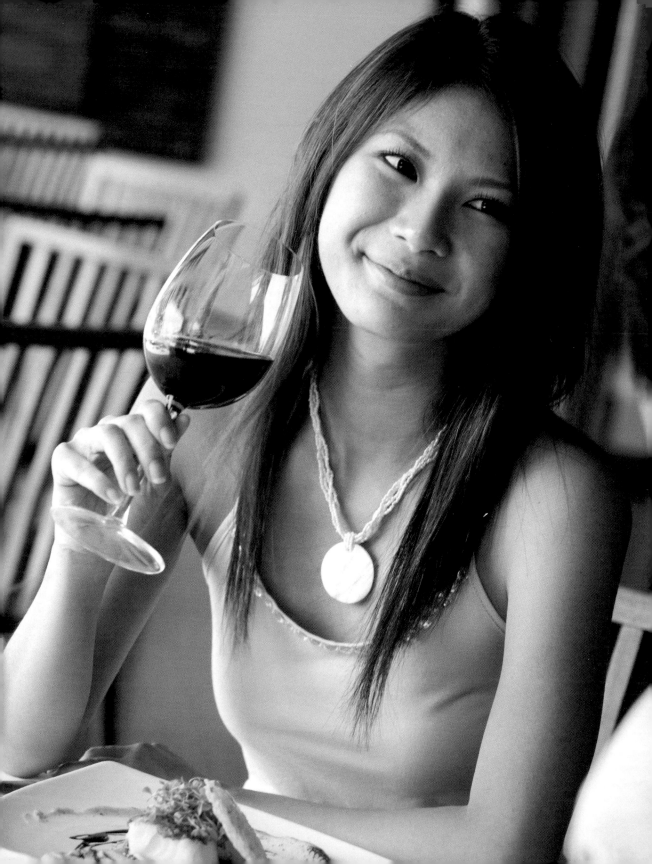

EATING CLEAN IN SOCIAL SITUATIONS

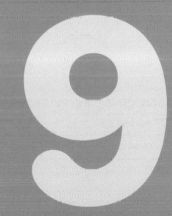

FOOD IS EVERYWHERE

You've started Eating Clean and you are already seeing results. Your clothes fit looser, your hair is shinier, your nails are stronger and your skin is glowing. Your self-esteem is on the rise, you feel great and start thinking to yourself, "This is a plan I can see myself sticking to for life!" You look in the mirror and smile.

The next day you walk past the office kitchen and notice that someone has brought in freshly baked cookies. They sure smell good – thankfully you've got the willpower to pass them by! Then your best friend calls and wants to go out for lunch to your favorite restaurant. Suddenly you start to panic. How are you going to Eat Clean at a restaurant, on a date or at parties? How are you going to cope when you are stuck in traffic or without your cooler?

Eating clean is easier at home where you have the luxury of purchasing and preparing your own meals. At home you know exactly what is going into each meal. That being said, you don't live your life out of your kitchen. Statistics show most North Americans eat out 33 percent of the time. Eating out has become a North American way of life, even a rite!

> "Statistics show most North Americans eat out 33 percent of the time. Eating out has become a North American way of life, even a rite!"

Social events aren't something to fret over. As long as you have a strategy to deal with social eating you will never have to worry about how to manage the Monday morning bagel meeting or the working lunch. Eating Clean in social situations is doable – it just takes a little know-how and a well-thought-out strategy. Food is everywhere, and the following pages contain your game plan to navigating the social food world.

THE OFFICE

Most of us work outside of our homes. This includes working mothers. Numbers show 55 percent of women are part of the workforce, but even a stay-at-home mom or dad is a working parent in my books. No matter where your workplace is: a typical office, a construction site, on an airplane or on a boat in the middle of the ocean, you've still got to eat. I've covered how to Eat Clean at work (by bringing a cooler) in my chapter on "Eating on the Go" (see page 140), but the idea of eating while in the workplace remains an area of great concern for many people.

Some offices have strict rules when it comes to eating. Many workers are not allowed to eat at their desks, as the smells and sounds of munching food can be distracting for colleagues. Eating is relegated to the office kitchen or cafeteria. In cases like this, it may be difficult to eat every two-and-a-half to three hours, or to heat up foods you brought from home. But Clean meals do not need to be an elaborate production. I suggest packing foods that are quick to pull out, easy to eat and quiet, so you don't attract undue attention. These meals might include such items as a pre-made protein smoothie in a stainless steel container, or a banana spread with nut butter in a whole-grain wrap.

At my office we are fortunate. We understand the need for consuming regular small meals throughout the day so employees are encouraged to bring cool-

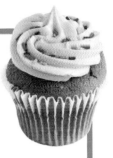

EATING CLEAN does not mean you can't have a slice of cake for the rest of your life, but indulging too frequently can add up to numerous unwanted pounds and then you will be back at square one again. I like to save eating cake for special occasions such as a family birthday or holiday. I bake my own Clean version of cake and savor every bite!

ers, stashes of food, beverages and more to sustain themselves while at work. As I look out of my office door right now I see someone munching on almonds and an apple, someone else is making himself a bowl of oatmeal and another is peeling a hardboiled egg. The kettle goes all day long as staff members prepare cups of hot tea. It feels a lot like home at the Robert Kennedy Publishing headquarters. We are indeed lucky. Tomorrow our book publishing team is having a meeting, which is guaranteed to go long. As nourishment we have decided to test out new Eat-Clean recipes. Each of us will bring a dish and make it a potluck working lunch session. I am making Ropa Vieja, from *The Eat-Clean Diet for Men*. We get creative about food because we are so passionate about the lifestyle. I recognize that many of us don't have this luxury, but I do include strategies in this chapter about how to restructure attitudes towards food in the workplace.

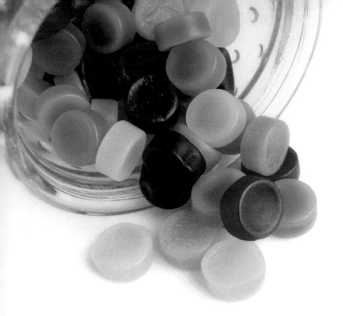

"If you can't resist temptation avoid mindless eating like the candy jar completely."

The office candy jar is a temptation for a lot of people. A few chocolates or pieces of candy add up quickly, especially when you grab a few each time you walk by. The next time you are faced with the candy jar, ask yourself if a few jellybeans are worth erasing the progress you have made by Eating Clean all day up until that point. The answer? Definitely not! If you can't resist temptation, avoid mindless eating like the candy jar completely. Take the longer route around the office. Without going into too much detail, explain your goals to your co-workers and ask them to keep their candy jars out of sight or in a cabinet so you won't be tempted each time you pass by. If they have to keep candy on their desks, ask them to use an opaque container with a lid so you can't see inside.

I have a friend who works at a company that celebrates everyone's birthdays with wine and cake in the boardroom. This happens several times a month! Usually the cake provided at these events isn't very good: store-bought, dry, with that sugary plastic icing. In my opinion, not worth it. To keep it Clean, you don't have to avoid the party and miss out on the fun. Bring your water bottle to sip on so you aren't empty handed. If you are pressured to accept a slice of cake, even after refusing, take one and hold it for the celebration and then throw it in the garbage. Half the people eat around the icing and throw most of it away anyway, so your indiscretion won't be noticed.

OUT ON THE TOWN

Many businessmen and women are expected to attend daylong conferences, or dine at restaurants to entertain clients and associates. Meetings take place over breakfast, lunch and even dinner. Attending conferences can make Clean Eating more difficult because your access is limited to what is set out on the corporate sideboard. You may feel trapped and frustrated to be faced with yet another bagel breakfast, but it is not impossible to fuel up with more nutritious options.

If breakfast is served buffet style, look for Clean options such as black coffee, hardboiled eggs and fruits. I like to pack a cooler in case there aren't any Clean choices but the circles some of us travel in for work may not support carrying an Igloo Cooler to the job. You can find my cooler plans starting on page 268 of this book.

In order to avoid those awkward situations I do something I like to call "pre-eating." This means I carry certain staple foods with me at all times (even on an airplane), so I can fill myself up in a pinch, avoiding less healthful food options. One of my favorite staple foods is Ryvita crackers. This crisp whole-grain flatbread contains four grams of fiber per two flatbreads (one serving – I checked the nutrition label on the box!) with much of the carbohydrates in the complex (healthy) form. Eating fiber-loaded foods like this helps to keep the tummy full and stabilizes blood sugar levels. If you pair Ryvita crackers with hummus, applesauce, natural nut butter, cot-

tage cheese or yogurt, you can survive the hunger crunch pretty well. Most breakfasts, no matter how meager or limited the options, will offer some form of fruit, so you can load up on that too. Being prepared is the best strategy for getting through difficult eating situations.

When entertaining clients in restaurants, stick to the Eat-Clean Principles and remember your goals. Let your guests know they can order whatever they like (including alcohol, if that is their preference) but be firm with your own choices if today is the day to stay firm. Obviously if you plan to celebrate something special regarding your work then live it up. I have never suggested that when living the Eat-Clean lifestyle you had to abstain from the pleasures of food altogether! Food is very much part of our culture and an established way of celebrating. There is nothing wrong with that – food does satisfy a need for humans, and that need is much more than simply filling a hungry tummy.

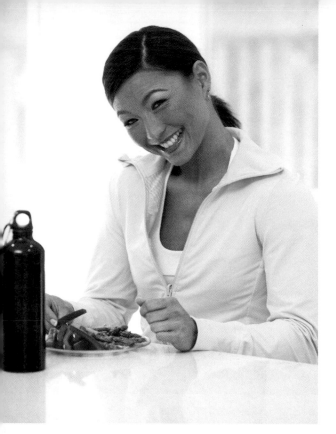

"Before a workout, eat for energy. After a workout, eat for muscle repair."

have just eaten. Clean meals are always full of the right nutrients to build a lean body anyway. That being said, if you are one of those people who need a more specific answer to the question, then here is the answer:

Before a workout, eat for energy. That means choosing readily digested complex carbohydrates from sources such as bananas, yogurt, applesauce or milk. After a workout, eat for muscle repair. Protein is the nutrient responsible for tissue repair so it makes sense to eat anything chock full of protein right after training. You can indulge in protein shakes or smoothies, fish, edamame, lean grilled chicken or fish, game or beef, tofu or virtually any other food that is rich in protein. Pair complex carbohydrates with your protein to round out your Clean meal.

Now you know to eat for energy before your workout and for muscle repair after. If you are working out first thing in the morning, it's still a good idea to eat something before hitting the gym. You haven't eaten anything all night; you need to break the fast to rev up your system. Some people suggest you burn more fat by exercising on an empty stomach. I believe that the energy you get from eating before your workout will fuel a more intense exercise session and let you

THE GYM

One of the questions I am asked most frequently is what should be eaten before and after a workout. If you are following the Eat-Clean lifestyle and eating every two-and-a-half to three hours, you don't need to eat special pre- and post-workout meals, because your regularly scheduled meals are frequent enough to nourish and replenish your body even through an intensive workout. My eating schedule always takes precedence over my workout schedule. In other words, if it is time to work out then it is time to work out and I rely on what I have already eaten to get me through the physical demands of my session. I will, however, wait 30 minutes to work out if I train harder, which ultimately will burn more fat. It's best to wait 30 minutes after your Clean meal before training. Don't forget to make sure your pre- and post-workout meals follow the Eat-Clean Principles by combining a lean protein with a complex carbohydrate. Some people like to eat a banana with a handful of raw, unsalted nuts before a workout and down a protein shake after.

RESTAURANTS

North American eating habits have changed noticeably in the past few decades and the trend is leaning toward eating out. Studies have shown an average of one out of every five meals is eaten in sit-down or fast-food restaurants. Since dining out is no longer reserved for special occasions, we have to pay more attention to what kind of food we order in restaurants and how it is prepared.

It is possible to Eat Clean in any restaurant, as long as you arrive at the table with a game plan in mind. A well-thought-out strategy will keep you in better control of your off-site nutrition than you may imag-

ine. Depending on your weight-loss goals and your mindset, you can be as strict or as relaxed about your food choices as you choose. If you are still in the process of trying to lose weight, it's best to pass up the breadbasket and glass of wine entirely, and the dessert too, while you are at it. If you are trying to maintain your lean, tight physique (already achieved through Eating Clean), it's possible to be slightly more lenient by splitting dessert with your dining companion and tossing in a glass of wine for the celebration too.

"Studies have shown an average of one out of every five meals is eaten in sit-down or fast-food restaurants."

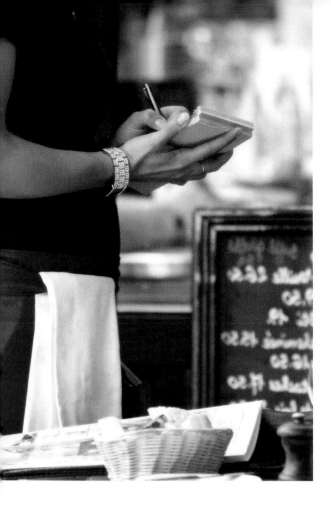

"No menu is written in stone and chefs are usually more than willing to prepare a meal with your dietary specifications in mind."

Scan the menu and think of it as a reference guide for what the restaurant has to offer. No menu is written in stone and chefs are usually happy to prepare a meal with your dietary specifications in mind. Be polite and make friends with your server. He or she is the gatekeeper to the Clean Eating kitchen. Once you have charmed your server, it will be easy to make special requests or send foods back if they are not prepared to your liking. Try to understand that ordering from a menu is like striking a deal with the wait staff and chef(s). Your attitude drives the outcome to a great extent. To quote an old saying,

"You get more flies with honey than with vinegar." Be pleasant and don't draw unnecessary attention to yourself. Instead, just order with confidence. If your order can't be done according to your request, decide to live with it or change it, but do it politely.

Let your server know you want your food prepared without added sauces, gravies, butters, fats and oils. Ask for meats to be grilled or ask for them "dry." Request that you would prefer your vegetables steamed and served without sauce or melted butter. If you run into resistance, explain that you have special dietary restrictions (food allergies or intolerances) and that's why you need your meal prepared a specific way. The chefs in the kitchen are certainly capable of preparing food any way you want it, since food preparation is their business. In fact, if their kitchen allows it, chefs will probably be pleased to make use of their culinary talents by deviating from the standard menu. However, not every kitchen is willing or able to deviate from the menu since some foods really do still come out of a box or a can.

❖ DECIPHERING THE MENU ❖

Use the following guide to help you with ordering off the menu.

Below are a few common menu words to seek and avoid:

LOOK FOR:

baked, grilled, dry-sautéed, broiled, au jus, roasted, poached or **steamed.**

AVOID:

breaded, au gratin (with cheese), **casserole, carbonara, creamy,**

sautéed, tempura, gravy, fried or **bisque.**

If the restaurant you are dining in offers brown rice, quinoa, sweet potatoes or whole-grain pasta, consider it a bonus and order away. I recently dined at a gorgeous restaurant in Portland, Oregon with my daughter Rachel. The restaurant was called "Andina" and specialized in Peruvian food.

I had never eaten this kind of food before, but the menu was beautiful and overflowing with many excellent Eat-Clean options such as:

❖ **Tabule de Cereales Andinos** (quinoa salad served with queso fresco, avocados and olives)

❖ **Esparragos Peruanos** (fresh asparagus brushed with olive oil and grilled)

❖ **Mixto Vegetariano** (sugar snap peas, beets, baby carrots and mushrooms)

❖ **Tuna Nikkei** (tuna, ají Amarillo, soy, pickled ginger and Japanese cucumber)

❖ **Quinoto de Hongos de la Montaña** (grilled market-fresh vegetables on a bed of golden beet and local mushroom "risotto" laced with truffle oil)

❖ **Corderito de Los Andes** (a succulent double rack of grass-fed lamb grilled to order, and served with a Peruvian yellow potato)

Look for restaurants like this that are happy to flex their nutritional and creative arms to feed you.

More and more restaurants are offering whole-grain choices such as wheat pastas, and brown rice in sushi restaurants. Look for other nutritional whole-grain heavy weights such as wheat berries, quinoa, amaranth and millet. If this is not an option, omit the starchy carbohydrates and ask for an additional serving of vegetables instead. I love that some restaurants are now regularly serving sweet potatoes. They are a personal favorite of mine.

The dessert menu strikes temptation and fear in the hearts of many, as this sweet last course is all about seducing the palette. We have come to regard eating out as a time for celebrating and treating ourselves. Dessert is an integral part of the celebratory mindset (as is alcohol). Last-course offerings in restaurants are usually fancier than what we serve in our homes – thus their allure.

I like to keep my dessert eating to a few limited occasions such as birthdays and special holidays or celebrations. If I am craving something sweet in a restaurant after my meal is over, I ask the waiter if there are fresh berries or fruits for desserts. Berries are often used as a garnish for other desserts and most kitchens keep them on hand. It may be bold to ask for something that isn't on the menu, but there is no harm in trying. I have always been pleasantly surprised when I ask for a departure from the otherwise heavy dessert selections on the menu. I've been handed some of the most beautiful and impressive fruit arrangements I've ever seen.

If you have met your physique and fitness goals and choose to order dessert, opt to split it with your dining companion or the entire group. One or two bites of something decadent is usually enough to satisfy any sweet tooth. You'll get the taste you crave while saving yourself a lot of needless fat and calories. I find that, having Eaten Clean for the last decade, I am quickly satisfied with just a few bites of a decadent dessert rather than the entire serving. I think that is because my palette has become more sophisticated to flavors, especially sweets.

Many restaurants serve food on 13-inch plates because it allows for better presentation. Unfortunately, portion sizes have increased along with plate sizes … and our waistlines! To put it in perspective, the average dinner plate in Europe is 9 inches and 11 inches in North America. A two-inch difference in plate size may not seem like much, but for every two inches, the surface area (amount of food) increases by 50 percent! No wonder North Americans are gaining weight.

A restaurant portion is often enough for two. My best advice here is to split your meal with your dining companion, or make two meals out of it for yourself. Ask your server for a doggie bag right away and put half of your food away before you begin. You are paying for your meal and deserve to take home the leftovers, so don't feel embarrassed — it happens all the time and servers are willing to accommodate you.

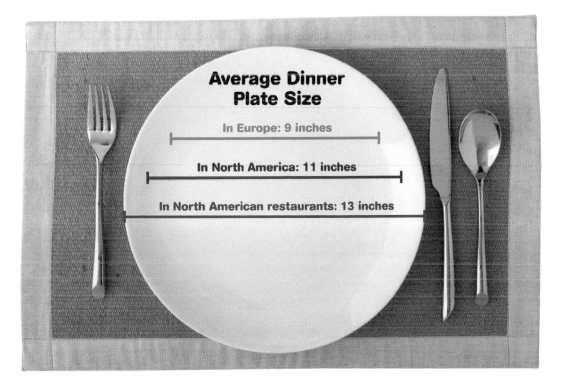

Average Dinner Plate Size

In Europe: 9 inches

In North America: 11 inches

In North American restaurants: 13 inches

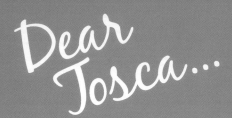
My name is Molly Peck. I am a chef from Austin, Texas. For the past six years of my professional career, I have been feeding people (to the max!) with the influences of French, Latin, Asian and Southern comfort. I packed each meal with cheese, butter and cream. Because I never typically ate that way myself, the impact of the food I made didn't quite hit me (until recently).

As I was walking with a friend, she mentioned to me how discouraged she was that she couldn't lose weight, had no energy, and was suffering through her dairy and gluten allergies. She is not a cook and felt that she couldn't make the switch to buying dairy substitutes and pre-made gluten-free products while staying within her budget. I felt horrible for her and vowed to do some research.

In the process I found your books. They have forever changed my approach to food and how I feed people. I am now implementing Eating Clean into my diet and the diets of my friends and family. I am two weeks into the process and I have already seen big changes – much happier and healthier bodies. I have also applied Clean Eating to a family that I was hired to cook for. They were extremely happy and I was happy to share my new inspiration with them!

I am now in the process of becoming a private chef and I can't wait to employ your cooking techniques for my prospective employers. Thank you for your hard work and dedication.

Thanks,
Molly Peck
Austin, Texas

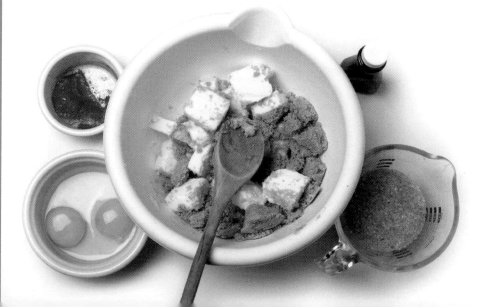

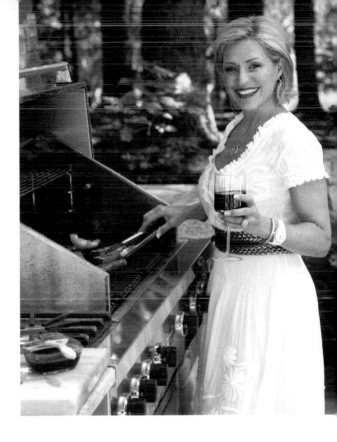

"Order wine by the glass, not the bottle, or have a spritzer instead."

PARTIES

Candied nuts, pigs in a blanket, bite-sized brownies, 7-layer cheese dip and fried hors d'oeuvres – does this sound like your typical party snack table? Buffet-style food tables and appetizers on display can spell trouble for your Eat-Clean goals. These are situations where mindless eating can lead to a serious case of overindulgence.

If I am faced with a banquet of food I surf the table first to see what there is. I can usually pick out foods that won't totally knock my Eat-Clean efforts out of the park. There are plenty of healthy party fare options. You will be in luck if you spot sushi or sashimi on the table. These are excellent nibbles! Look for shrimp and load up on them since they are pure protein. Partner your selection with raw vegetables, vegetable-based dips and whole-grain crackers or cracker bites. If an appetizer looks gooey and cheesy you probably want to avoid it, since the main ingredients betray themselves.

If I know the host well and it's appropriate, I offer to prepare and bring my own Clean dish for the group

to enjoy, such as whole-grain pita triangles and raw crudités with yogurt-cheese dip and hummus.

I am often asked if alcohol is permitted in my Eat-Clean lifestyle. Alcohol is a form of sugar with as many unnecessary calories as any dessert, so it's best to avoid or limit alcohol intake. At a party or in a restaurant, this is an instance where you must ask yourself where you stand in terms of your goals. If I am preparing for a photo shoot, contest or other special occasion where I want to look my best, I'll choose water as my drink of choice. I occasionally indulge in a glass of wine or a light beer, but I limit myself to one only. Order wine by the glass, not the bottle, or have a spritzer instead. On the

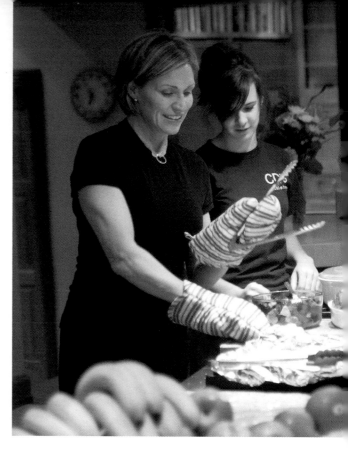

> "When I host a dinner party I always make more than one main course and several accompanying dishes that span the interests of my guests."

subject of wine, there have recently been many positive discoveries about this fermented drink. The phytochemicals in wine are potent cancer-fighting agents, which may well serve a positive purpose in your nutritional regime. I love red wine and this is what I enjoy most often.

When I host a dinner party I always make more than one main course and several accompanying dishes that span the interests of my guests. I depend on fresh ingredients, sometimes from my own garden and often from the local farmers market. This way everyone's palette is served. Attending a dinner party hosted by someone else may be more diffi-

cult to navigate if you wish to stick to the Eat-Clean Principles. Let your host know your dietary concerns before attending. Don't feel you are overstepping your boundaries here. If you were a vegetarian or had severe allergies, you wouldn't think twice about speaking up. Politely and privately explain that your goals are very important to you. Your host doesn't need to prepare an entirely separate meal just for you. Compromise and ask for your food to be served without added butter or sauces.

Keep birthday parties simple. Focus on the fun, not the food. I used to stress myself out trying to plan perfect birthday parties, fretting over tiny details.

Plan an active birthday by coming up with an easy theme such as swimming, skating, bowling and dancing, or play traditional party games and have a scavenger hunt. Devise a menu appropriate for your guests and keep it manageable. Children and adults don't like the same types of food, so plan accordingly. Whereas most adults enjoy trying new or exotic flavors, children are attracted to simple, standard fare. They don't want to eat anything that has a funny texture or "looks weird."

I have learned from experience to offer a variety of foods that are neither fussy nor complicated. The more I fuss with things the less success I seem to reap. Parties are the time when I depend on foods that are in season — simple, nutritious offerings. At the last party I had (for 50 people!), I decided to go for a dish I like to call "Mixed Grill," which is an array of grilled meats including jumbo shrimp, chicken, beef tenderloin and homemade sausage. The meat offering was served with numerous vegetable- and grain-based salads and a delicious sangria. The simplicity kept my prep stress down. What stood out about the menu was the excellent quality and variety of delicious, satisfying foods.

Every celebratory meal at our home ends with an enormous bowl of mixed fresh berries. When I put the bowl together I always think that there will be leftovers but there never are. Everyone seems to love them. I see guests piling mixed berries on to carrot cake, chocolate tofu mousse and popping them into their mouths.

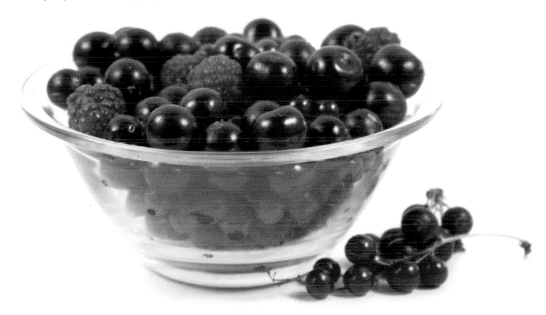

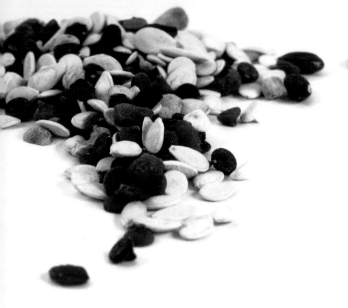

ies and tuna or other lean proteins wrapped in foil. I know I have mentioned this before, but the meal I depend on most when traveling is a pre-mixed container of dry oatmeal with flaxseed, bee pollen and wheat germ, an added scoop of protein powder, and some unsweetened dried fruits like apricots, raisins, cranberries or cherries. Wherever I am, I get a cup of hot water, mix it in and have an instant meal. It really is so simple and satisfying I had to tell you about it twice!

ON THE GO

We live in a hectic go, go, go atmosphere and it's not always possible to sit down for proper meals six times a day. Although I like to eat at least once a day surrounded by my family at the kitchen table, the rest of my meals are often eaten on the run, anywhere from in my car or at my desk to at the airport. You can Eat Clean and maintain a busy lifestyle, especially when you travel with a cooler like I do. It just takes a little thought and preparation to make it work.

When I'm in a rush, I pack foods that keep well and are easy to eat, like a container of premixed nuts and seeds, hard fruits like apples and pears, fruits with peels such as oranges and bananas, containers of nonfat or low-fat cottage cheese, nonfat or low-fat plain yogurt and a small container of nut butter. Whole-grain wraps and Ezekiel breads are great for eating on the run, as are pre-chopped vegetables, hardboiled eggs, pre-mixed protein smooth-

There may be times (and this happens to the best of us) when we find ourselves out and about, hungry and without our handy cooler. There isn't a grocery store or restaurant in sight and the only option is fast food. The phrase "fast food" should not be synonymous with fat. We typically associate fast food with unhealthy eating habits because the majority of options are not good ones, however there are still Clean fast-food choices available. Many fast-food restaurants have jumped on the "healthy choices" bandwagon and now offer options such as low-fat milk, grilled chicken and salads. For times like these, it's best to make do with what you've got. Order the grilled chicken, ask for no sauces, skip the bun and eat the salad dry, without dressing. Fast-food places are usually willing to make adjustments to your meal. Making a special order will also ensure you receive the freshest ingredients possible.

THE BEST FAST-FOOD CHOICES AT EACH RESTAURANT

I mentioned some of the best and the worst fast-food options in the previous chapter, but here is a little more inside info to make the best possible choices when you are out and about in a pinch. You can visit each establishment's own website for nutritional stats.

- ❖ **MCDONALD'S:**   **Asian Salad with Grilled Chicken** (without almonds or orange glaze)

- ❖ **BURGER KING:**   **Tendergrill Chicken Garden Salad** (without croutons, dressing or cheese)

- ❖ **WENDY'S:**   **Mandarin Chicken Salad** (without roasted almonds, noodles or dressing)

- ❖ **SUBWAY:**   **6" Oven-Roasted Chicken Breast with Vegetables** (without sauce)

- ❖ **TACO BELL:**   **Chicken Ranchero Taco, Fresco Style** (without cheese or avocado dressing)

- ❖ **HARDEE'S:**   **Charbroiled BBQ Chicken Sandwich** (without BBQ sauce)

- ❖ **SONIC:**   **Grilled Chicken Sandwich** (without honey mustard sauce)

- ❖ **CHICK-FIL-A:**   **Chargrilled Chicken Garden Salad** (without croutons or dressing)

- ❖ **JACK-IN-THE-BOX:**   **Asian Grilled Chicken Salad** (without dressing)

Get in the habit of visiting the websites of restaurants and fast-food places before you go. Many companies post nutritional information online and you can rest assured that you are sticking to your Eat-Clean goals by making the best choices possible!

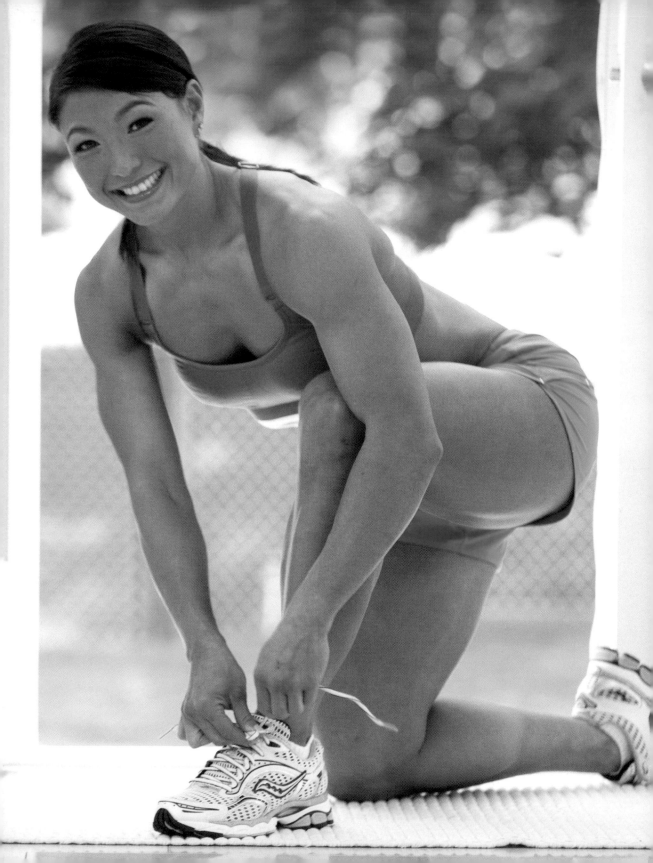

GETTING STARTED WITH EXERCISE

10

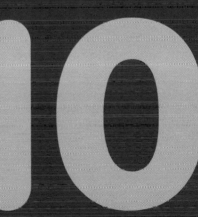

MAKING THE DECISION

You're sitting on the couch on a sunny afternoon with the TV blaring. You can't remember the last time you spent the day outside enjoying it. Worst of all, you don't even know if you could make it through a bout of physical activity without gasping for air, aching or hurting yourself. Sound familiar? It did to me when I first started up again. Although I had played soccer in my high school and university years it had been some time since I had been legitimately physically active. At the beginning of my own Physique Renovation I couldn't even make it up the stairs without panting. To me, exercise felt like intimidation

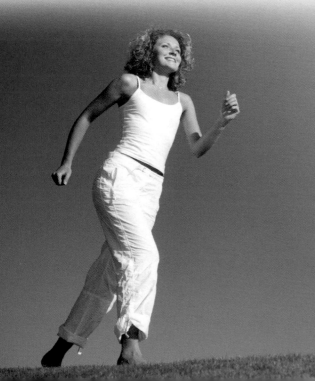

and punishment. I did not have the confidence to push past my weaknesses then. Now, knowing what I do and what I am capable of, I can't imagine my life without it.

Becoming physically active again or for the first time can be a daunting task, especially if it's something you have never been introduced to before. Making it a regular part of your life seems as plausible as striking gold in your backyard. Some of you may have been serious athletes in your earlier years and although you may have sported trim limbs back then, you don't think you could ever get back to your best shape again. As with so many things in life, the key to success is taking baby steps. Congratulate yourself for taking a walk around the block each night; a small triumph in being able to lift five-pound dumbbells for 12 repetitions and three sets becomes noteworthy, and so on. Small successes, celebrations and changes are far more interesting and easier to sustain than the big enchilada all at once.

The first baby step you need to take is making the decision. Apparently you are ready to make it – look at the title of this chapter! Getting your body moving is a critical part of living a healthy life. You may think moving around doesn't matter much – I bought into that kind of flawed thinking once too – but physical activity is necessary for optimum health. I believe it is also part of being human. The body was meant to move and nothing is more stunning to watch than a sleek, trained human body in motion.

Whether it's as simple as looking great on the beach or as important as making it to your child's wedding, there is a reason deep down inside of you to get active. Personally, I love to move my body around now because it feels joyful for me. Knowing that strong legs can now carry me up a big mountain or pedal me along a boardwalk gives me a whiff of the power superheroes must feel – I think they call it confidence. It literally propels me through my days.

Take a few moments right now to close your eyes, shut out your negative thoughts and really focus on why you want to get moving. Is it because you are fed up with hurting? Can't make it up or down the stairs? Embarrassed because you don't fit in one airplane seat anymore, you now need two? No one but you will see these reasons, so go ahead and purge on paper. Write it all down! You can write your reasons in the margin of this book if you like. I think a book with notes written all over the pages is an indication you are sucking up every word and, better still, are really processing what you are reading. Keep your notes in a place where you can see them and remind yourself what you are up to. Now, read on for no-nonsense steps to get going and get healthy.

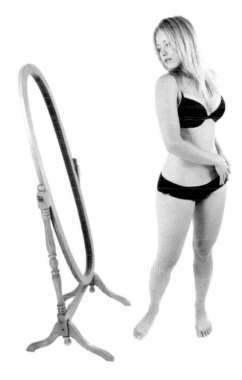

MEASURING UP

One of the best ways to figure out your plan of attack is to measure up. The first thing I did when I couldn't stand myself anymore was spend a few moments with myself behind a locked bathroom door. I stripped down naked in front of the mirror and took a good, long look. Don't doubt that this is difficult to do. There you are, all alone with yourself and the evidence of numerous ice cream binges pasted onto you! There were days when I didn't even want to turn the lights on while getting dressed, let alone stare in the mirror at my gelatinous self, but I knew it was time to get good and serious about what I was facing. I also knew I could not carry on feeling unwell. Things would only get worse if I didn't make a change.

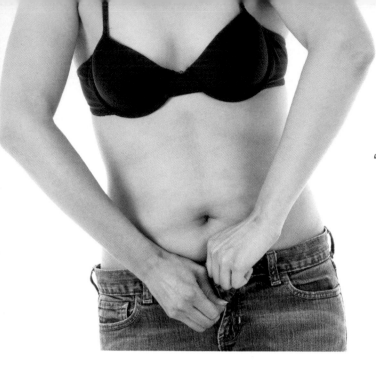

"You could also pull out a pair of your favorite 'skinny jeans' and use these as a measure of your fat-loss progress."

Make mental notes about the things you like and the things you don't like about your physique. Let me repeat: **things you like!** This isn't a body-bashing session. It's about being real. I love my eyes, I love my hair, I love my toes, I don't love my thighs. For every negative thought, balance it out with at least three positives.

Next, grab a measuring tape. The scale can be a nightmare when it comes to weight loss. Our body weight fluctuates regularly, based on hydration levels, hormone levels, the food and liquid in our stomach at that exact moment, etc. Furthermore, muscle is much more dense than fat so there will be times early on when your weight won't change much but your body will. Like a handful of lead compared to a handful of feathers, one cubic inch of muscle weighs more than one cubic inch of fat. A measur-

ing tape is a much more accurate way to record these changes. Write down the size of your waist, hips, thighs, calves, chest and arms. You could also pull out a pair of your favorite "skinny jeans" and use these as a measure of your fat-loss progress. The latter is most reliable for me.

If you must use the scale, I encourage you to wean yourself off of it. Start by weighing yourself once a week, then down to once every two weeks, and eventually limit it to once a month or less. Soon enough the results of Eating Clean will start showing up: improved energy levels, mental clarity in place of afternoon fog, great skin and TAH-DAH! Weight loss!

Now that you are measured up, it's goal-setting time!

SETTING GOALS

You've made the decision to get moving and found your starting point; now what? It's time to set your goals. As with any aspiration in life you have to take small steps toward achieving it. The same applies to shaping up. It's exciting to set your mind toward achieving a major goal, such as losing 100 pounds, but it's important to set smaller goals along the way so you feel motivated to keep going. As the age-old proverb goes, "How do you eat an elephant? One bite at a time." This applies to weight loss too – one pound at a time folks, one pound at a time. If you follow the Eat-Clean lifestyle you will never see those extra pounds again. Good riddance!

My overall goal was to lose sufficient weight to regain my health. I wanted to walk up the stairs without gasping for air and I wanted to be a healthy, physically active mom for my daughters. Of course, I wanted to look good in a bathing suit, too. But before I reached this goal I had to set smaller ones along the way.

BODY-FAT PERCENTAGE MYTHS

Your body-fat percentage is an important measure of how much fat you have on your body in comparison to lean body mass (think organs, bone and muscle). The methods of measuring body-fat percentage vary based on accuracy and practicality. Those fancy body-fat scales may wow you at your gym, as might the hand-held tools you can buy at the store, but they are among the most inaccurate tools. The golden standard to date is either an MRI scan or hydrostatic weighing. However, these are both costly and impractical. Your best bet? Calipers! These tried-and-true tools that look like medieval pinchers are easy to use and highly accurate when used properly. Better yet, they are cheap. Invest in a pair of these instead of buying a fancy digital tool.

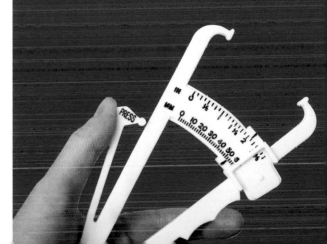

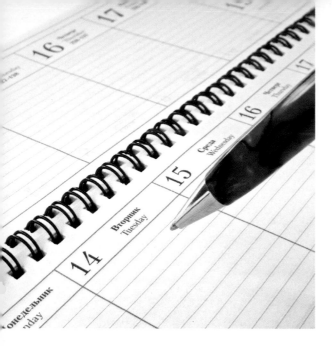

"Choose a goal to reach one week from your start date. Set a new goal each week, but be sure to stick with the habits adopted from the previous week."

Grab a piece of paper and let's get started:

1) Decide on your overall goal: Write it down in a place where it will never be out of your sight.

2) Decide on smaller goals:

a. Choose a goal to reach one week from your start date. It could be losing two pounds, ditching cream and sugar in your coffee or going for a walk each evening. Set a new goal each week, but be sure to stick with the habits adopted from the previous week.

b. Set a goal for one month from your start date, then a goal for one year, and so on, until you reach your target.

Add progress pictures, workout hurdles mounted, race dates and whatever else you need to get going. If you plan on being *Oxygen*'s or *Maximum Fitness*'s next cover model then post that up too. I help people accomplish their weight-loss goals and I find it particularly helpful to make a "Dream Board" full of pictures that represent those goals you are seeking to reach. Some of you want to run marathons, compete in fitness competitions or simply feel well enough to go for walks with your kids. All of these are laudable goals.

I keep my goals in my workout journal where I see them every day. I can make adjustments as I need to and keep myself motivated at the same time. Here is where I record my tough times, mistakes, tiredness or thrills, like when I could finally leg press 500 pounds! Use that space to record the details of your journey.

BE PREPARED

In order to enjoy exercise it's important to be comfortable. With the wide range of athletic apparel available, it is not difficult. Here is a checklist of important things to have with you when you work out:

- ✪ Good-quality shoes. They may need to be changed every few months based on the amount of wear you give them.
- ✪ Comfortable clothes. Choose items that are comfortable and breathable. If your clothes are too loose they can interfere with the machines. Keep them close fitting.
- ✪ Water. I have my stainless steel water bottle with me wherever I go, especially at the gym.
- ✪ Gloves. Once you hit the heavy weights I highly recommend training gloves for a better grip on the weights and to avoid calluses.

I know you're feeling better already and we haven't even gotten off the couch yet. Let's get moving!

Dear Tosca...

TESTIMONIAL

I lost three more pounds and several more inches this month. I shaved five minutes off my mile and 10 beats per minute off my heart rate. I can now run at least four miles without a walk break and I'm competing in a 5k on March 15th, 2009 and working toward a 10K on May 15, 2009.

Still no sweet tooth, no alcohol, no caffeine, no processed junk food and only occasional white flour consumption. My stress is down, my joy is up and I'm sleeping through the night every night.

Life is good!
Cindy Miller

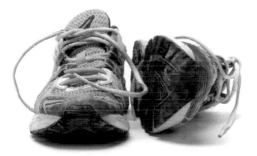

> *"Cardio can be your worst nightmare or your best friend, depending on how you tackle it."*

CARDIO

Cardiovascular fitness refers to the strength and efficiency of your heart. This powerful muscle is about the size of your fist, and it needs to stay strong and healthy in order to pump blood throughout your entire body every second of every minute of every day that you are lucky enough to be living here on this giant spinning mud ball.

Cardio can be your worst nightmare or your best friend, depending on how you tackle it. Either way, it's important for your overall health and for accelerated weight loss. Treadmills, stair climbers, ellipticals, jump ropes, step classes, swimming and cycling are just a few of the ways in which to become a body in motion rather than a body gone dormant. The list of cardio equipment and cardiovascular activities goes on and on, and can be daunting especially if you are a beginner. Relax! Start by getting outside. You'll get fresh air and exercise all at once. Your neighborhood sidewalk can be much less intimidating than the gym. In this tough economy, it may well be your least expensive option.

Once you're ready, you can kick it up a notch by trying a class at your local gym or teaming up with a buddy to run laps around the track at the local high school. It's really important to choose an activity or several activities you enjoy, otherwise it will just feel like work.

For weight loss, I recommend five or six cardio sessions weekly, for at least 30 and up to 45 minutes each. If you can't get through a full 30 minutes right away, that's okay. Even walking is cardiovascular exercise, so do what comes naturally and walk. Start short and work your way up to a steady pace. Don't forget to throw in a five-to-ten minute warm up at the beginning of your workout to introduce your heart and muscles to the movement.

One of the most important things to remember with cardio is to make sure you are working within your target heart rate zone. It will change as you get older and as you become fitter, so make sure to adjust your training sessions accordingly. You can also measure how hard you are working by using the rate of perceived exertion (RPE) scale. Turn the page for more information on both the target heart rate zone and the RPE scale.

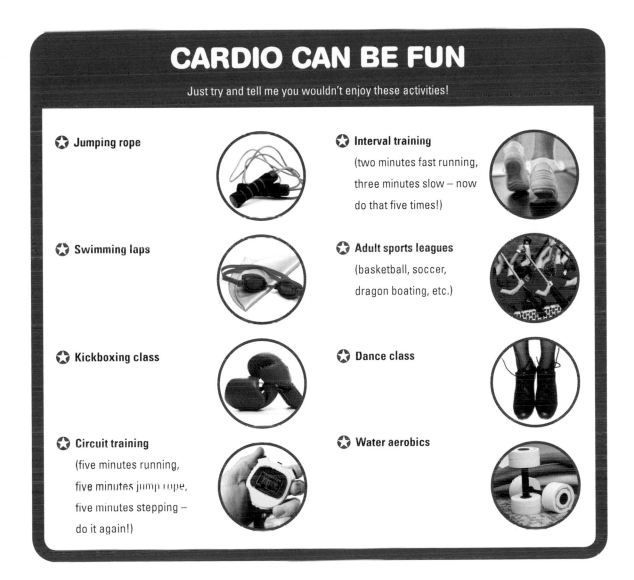

CARDIO CAN BE FUN

Just try and tell me you wouldn't enjoy these activities!

⭐ **Jumping rope**

⭐ **Interval training**
(two minutes fast running, three minutes slow – now do that five times!)

⭐ **Swimming laps**

⭐ **Adult sports leagues**
(basketball, soccer, dragon boating, etc.)

⭐ **Kickboxing class**

⭐ **Dance class**

⭐ **Circuit training**
(five minutes running, five minutes jump rope, five minutes stepping – do it again!)

⭐ **Water aerobics**

ARE YOU IN THE ZONE?

Calculate your maximum heart rate by subtracting your age from 220. For example, if you are 50 years old your maximum heart rate is 220 - 50 = **170 beats per minute (bpm)**.

220 - (YOUR AGE) = MAX. HEART RATE

Beginners should stay within 55 to 65 percent of their maximum heart rate. To calculate this, multiply your maximum heart rate by 0.55 and 0.65. For example, if your maximum heart rate is 170 bpm, your range would be between 170 x 0.55 = **93 bpm** and 170 x 0.65 = **110.5 bpm**.

An **intermediate** should train between 65 to 75 percent of his or her maximum heart rate, while an **advanced** trainer will work out within 75 to 85 percent of their max.

How do you measure your heart rate while you're working out? You can use the readers on the cardio equipment, but they can be inaccurate. Your best options are using a strap-on heart rate monitor or taking your heart rate yourself. To do this, with your index and middle finger, find your carotid pulse located on either side of your trachea (windpipe). Press gently and measure your pulse for 10 seconds. Multiply this number by six to find your bpm.

RATE OF PERCEIVED EXERTION

Rate your exercise level using this scale. Stay between level 4 and 6 for steady state exercise. For interval training, stay at level 8 or 9 for your fast pace, and level 3 or 4 for your slow pace.

LEVEL 1: Easiest. It's like I am sitting on the couch.

LEVEL 2: Easy. I could stay like this for a while.

LEVEL 3: Less easy. I am breathing harder.

LEVEL 4: Moderate. I'm breaking a sweat, but I can still talk.

LEVEL 5: Moderately hard. I'm sweating, but I can still talk.

LEVEL 6: Hard. Okay, this is getting tough, and my conversation is waning.

LEVEL 7: Really hard. I'm sweating profusely and can't keep up a conversation.

LEVEL 8: Insanely hard. I'm panting and grunting.

LEVEL 9-10: Too much! I can't keep this up.

WEIGHT TRAINING

When I started working out I did cardio all the time, simply because I did not know what else to do. The treadmill and I were best friends then, and for me it felt wonderful to run off the day's stresses listening to dance beats, forgetting myself as I ran. Unfortunately, a few months later I realized I was just a smaller version of my formerly flabby self. Something had to be done to tighten up my saggy muscles. While I continued to work up a sweat on the treadmill or the elliptical – my two favorite machines – I also worked up the courage to try my hand at weights. Yes, strength training!

The idea of pumping iron can be terrifying for the beginner. Walking into a gym for the first time is an experience I'll never forget. Everywhere I looked there were grunting, hulking men and machines I had no idea what to do with. I stuck to the cardio

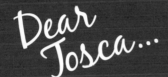

TESTIMONIAL

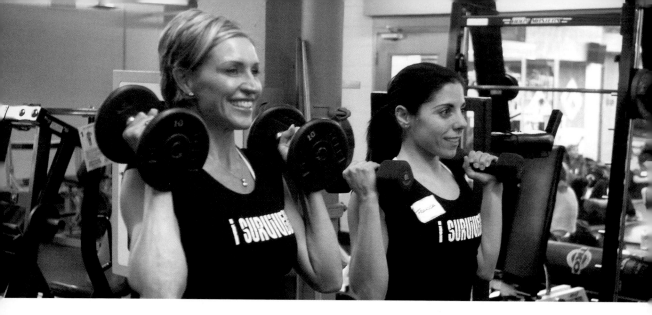

machines out of fear and ignorance – I had no idea what to do with a barbell let alone the Gravitron! At least I could figure out a treadmill; it's one foot in front of the other, right?!

When I was issued the challenge to compete in a bodybuilding contest I had to get over my fear of iron. I organized a few training sessions with a personal trainer at my local gym and received an introduction to the Iron Game. Together we built a program and I admit I depended on him to buffer me from stares and silliness in the weight room. But I will hand it to him; he shaped my fears into enthusiasm and took my body from skinny fat to muscle. I worked hard and regained a level of confidence I hadn't seen or felt in years. Soon I had a plan to re-shape my physique and I did it with determination. When I got to the gym I plugged my buds into my ears, pulled down my cap and got to work. Believe it or not, this is when the magic happened.

I no longer work out with a personal trainer at the local gym. I lift with my husband and personal coach, Robert Kennedy, in our own gym. It was more efficient for us to set up a gym in our home because both of us have intense schedules that might otherwise prevent us from making it in. Since our gym is right in the house, I can never say I am too tired to get there.

If you're just getting started lifting weights, I highly recommend booking an orientation session at your local gym. The experts there can walk you through each and every machine. If you're confident enough, pick up a book and put together a program for yourself. If not, hire a personal trainer for a few sessions. You'll be amazed at what you can do. That personal trainer may be just the person to help you overcome your fear of crossing over to the "other side" of the gym – the weight room. But you will definitely want to get there, because this is where the real transition to your body happens.

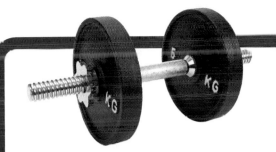

GETTING STARTED WITH WEIGHTS

Here are a few tips for getting started:

⭐ **Start on machines.** Core strength is an important part of free-weight work. Beginners often struggle with this and wind up discouraged and injured. Machines are designed to help your core stay stable.

⭐ **Make sure you work opposing muscle groups.** Don't just train your biceps; you have to work your triceps, too. Men often like to train their upper body only, but lower-body strength is equally important. Training the entire body ensures the development of a balanced physique.

⭐ **Start light and long.** You don't want to injure yourself on your first day. Start with light weights and longer sets. More information on sets and reps are on the right.

⭐ **Challenge yourself.** Be sure the weight you are using isn't *too* light. Your muscle should be tired at the end of your set but not so tired that you lose your form.

⭐ **Switch it up.** Every four weeks you should reassess your workout plan. Your body adapts to exercise quickly and this is why we find ourselves at a plateau. In order to keep seeing changes you have to change your program frequently.

REPS AND SETS

REPS (REPETITIONS):
doing each movement one time

SETS: a group of reps

FOR MUSCLE ENDURANCE:
⭐ **Light** weights
⭐ **Reps:** 14 to 20
⭐ **Sets:** 2 to 3

FOR MUSCLE STRENGTH:
⭐ **Medium** weights
⭐ **Reps:** 8 to 12
⭐ **Sets:** 3 to 4

FOR MUSCLE POWER:
⭐ **Heavy** weights
⭐ **Reps:** 5 to 8
⭐ **Sets:** 4 to 6

Note: *You should find it challenging to finish a set. If it is not, you need to use heavier weights.*

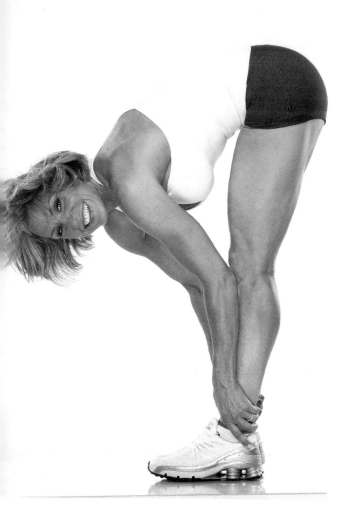

> "Stretching is a great way to encourage blood flow to your muscles, which removes toxins and reduces soreness."

KEEPING TRACK

So how on Earth are you supposed to keep all of this straight? My trick is a journal. Just like the one you use to watch your food intake, a workout journal is the ideal tool to track your progress. I keep my measurements, goals and daily activity all at the ready. Each day you can mark down what you've done for the day: your cardio, your weight training, how you're feeling, etc. You can also use your journal to store new workout ideas from the latest magazines. With a flip of the pages you can tell when it's time to change your routine to keep motivation up and progress flowing.

STRETCHING

Stretching is the best way to cool down after a workout. It's also a great way to encourage blood flow to your muscles, which removes toxins and reduces soreness. Flexibility is also key for avoiding injury as you age. Stretch the muscles you've worked that day. Hold your stretches for at least 30 seconds. You can also try yoga as a method of increasing your flexibility. You'll be amazed at the advances you make in a short period of time.

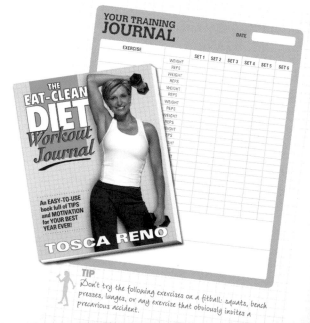

TIP
Don't try the following exercises on a fitball: squats, bench presses, lunges, or any exercise that obviously invites a precarious accident.

YOU'RE READY

You've got the motivation, you've got the tools and you've got the know-how. Now it's time to put it into action. Take it slow and listen to your body, and don't miss an opportunity to get active each day. Taking the stairs, riding your bike and playing with your kids outside really does make a difference — in more ways than one.

PROTEIN BAR DILEMMA

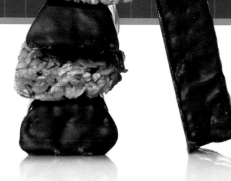

QUESTION:

When is a good thing no longer a good thing?

ANSWER:

When that good thing becomes your default meal and you are eating too much of it.

This is the trouble with protein bars. Out of laziness or convenience, many of us assume that a protein bar is The Answer to every "What to Eat?" emergency. While protein bars do serve a purpose, it is dangerous to depend on them entirely as a meal substitute, not only because they contain a lot of foreign ingredients, but also because we eat too many and too much of them.

My own rule of thumb is that I eat a store-bought protein bar only in hunger emergencies when I'm without my trusty cooler, which usually amounts to only one or two times each year. Here's why: If it tastes too good to be true, it probably carries a whopping dose of sugar and other strange ingredients (which I cannot pronounce and which my body can't easily process).

In theory a protein bar is a good idea. Packaged in a readily transportable bar format and loaded with good-for-you protein, the bar at a glance seems to be the ideal energy food. In practice, however, many bars are the antithesis to healthy nutrition. Unscrupulous manufacturers have recognized the massive market potential of bars and often stuff them with anti-nutrients and poor-quality filler ingredients, contradicting the original purpose of the bar. In other words, all energy bars are not created equal.

A good-quality protein bar can act as a convenient supplement in an otherwise poor diet, but once you start Eating Clean you will discover that these bars have limited place in your eating regimen (unless you are in a pinch). One of the wonderfully liberating facts of living the Eat-Clean lifestyle is that you

> "Steer clear of most bars, approach others with caution, and, if in doubt, head for natural, unsalted nuts and a piece of fruit."

are now consuming protein at least six times per day – it is programmed into your nutrition. It would be very difficult to find yourself in a position of not eating enough protein, so be cautious about bars. Many North Americans already eat too much protein, anyway.

If you are physically active, doing either cardiovascular exercise or resistance training on a regular basis, you will need to be cognizant of consuming sufficient protein. That being said, the ultimate fuel for creating a lean, nicely muscled physique is the super-combo of lean protein and complex carbohydrates eaten together. You could just as easily eat an apple and a handful of raw, unsalted almonds as you could eat a protein bar. The difference is that by eating the apple/nut combination, you know exactly what you are consuming. Compare that to eating the bar – what really is in that bar?

Therein lies the problem. Many bars contain unhealthy trans and saturated fats, loads of high fructose corn syrup (read – sugar), artificial sweeteners (which are deadly) and a laundry list of ingredients that have no place in a healthy body. You might as well be eating a chocolate bar instead! The most detrimental of the listed ingredients is sugar. Yes, sugar! (For more information on this white poison, see page 216.)

On every level, sugar is a destructive "anti-nutrient" (as I prefer to call it). You can't eat sugar and think that it is only something sweet. The sweetness is a disguise for the stealthy devastation sugar inflicts inside us at the microscopic level – from the very first bite. Most bars are heavy with sugar or sugar alternatives, which is why they taste so good. Buyers beware!

When Eating Clean, I advocate consuming foods in their most natural state. Why ignore this healthy habit by loading up on a quasi health food? Steer clear of most bars, approach others with caution, and, if in doubt, head for natural, unsalted nuts and a piece of fruit. What's not portable about a crisp apple and a handful of unsalted almonds?

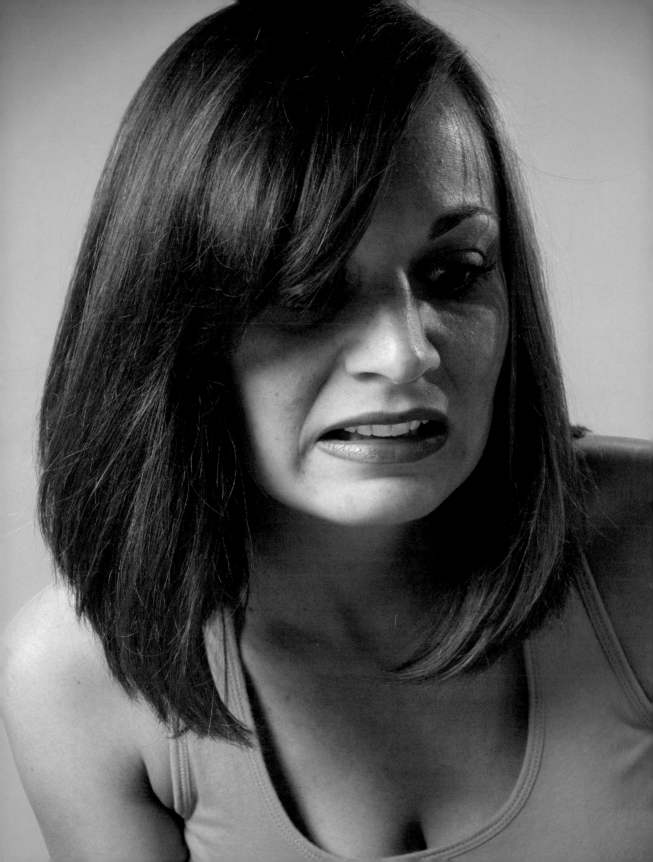

CELLULITE, LOOSE SKIN & SAGGY BITS

11

THE FAT IS GONE AND SO IS YOUR SHAPE!

It's wonderful! You've stepped on the scale and you are down 40 pounds. Congratulations! The weeks of Eating Clean have paid off and you look … better, but a little bit strange. Where there was previously fullness, namely your breasts, your butt and your face, you now have little more than Socks and Rocks, as I like to call what is left of your bust, an Old Lady Face, which seems to occur once your face loses fullness, and Saggy Butt Syndrome you know where! Yikes!

You didn't bargain for this. Why didn't someone tell you this unusual topography might result, even in the face of doing a good thing for yourself? It's a bit like having a baby. It is all very nice being pregnant and you know the baby has to come out sooner or later, but no one gives you the gory details about the pain and the sloppy pouch you would be left with.

Fat loss can be a bit daunting that way, and not just for women. (Men – there are tips for you in this chapter, too!) You want to lose weight, and for a little while it is unbelievably exciting to see the pounds slipping away, but then you have to reconcile your-self with the "new body" you have unveiled. Who is that person staring back at you in the mirror? That person looks like a smaller version of you but some-thing is amiss. Skin is loose and flabby and lacks full-ness – the fullness that was previously achieved by fat. Virtually everyone who has ever lost weight has faced the same problems and, judging by the scores of letters and emails I receive, you want answers.

THE FAT IS GONE BUT THE TIRE IS STILL THERE!

I am most commonly asked what to do about flabby skin, particularly in the tummy area. Skin is an incredibly forgiving structure. It can take years of poor eating, gallons of Chunky Monkey, hundreds of pounds, pregnancies carrying one to eight babies (think OctoMom!) at a time and anything else you can throw at it, and often skin will rebound if you give it heavy duty nourishment and a serious train-ing regimen. I have seen people lose 45 pounds and still have beautifully taught skin at the finish line. On the other hand, I have seen similarly heavy people slim down, and then end up with a flap of flesh they would like to get rid of. Hence the empty tire around your waist. There are answers.

SKIN – A BIT LIKE MOM AND A BIT LIKE DAD

Your skin is genetically predisposed to be a bit like Mom's and bit like Dad's, sometimes more heavily in favor of one than the other. Have a good look at your parents and you will get an idea of what your skin will look like too. You will have to accept the genetic condition of your skin, although you can work magic on it through proper nutrition. I have had three babies and I have shed nearly 70 pounds, and I do find that my skin has improved greatly with consistent Clean Eating.

The biggest change I noticed is what happened in response to cutting sugar out of my diet. Fasten your seatbelts! I am about to give you a huge tip: avoid refined sugar and refined flours at all costs. Sugar is a killer and it is a skin destroyer. Don't ever underestimate the deadliness of this dazzling poison. Sugar, like cocaine, is a pure substance, but a thousand times deadlier because it is not considered illegal. I think it should be, but that is topic for another book.

With respect to skin, think of your fleshy outer envelope this way: your skin is a dense tissue composed of layers of elastic proteins called elastin and collagen. These delicate protein fibers interweave to create a thick mattress-like layer, which is how skin achieves both its resiliency and its barrier-like qualities. The entire elastin/collagen mattress-like layer is bathed in a watery fluid called "ground substance,"

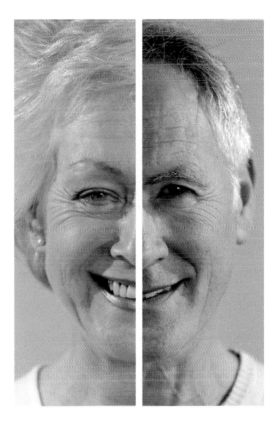

"Nutritionally you can work magic on your skin."

> "Sugar attacks your skin, making the elastin and collagen glob together."

a predominantly aqueous liquid containing an array of nourishing ingredients thrown in for healthy skin measure. When we consume sugar, the entire beautiful array is doused with stickiness only sugar can deliver, and the whole business gums up.

Try this little experiment at home. Pour something sweet like orange juice or soda on the counter. Let it sit until it begins to dry. Then touch it with your finger. What happens to the liquid? It becomes a hard, sticky blob on the counter. Close your eyes and imagine the beautiful, willowy strands of collagen and elastin underneath your skin. That Coke you just drank is attacking your skin and making the elastin and collagen glob together. Now the fibers can no longer do their job because they have lost their

flexibility. The result? Over time the skin begins to look sallow, haggard, less resilient and even grayish in tone. Make no mistake – sugar ages the skin!

THE FORGIVENESS OF SKIN

After the loss of a great deal of weight, skin will recover to some extent. Women go through this all the time during and after pregnancy. The skin not only stretches to make room for the growing fetus, but it then tightens up after the child is delivered, and that can take up to a year or longer.

Elasticity gives skin its main identifier as a resilient, protective barrier. The stretch factor in skin is sorely tested during any period in human life when the body is changing rapidly – adolescence, pregnancy, weight gain and subsequently loss. Keep the idea in your mind that your outer layer may be able to accommodate you only up to a certain point before it starts to show signs of trouble in the way of damage, decreased suppleness, stretch marks, wounds, bruising and more. Being aware of this may help you avoid developing these problems as you navigate through life. Awareness accounts for at least 50 percent of a person's change in attitude.

Let's not forget that age also plays a role with respect to skin tightening. With advancing years, skin becomes less and less resilient as collagen and elastin break down, a natural side effect of aging. There is little that can be done about this except to be vigilant about diet and exercise, and to be comfortable and confident in your own skin, knowing you have done your homework and that you have taken good care of your outer layer. This is where following an Eat-Clean lifestyle is very much in your favor.

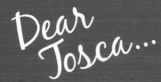

Dear Tosca...

TESTIMONIAL

I am so excited! I'm not very big, only 5 feet tall. I'm 46 years old, started my journey at 138.8 lbs and today weighed in at 126.8 lbs!

I have been trying my whole life to lose weight. For almost 30 years now, I've been on some type of program - successful at times with a 5-lb loss here and there but nothing significant.

Eating Clean has changed my life. I got serious in November after booking a trip to Mexico. Cooler 1 set me straight in a big hurry and I saw a 5-lb loss

within two weeks. The other weeks have been a mix of Cooler 1 and 2 and I must say I feel fabulous.

My belly is almost flat. To be honest I thought I was born with a belly!

We leave for Mexico on Friday and I have three bathing suits packed. I am so excited for being successful. When I return it's back to Cooler 2 and toning up!

Go me!

Helen Parc

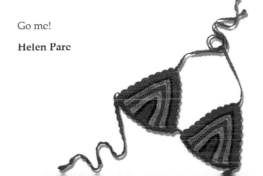

FEED YOUR SKIN

Skin, on any part of the body, responds well to proper nutrition. Sugar is not the only facet of your diet that needs to be addressed. Your outer covering is the largest organ in the body, performing numerous tasks at once – consider it the supreme multitasker. Not only does skin act as the envelope that contains our inner workings, it also acts as an air conditioner, cooling us off when too hot or keeping us warm when necessary. It also flushes out toxins and protects us from potentially threatening agents. Organs, including your skin, require plentiful minerals, vitamins, protein and water to maintain optimal health and thus offer maximum functionality.

Eating Clean is a lifestyle that prescribes consuming foods in a natural state. Each meal should contain both complex carbohydrates from fresh fruits, vegetables and whole grains along with lean protein, so it is straightforward that this lifestyle will go a long way toward helping you revitalize your skin, even if you have previously abused it. Every healthy food group constitutes the Eat-Clean platform. Such nutrient-dense foods as apples, eggs, nuts, beans, fish, asparagus and so on contain the bounty of the earth, which ultimately ends up in you. These nutrients, including vitamins, minerals and more, are essential to building a healthy, resilient skin layer.

Consider the opposite. Anyone suffering from diabetes knows the condition, which can often be managed by improved diet, can lead to dangerous openings in the skin, which can then lead to infection and ultimately amputation. If you doubt that nutrition makes a difference, doubt no more!

The idea is to reinforce the toughness of the outer layer by giving it every nutrient possible at every meal of the day. Over time your skin will respond by reestablishing its suppleness, resilience and luster. In as little as three weeks you will notice your skin looking brighter and more glowing. Proper nutrition is the surest and ultimately least-expensive approach to achieving and maintaining healthy skin. It is as simple as making more informed food choices – that is what the Eat-Clean lifestyle is all about.

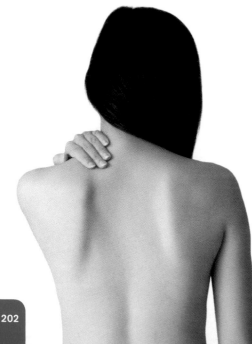

"If you doubt that nutrition makes a difference, doubt no more!"

EXERCISE

Technically, skin does not respond to exercise by toning – it is the muscle that responds to exercise. As a muscle grows and becomes fuller and more toned, the overlying skin sits upon it more tightly. This is one of the most common misconceptions about training. People will write to me telling me they do hundreds of sit-ups and crunches each day, but they still have a flap of skin on their belly, which they abhor. Sit-ups keep the abdominal musculature toned, but they won't help with loose skin. However, I won't tell those people – or you – to stop exercising, since there are so many benefits to be enjoyed from it. Instead, I try to correct their thinking and encourage proper nutrition.

INVASIVE AND NONINVASIVE PROCEDURES

If genetics, proper nutrition and training do not yield the taught physique you desire, there are alternatives for you to consider. Many of us are not so lucky as to have our tummies tighten up like a drum after either weight loss or childbirth. If you have lost quite a bit of weight, the story is more complicated still. Skin has only so much forgiveness. After it's done all it can naturally do, you may need some help. It's a bit like an elastic band that has been overstretched. Once the elasticity of skin is gone, you might want to consider other options.

Fortunately we live in an age when anything is possible. Not only can we clone genetic material to make a copy of a living being, create embryos in test tubes, map DNA, use stem cells to generate new tissue and so much more, we can now also address certain skin problems without the need of surgery. These are called noninvasive or nonsurgical procedures and are often delivered at the hands of skilled and accredited dermatologists. Such procedures include a myriad of bewildering agents from lasers to chemical peels and can often be accomplished in minimal time right in the doctor's office, without being exposed to the risks of surgery.

This book is not meant to be a comprehensive study on procedures such as these, but I will provide some direction and the rest will be up to you and your doctor.

LASERS AND SKIN TIGHTENING

Lasers are key players in the aim to tighten lax skin, particularly on the lower face and neck, triceps area and tummy. According to David J. Goldberg, MD, JD, FAAD, clinical professor of dermatology and director of laser research at the Mount Sinai School of Medicine in New York, N.Y., "The monopolar radiofrequency (RF) technology, which was introduced five years ago and which is credited as the first nonsurgical skin-tightening device, has been the catalyst for what is now an explosion in noninvasive skin tightening with different technologies and areas of the body that we can treat." This technology is relatively new but already findings are positive, with many patients responding by showing signs of increased tightness even after the first treatment. Laser treatments will stimulate collagen

> "Laser treatments will stimulate collagen production and produce a visible firming effect in lax skin areas."

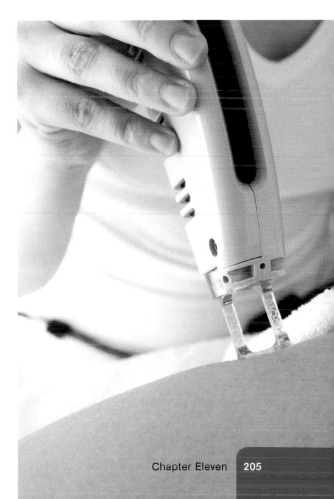

production and produce a visible firming effect in lax skin areas. You will notice that your skin will become smoother, tighter and more elastic, and that fine lines will disappear.

Apparently skin doctors like to have an array of light strengths or wavelengths at the ready. It is the powerful light wave, for example a wavelength of 850 to 1800 nanometers, which is able to penetrate the layers of the skin and "heat" the collagen/elastin mix in the lower levels of the skin. In so doing, these wavelengths cause the fibers to become, in a sense, reactivated and able to regenerate themselves to some extent. Of course, repeated treatments are required for best results. The outer skin or epidermis is not burned because these powerful devices come equipped with cooling devices to prevent this.

Physicians using laser correction procedures such as this are enthusiastic, because as long as the skin being treated is loose and the muscle beneath is toned with no underlying fat, any part of the body can be tightened this way. The key is to do your homework and look for a reputable, certified dermatologist. Do not hang your hopes on a charlatan. In the right hands, skin-tightening techniques can work wonders on previously over-stretched skin, although you do have to keep in mind the costs associated with this kind of approach. Also, remember that the effects of laser treatments are not permanent, they last for several weeks or months only.

CELLULITE

The French coined this term in the early 1970s to describe the dimpled, orange-peel appearance of what women see on their hips, butt and thighs — those biologically telling areas in those with the double X chromosome tend to collect fat in preparation for that greatest of female endeavors — motherhood. The medical term for cellulite is lipodystrophy and a new field of study called Aesthetic Endocrinology has blossomed around how femaleness — hormones — may predispose women to developing cellulite.

There are two kinds of cellulite: hydric and lipidic. Hydric cellulite is mostly water, as the name suggests, with a bit of fat. This kind of cellulite seeps into tissues and saturates them. Lipidic cellulite tends to collect in localized areas and is predominantly fat. This is the kind that gives the skin the orange-peel look associated with cellulite.

We are obsessed with this bubbled flesh, probably because so much of our body is on display in our clothing. Regardless, you don't like cellulite (I don't either), and every other email I receive begs for a solution to the problem. North Americans spent almost 12 million dollars on department-store get-rid-of-cellulite potions in 2008, and liposuction became more popular despite its risks (think Kanye West's mother Donda, who died on the table while undergoing this procedure). I can think of at least a dozen people I know who have had it done, and those are only the ones who are fessing up!

Doctors have a tough time describing what cellulite is in clear terms. You and I describe it as "that cottage-cheese-like stuff that peppers our girly bits." Cellulite seems to have a genetic factor. If your mother and hers before that and so on had it, you probably will too. In fact, hardly a woman escapes having some part of her topography riddled

> "The tighter you keep your diet and the Cleaner your food choices, the less pronounced your cellulite."

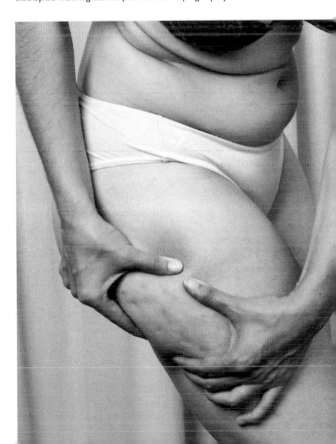

with the stuff, from the obese to the skinny. Yes, even the skinny! Cellulite affects more than 85 percent of women, particularly those who are overweight or obese.

I am not a skin doctor but I have noticed something. The tighter you keep your diet and the Cleaner your food choices, the less pronounced your cellulite. My favorite saying is, "Keep it tight!" By that I mean, keep your diet in check. Don't stray from the Eat-Clean Principles and for goodness sake, don't load up on engineered quasi-foods. The stuff will kill you if it doesn't deform you first.

Cellulite develops gradually, but is helped by certain conditions that we inadvertently set up in the body. Part of our waste-clearing machinery includes the lymphatic drainage system, which is a system similar to the circulatory system, branching throughout all parts of the body and equipped with a series of valves. Lymph is a colorless fluid containing lymphocytes or immune cells and is the primary component of our immune system. The lymphatic system's job is to remove excess fluids and waste products from tissues, and to transport nutrients to cells. When

damage occurs to the lymphatic system and waste products begin to accumulate in tissues, cellulite can result. Poor diet and digestion, insufficient protein, hormone imbalance, repeated weight gain and loss, lack of exercise, accumulation of waste and toxins, and a toxic liver are contributing factors to the development of cellulite.

For those who want a clearer picture of what cellulite is, try this one. One of my favorite simple recipes is Yogurt Cheese. To make it, you have to layer a fine mesh sieve with cheesecloth – a loosely woven fabric – and place this arrangement over a deep bowl. Then you dump the contents of a 750-gram container of plain natural yogurt into the sieve and let it drain. What does this have to do with cellulite? After an hour or two look at the bottom of the sieve. You will see the cheesecloth bulging out between the metal strands of the sieve and that is what cellulite looks like, in my opinion anyway. In the body it is much the same. Fat pushes against bands of connective tissue and ultimately skin, making the tissue look like unsightly dimpled orange peel. Genetics, hormones, inflammation and diet contribute to the proliferation of cellulite.

WHAT IS THE FIX?

That is the 64-million-dollar question! There is no absolute cure for cellulite. However, thanks to today's modern technology, there are ways to mitigate the look of these fatty bumps. Most of these require a visit to your nearby dermatologist or plastic surgeon where you can sample his or her noninvasive potential cure. I say potential because there has not been anything devised yet to guarantee the obliteration of cellulite.

The treatment for cellulite is much like that for treating loose skin. A hand-held unit combining radiofrequency and infrared technologies, along with a suctioning massage feature, helps to loosen fatty deposits beneath the skin in the affected areas and then stimulate the weakened collagen fibers to produce new, healthy, flexible fibers in their place. Called the VelaShape, the machine also metabolizes fat collected beneath the skin. Several weeks of treatment are needed to produce a visible result, which may include a lessening of the appearance of cellulite and a tightening of the

skin in the area. The cost is significant. Remember that there is no complete cure for cellulite, so your best bet would be to avoid developing it in the first place by sticking to a Clean diet and healthy lifestyle. (Come on! You knew I was going to tell you that!)

UNIPOLAR RADIO FREQUENCY FOR CELLULITE

A great deal of study with a new unipolar, volumetric radiofrequency (RF) device has been conducted recently to determine its effect on treating cellulite. This kind of technology works by releasing a high-frequency electromagnetic radiation rather than a laser.

CREAM ANYONE?

There are numerous topical creams claiming to improve cellulite, but it is difficult to gauge if any of these are successful, since most of them aren't. If there really was a miracle cure, I wouldn't have to write this part of the book! One interesting cream is called Alpha-Cell and was developed by a Russian doctor. The product, through facilitating the mobilization of fat, claims to reduce the appearance of dimpling and wrinkling in affected skin. I will still caution you to be suspicious about "snake oil" products. As I said before, the best advice I can give you is to try to avoid developing cellulite at all by keeping your diet nice and Clean.

GOING UNDER THE KNIFE – INVASIVE PROCEDURES FOR REMOVING AFFECTED SKIN

You may be at a point with your physique renovation where you just want that extra flap of loose skin around your middle gone! Sometimes excess skin does not respond to diet, nutrition or exercise. This is the time to consider a more invasive or surgical procedure. I am not advocating plastic surgery by any means, but if you are unhappy with the way your body looks after any amount of weight loss and you just can't live with a baggy excess of skin anymore, then you may choose some kind of corrective surgery.

You need to consider this kind of surgery as something you are doing for yourself, not for others. Undergoing a tummy tuck because your husband can't stand you unless your belly is flat is not a sound reason. I say this because surgery can only do so much. It is effective but it cannot make you "perfect," which is an ideal you may have percolating in your mind. Your reasons for having any sort of corrective surgery must be your own.

THE TUMMY TUCK OR ABDOMINOPLASTY

The work "tuck" defies the severity of this abdominal procedure. To remove excess skin, incisions are made in the lower abdomen along an easily hidden line, usually a panty line, ostensibly to hide the resulting scar. Fat, if any of the offending material remains, is "Hoovered" out. The navel, which is the scar remainder of your connection to your birth mother, is loosened from its anchor to the abdominal wall and repositioned. At this point the surgeon asks for his scalpel or laser tool and cuts away excess skin and fat. Finally, the wound is closed with sutures and you are left to heal over a period of months. It is a radical surgery yielding a striking result.

Tummy tuck surgery or abdominoplasty is a nifty solution for the dreaded post-pregnancy, post-weight-loss skin mess that often remains long after either of these events are over, but it is not a walk in the park. You will require several weeks of healing and you will also foot the decidedly hefty bill for this type of corrective surgery, little of which is covered by health insurance.

IN SUMMARY

I recently had the honor of standing on stage with a woman at a physique contest; I don't know her name. She blew me away and it was not because she had the winning physique. Rather, what caught my attention was her poise. She was the 58-year-old mother of eight children, all born in the usual way, and she was also previously overweight. I don't know how much; I didn't ask her. She was competing, as I was, in the Miss Bikini America contest in the Masters Class. She was in shape and her body looked great, but I could see that she had carried multiple pregnancies and maybe some excess weight at some point. Her tummy still showed the evidence of that. The skin around her belly button was dimpled and loose. Despite that, she had a sense of magnificence about her that I couldn't help but admire. I can still remember her beautiful smile and the strength that emanated from her.

This is what I mean about confidence. This gal was confident in her own skin. She had lived life and made no apology for herself as she incredibly put herself through the scrutiny of competition. In my mind she was a winner because she did not choose to hide who she was, dimply skin and all. She was a mother, a fighter, a winner and one heck of a classy lady. I admire that incredibly.

CELLULITE BUSTERS

- Exercise five days a week for at least 10 minutes, but up to 60 minutes
- Avoid sugar and all refined foods
- Eat enough lean protein
- Stop smoking
- Avoid excessive alcohol consumption
- Drink plenty of water each day – at least two liters
- Start each day with a glass of hot water mixed with the juice of one lemon to cleanse the liver.

Note: these tips are notoriously similar to the Eat-Clean Principles. What a coincidence!

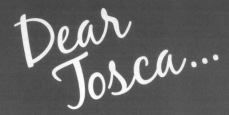

I started this diet because my body was falling apart and I was feeling terrible about myself. When I turned 50 a couple of years ago, I was in a downward spiral. I was going through menopause, putting on weight and my body was doing something I had no control over. I've always been a small person but when I gained 10 lbs in the year before I turned 50 and another 10 after, I knew I had to put a stop to it. I was ballooning out of my clothes, nothing fit. I told myself I wouldn't buy any new clothes for a bigger size. I've been a runner over the last 20 years but that wasn't helping anymore. I added strength training but that didn't seem to help much either. So on January 1st, 2008, I decided it was time to get *The Eat-Clean Diet* book and change my eating program. I was getting *Oxygen* magazine and always read about this diet. I knew one day I would get serious about my weight and when I did I knew this was the way I wanted to eat.

By the beginning of summer 2008 I had lost 15 lbs and just over 30 inches. My clothes were falling off. I was actually having trouble finding clothes to fit. I sure didn't mind because it felt great. Within two months of starting I had changed what my body used to look like. I haven't had any urges to eat sweets or any simple carbs. I feel trim and fit. I still have more to lose for my goal. I've always felt comfortable at 115-120 lbs. Before I started, I weighed 135 lbs. I'm now down to 120 lbs less 30 inches. And even though the pounds aren't a lot, the inches make up the difference. I've also included cardio and strength training every day for 45 minutes to 1½ hours.

I see this as a life change. Once I achieve my goal I may enjoy a little something sweet but that will only be on occasion. I will monitor my weight from here on out.

Thank you again for the support. I find myself rereading the books. It keeps me motivated.

Sandi Wright

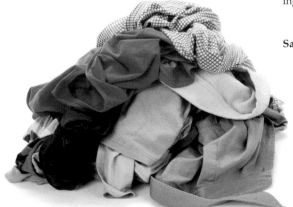

AND NOW FOR THE BOOBS!

I have been very blunt about my own physique transformation – I like to call it my RENO-vation. Why not? During my adult life I was always a nicely endowed 36C. With successive pregnancies, nursing of the resulting children, weight loss and gain and of course age, I lost the once full bustline I used to own. The story gets worse. As I embarked on the weight loss/body transformation of a life time, any semblance of breasts was now reduced to Socks and Rocks, or Nipples and Pockets, as the fatty tissue melted off of me. I chose to enhance my bustline, undergoing implant surgery for the first time in 2001. I underwent a reduction in 2006 and now I'm happily back to where I was when Mother Nature first stepped in: 36C, although an enhanced version thereof.

My reasons for opting for breast implants were initially more for the competitive stage than vanity. When competing in a physique contest of any caliber, the judges look for symmetry, balance and fullness of muscle. Symmetry measures how well the left and the right side of the body match up. That is purely related to training and partly genetics. Fullness of muscle is all about nutrition and training. Balance measures how the body flows from one part to the other.

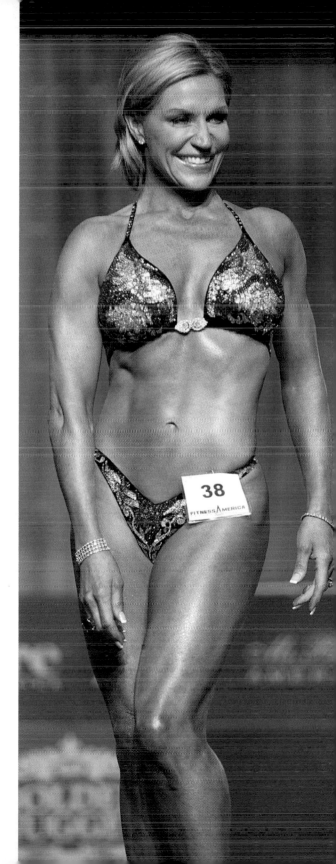

This is where breast implants come in. In nature, the curve attracts. On the human body, replete with sensual curves, the buttocks are the most generous of these. The curve of the hamstring and the round of the breast in women balance the buttocks. Nicely implanted breasts have the effect of creating a beautifully balanced physique, which is pretty close to the human ideal of a perfect body shape. Implants need not be trashy accoutrements to a well-trained body, although many less-informed folks feel they are strictly the domain of strippers.

Not so in North America! Implant surgery is the most common cosmetic procedure practiced each year. According to the American Society of Plastic Surgeons, the number of breast augmentation surgeries in the United States increased by 45 per-cent from 2000 to 2008, from 212,000 to 307,230 surgeries respectively. It has become so routine, hospitals have had to come up with a different way to perform mammograms since implant material is not easily surveyed.

Implant surgery is highly personal. Like any other corrective cosmetic procedure, it must be done for your reasons alone, since you will be living with the result. I feel the biggest decision to make is about the size. Most of us overestimate what a good implant should be. There is nothing more unbalanced than an enormous set of watermelons, especially on a lean, trained physique. I think it is always best to be modest, since any enhancement will look and feel bigger than the breasts you may own now.

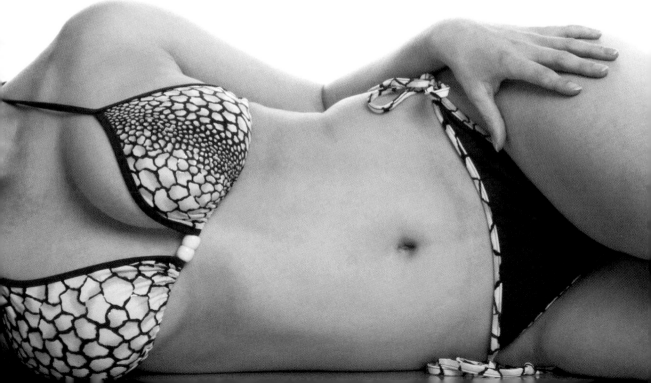

Your surgeon will help you select a possible size by letting you experiment with the implants during an early consultation. Here you can judge what the outcome of surgery will be and also decide if you want saline or cohesive gel implants. Make absolutely certain your surgeon is not looking at your breasts as a healthy donation to his bank account. The more cuts a surgeon makes, the more expensive the surgery. I went for three consults with various highly recommended physicians and I finally decided on an accredited surgeon who would give me a modest but very successful result. No watermelons for me! I also did not want numerous incisions. These were my breasts and I have to live with them whether the lights are on or not. I insisted on this well before the surgery, too.

Today I am happy with the implanted breasts I have and make no apology for them. If I need to correct the implants down the road some time, I will probably go smaller again, but that is for another time.

IT'S YOUR TURN

Ladies, I know that every one of you mourns the loss of full breasts. It is as if you are saying goodbye to your youth in some way. Full breasts are youthful! You have written to me with your complaints. "Tosca, what am I going to do? My nice full breasts are now gone, gone! What can I do?"

There are only two answers. You must either live with what you have left or enhance. One involves nothing more than perhaps placing the very handy "cookie" into your bra to give it a lift. Victoria's Secret can help you out, too. Try the engineering miracle called the push-up bra – now that is what I am talking about! Push-up bras and enhancing gel inserts are all good and well if you don't need to remove your clothing. But when the lights go down and your Nipples and Pockets head south, well, the illusion backfires somewhat and you may want to consider implant surgery. Either way, the decision is in your hands (or your breasts?) Just remember, bigger is not necessarily better when it comes to The Girls.

SUGAR

WHAT IS SUGAR?

Sugar, also known as carbohydrate, is an essential macronutrient in our diet.

Dietary sugar comes in three forms:

1. **Monosaccharides** – simple sugars (includes glucose and fructose found in fruit, corn, corn syrup and honey)
2. **Disaccharides** – complex sugars (includes sucrose, lactose and maltose, found in table sugar, milk and beer respectively)
3. **Polysaccharides** – complex sugars (includes starches from plant sources found in grains, legumes and vegetables)

These sugars are metabolized (broken down) in the body to create glucose, which is then further metabolized to produce loads of energy for our bodily functions, including exercise and brain function, among other things.

Glucose is the preferred fuel source of the brain. Ever had that foggy feeling when you are low on carbs? That is your brain in a sugar slump. The grogginess comes from lacking this high-powered energy source called glucose. Complex carbohydrate fuel is a necessary source of non-fattening energy, regardless of what you have been told. We don't get hung up on calories when Eating Clean, but FYI: one gram of carbohydrate = four calories (same as protein) while one gram of fat = nine calories. However, when carbohydrates are consumed in excess amounts, what your body does not utilize will be converted to fat and stored in your fatty tissue.[1]

[1] *Lippincott's Biochemistry 4th Edition*

WHY AREN'T ALL SUGARS CREATED EQUAL?

If sugar is necessary for your body to function properly, why are some sugars better than others? It makes sense to assume that simple sugars would be the optimum fuel source, particularly for your brain, because the body converts sugars into glucose. However, that logic is incorrect.

Here's why: Past theories have stated that simple sugars cause dramatic spikes in your blood glucose levels. This is the idea behind the Glycemic Index, which is a system that associates a "sugar content number" with each food. Many people believe that eating foods low on the Glycemic Index will keep you fuller longer, thereby decreasing your caloric intake overall.

It turns out that a teaspoon of table sugar may cause the same glycemic reaction as a potato. So why eat a potato instead of a teaspoon of sugar? Sugar is a pure substance, but it is an anti-nutrient, containing nothing of use toward building and maintaining a healthy body. A potato, on the other hand, contains fiber, vitamins and minerals, which contribute significantly to human health. The potato is the entire package while sugar is but one element.

Carbohydrates consumed from vegetables, grains and legumes will contain many more nutrients than a teaspoon of table sugar (which contains none of these things) because their delivery system is complete. Your body will use the vitamins and minerals from a potato for dozens of cell processes, and the fiber in the food will slow down gastric emptying to make you feel fuller for longer. This is the Clean-burning fuel I've been talking about — the good stuff that will keep your body burning like a well-tuned, sleek and perfectly running machine.[2]

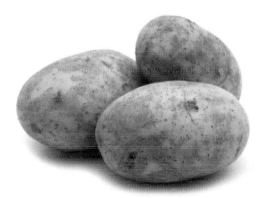

[1] Lippincott's Biochemistry 4th Edition

HOW IS SUGAR CONTRIBUTING TO DISEASE?

While the jury is still out on some of these issues, simple sugar consumption has been linked to a variety of diseases, mentioned below. Simple sugars are refined and tend to go unrecognized by the body, thereby leading to their harmful effects.

■ Simple sugars have been linked to immune suppression. This means your reactions to bacterial and viral infections are blunted and you run the risk of contracting disease much more easily.[3]

■ Simple sugars have also been linked to inflammatory conditions. Similar to the over-consumption of omega-6 fatty acids, eating too many simple sugars can cause more blood flow, more constriction and more scar tissue in your blood vessels. These are all factors that can lead to heart problems.[4]

■ Eating foods high in simple sugars and low in other nutrients can lead to dramatic spikes in blood sugar levels, generating a correspondingly high insulin response. This can lead to liver fatigue and possibly diabetes. This is also responsible for that "crash" feeling you have after eating a candy bar in the middle of the afternoon. High-fructose corn syrup products, which are readily used in most processed foods, are closely linked to pre-diabetic conditions.[5]

■ Simple sugar consumption has been linked to cancers of the intestine among other cancers. These sugars provide your healthy intestinal bacteria with a quick fuel source (simple sugar), allowing for the intestinal bacterial to overgrow. This causes damage to your intestines, leading to tumorigenesis (formation of new tumors).[6]

■ According William Dufty, author of the cult classic, *Sugar Blues*, sugar addiction is a widespread problem and has been since the refinement of complex carbohydrates during the Industrial Revolution. Dufty explains the phrase "sugar blues" as the mental and physical miseries caused by eating refined sugars. In this book, Dufty writes that excessive consumption of refined sugar is the cause of many neuroses we see today.[7]

■ Over-consumption of sugar can lead to excessive uric acid production in the body, which leads to the development or exacerbation of gout.[8]

[3] *Curr Atheroscler Rep.* 2007 Dec;9(6):479-85. The glycemic index and cardiovascular disease risk. Brand-Miller J, Dickinson S, Barclay A, Celermajer D. Human Nutrition Unit (G08), University of Sydney, Camperdown, NSW, 2006.

[4] *Nutr Rev.* 2003 May;61(5 Pt 2):S49-55. Glycemic load and chronic disease. Brand-Miller JC. Human Nutrition Unit, School of Molecular and Microbial Biosciences, University of Sydney, NSW, Australia

FUN FACTS ABOUT SUGAR

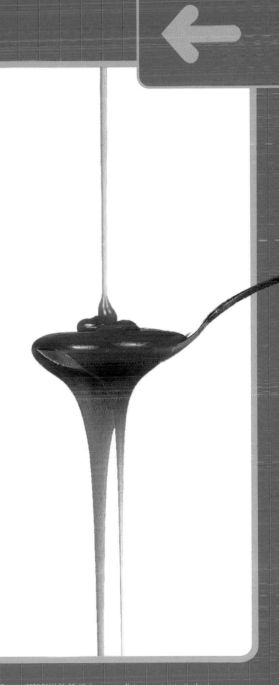

- The official sugar website (www.sugar.org) markets sugar as a healthy sweetener that comes straight from nature. Don't always assume something natural is something healthy. Tobacco is natural and it certainly isn't good for you! The same goes for cocaine, opium and heroin.

- When it comes to any sweetener, the key is moderation. Even "natural" sweeteners such as those made from honey, maple syrup, rice and the agave plant need to be consumed in limited amounts. Too much of a good thing is still too much.

- A teaspoon of white sugar contains 15 calories and 15 calories are easily burned after two minutes on the treadmill, but how often do you have only one teaspoon of sugar in a day? And how do you erase the microscopic damage that occurs in your body after its consumption?

- Artificial sugars are linked with weight-loss sabotage. You continue to battle your addiction to sugar AND you are tricked into believing you can still eat super sweet stuff, even though it remains stored in your fat.

[5] *Curr Opin Gastroenterol.* 2008 Mar;24(2):204-9. Dietary fructose and the metabolic syndrome. Miller A, Adeli K. Molecular Structure & Function, Research Institute, The Hospital for Sick Children, and Department of Biochemistry, University of Toronto. Toronto, Ontario, Canada.

[6] *Nutr Cancer.* 2009;61(1):81-93. High sucrose diets promote intestinal epithelial cell proliferation and tumorigenesis in APC (Min) mice by increasing insulin and IGF-I levels.

[7] Dufty, William. *Sugar Blues.* New York: Warner Books, 1975.

[8] Nagel, Rami. *Is Agave Nectar Harmful?* 2008

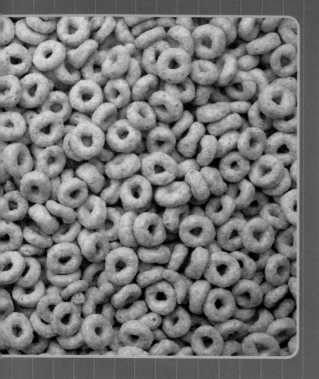

HIDDEN SUGARS

Here are just a few places that you wouldn't expect to see simple sugars. Beware! Even the French fry is often dipped in milk sugar (lactose) before frying!

- Starbuck's latte
- Cheerios
- granola
- granola bar
- white bread
- peanut butter
- ketchup
- deli meats
- alcohol

TYPES OF SWEETENERS

- White and brown sugar
- Honey
- Maple, brown rice, corn and cane syrup
- Agave nectar
- Stevia
- Truvia
- Molasses
- Rapadura
- Turbinado
- Demerara (Guyanese)
- High Fructose Corn Syrup

TYPES OF ARTIFICIAL SWEETENERS

These sweeteners should be kept off your shelves and out of your reach. They are linked to cancers, dental problems, and other major health issues.

- Sweet 'N Low (saccharin)
- Nutrasweet (aspartame)
- Equal (contains aspartame)
- Sugar Twin (cyclamate)
- Splenda (sucralose)
- Sorbitol, mannitol, xylitol

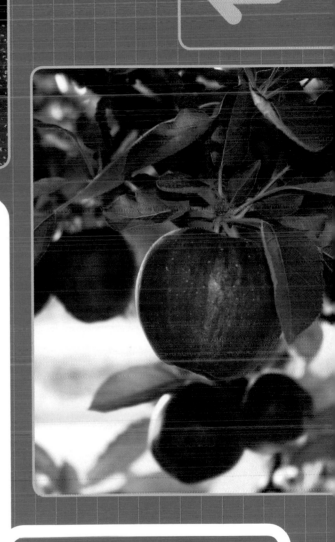

HEALTHIER SWEETENER OPTIONS

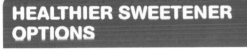

While your ultimate goal should be to kick the sugar/ sweetener habit altogether, in a pinch these options should be chosen over the others:

- Sucanat
- Agave nectar
- Rapadura
- Fruit sugar
- Unsweetened applesauce
- Brown rice syrup

There has been some evidence suggesting that the processing of agave nectar leaves it full of refined fructose, which, as you have just learned, is a simple sugar linked to many detrimental health concerns. The most important thing to remember when purchasing and using sweeteners (healthy or not) is that they should be used in moderation regardless. Even xylitol (a sugar alcohol) has been linked to diarrhea because of its diuretic qualities.[9]

BOTTOM LINE

If you are craving something sweet, grab an apple or a bowl of berries before reaching for a sweetener. Eating sugar (including "fake" sugar) all day long is not an option!

[9] *Agave Nectar, the High Fructose Health Food Fraud* by Rami Nagel 2008

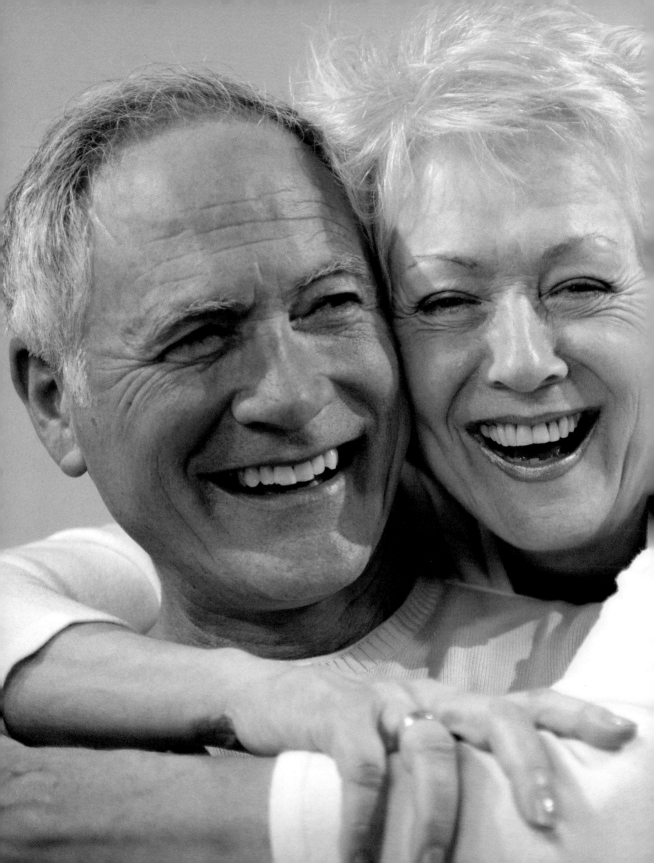

LONGEVITY

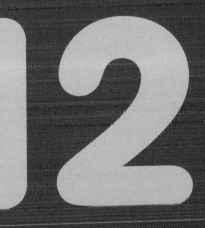

12

It is the rare genetically blessed specimen who can smoke, drink, party with the band and still live in good health until the age of 103. (Is Mick Jagger one of these?) We enjoy hearing the stories, but most of the time a pot-smoking food abuser doesn't make longevity news because the lifestyle doesn't let it happen. Most people pursuing unhealthy habits live shorter lives – and those short lives are often marred by illness, reduced energy and even reduced productivity.

To state the obvious, the better care you take of your health, the longer your life will be. In my mind, the aspect of living a life of quality is far more important. These statements are not groundbreaking. They are probably just this side of boring since we read them all the time. The only time words like these have an impact on our gray matter is when you or someone close to you has been affected by health and overweight problems. That is when you say, "I should have" and "Why didn't I?" Good question!

MODERN HEALTH

The above subheading is almost an oxymoron. While advances in medicine allow us to fight diseases that once would have been death sentences, we seem determined to shorten our life span. Eating antifoods will surely lead us to an early grave. Society's propensity toward eating junk food is being blamed for the fact that children are now getting diseases that used to be unheard of in those below middle age: kidney stones, high blood pressure, type 2 diabetes and fatty liver disease, certain cancers and heart disease.

The belief is that eating foods high in sodium, consuming too few vegetables and other complex carbohydrates, and not drinking enough water can cause kidney stones. And yet potato chips, processed meats and cheeses, crackers, hot dogs, fries, burgers and sodas make up a familiar-sounding list of modern "foods" constituting a typical North American child's diet today.

"Today, around 70 percent of the population is overweight or obese."

> "This is the first known generation of kids whose life span is not expected to exceed that of their parents."

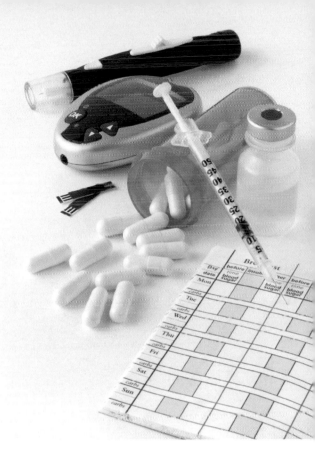

This nutrition-void diet isn't just causing painful kidney stones. It's causing a host of other life-shortening illnesses and ailments. Type 2 diabetes used to be known as adult-onset diabetes because it was rare in children, but this is no longer the case. Risk factors for developing this disease simply did not threaten children 20 or 30 years ago, but now they are common. These risk factors Include obesity, high blood pressure and lack of physical activity along with unhealthy eating habits, obesity being the number-one predictor. The more fat you have (especially abdominal fat), the more likely it is that you will suffer from insulin resistance, because excess fat reduces the body's ability to use insulin.

This is the first known generation of kids whose life span is not expected to exceed that of their parents. We know the reason and we are not preventing it. In fact, we are perpetuating it, in record numbers. Children are not alone in their health troubles — again in record numbers, we are living exactly as our children: eating junk food and not exercising. Today,

around 70 percent of the population is overweight or obese. Children and their parents are rapidly developing obesity related diseases. The Overfed and Dying malaise is spreading to other societies as they embrace our fast-food outlets and soda-manufacturing plants throughout the world.

How is it possible to develop such grave (and preventable) illnesses so early in life? How can we think the lifestyle factors leading to these illnesses are somehow acceptable? How can we think we will not be shortening, and worsening, our lives by eating this way? These are numerous questions that need sound answers.

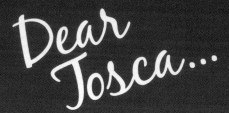

Dear Tosca...

My husband and I have been Eating Clean for a little more than a year now. I was overweight and feeling drained as a new mom, and my husband had just been warned by his doctor that if he didn't lower his cholesterol on his own, in three months he would need to start taking Lipitor [a cholesterol medication].

My parents bought your first book and had it sitting around. I "borrowed" the book, read it cover-to-cover, and we began Eating Clean and exercising. We both dropped pounds and inches, gained lots of energy and confidence, and I know it made our relationship stronger too. Just when I was feeling my greatest and reached my goal weight, I got pregnant again ... surprise!

I love how your program is not really a diet. I was afraid to "cut calories" because I was still nursing. By Eating Clean, I was able to continue nursing Mariella for 13½ months, go through a very healthy pregnancy, and I am now nursing Vivianna. (Yes, I was pregnant and nursing at the same time.)

I did overindulge every now and then while I was pregnant, but I was about 10 lbs lighter at the end of my second pregnancy than I was at the end of my first. My daughters are now 24 months and five months old, and I am almost back to my goal weight.

The best and most exciting news is that my husband just went for his physical and high cholesterol is no longer an issue for him! We are much more active as well. We have done a couple of 10 km runs together this summer, and we take turns running 10 km every Saturday morning. I meet a good friend at the gym once a week, and then we enjoy a homemade Clean lunch together with our kids. I stick a third workout or run in during the week as well.

It is amazing how running 10 km felt like such a challenge at first, and now it is pure joy. My husband has committed to running almost every morning. He lost his father at a young age, and with his two baby girls, he does not want to "check out early" as he puts it. Thanks again Tosca!

Yours in good health,
Jennifer Doria & Karl Fernandes,
Mariella & baby Vivianna

THE COMMUNITY WITHIN YOU

Your body is not just one organism. You are a community, made up of literally trillions of cells. Each one of these cells has an individual lifespan and each of these cells needs specific nutrients to function properly. If the cells don't function properly, illness results.

Think of a city. Each person living in that city requires food, shelter, love and other basic human needs to thrive. If a few individuals don't manage to obtain these basics, it doesn't greatly impact the viability of the city. But the more people there are without work, a place to live, food, family … it soon becomes obvious the city would not prosper. You might say that the population, and thus the city, is functioning at a very basic and barely sustainable level.

When you feed your community of cells – your body – inferior nutrition, you are keeping them at this same basic and barely sustainable level of functioning. This means you are keeping yourself in this state as well. A community functioning at this level for a long period of time, whether that community is a city or your own body, cannot prosper or thrive. The longer you keep yourself in this state, the shorter your life will be. Besides, is "barely functioning" really the type of life you want for yourself? Wouldn't you rather function at an energized, productive, vibrant and even superior level?

"All you have to do is feed your cells, your own community, with nourishing, Clean food."

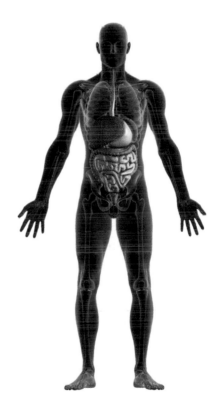

You can! All you have to do is feed your cells, your own community, with nourishing, Clean food. When you feel the urge to eat a gooey dessert or a plate of fries, don't just think of your taste buds. Think of your community of cells – in your heart, your brain, your blood and your lungs – all relying on you to think of them, too.

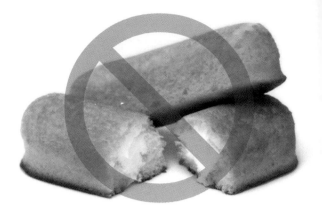

> "If you want to live a long, healthy, vibrant life, then you will have to eat life-giving foods."

DEAD FOOD/LIVING FOOD

Processed, chemically charged, sugar-fortified, partially hydrogenated foods are more common than ever and it's easy to see why eating these pseudo-foods does nothing to improve the length and quality of your life. In fact, the effect is quite the opposite. Lately, such foods have been called "dead foods" or as I like to call them, anti-foods.

Foods that have had their natural nutrition removed and have then been subjected to refining, processing and further manufacturing lose whatever potential they originally possessed. Now throw in a few chemicals to increase shelf life and seduce the customer with added sugar, salt and hydrogenated fats (to make you think this stuff tastes good), and you are left with marginally beneficial anti-foods. These are dead foods. Agri-business spends a lot of money marketing such foods, and if you're like most North Americans, it's what you buy. It's fast, it's readily available, it's cheap and it's everywhere. If we don't think about it too much, that's what we feed our families and ourselves. It's a slippery slope once you begin to lean on such nutrient-devoid foods.

EAT LIVE FOOD

Contrast anti-foods with fresh, still-living produce. When you pick a fresh head of lettuce it is actually still alive, nutrients bursting through its leaves. Most fresh produce is living. If you allow a potato to grow an eye and then plant it, a potato plant will grow. If you take the seeds from your tomato and put them in soil, you can grow a tomato plant. If you throw peels and flesh in the compost, every last bit will be broken down to nourish the earth.

Try that with a Twinkie! The thing will still be sitting there, "good" as new, weeks later. Now imagine what happens when you put that Twinkie in your body. Your mouth and stomach do their job and break it down, but then what? When your body encounters a molecule of polysorbate 60, otherwise known as polyoxyethylene (20) sorbitan monostearate (a common ingredient in processed foods such as the Twinkie), what will it do with it? In what way will that molecule aid in the health and longevity of your cells?

Your body has no idea what to do with many of the chemicals common in foods today, but the body's pretty smart, so it has a storage mechanism planned to deal with the unexpected. When it can't figure out what to do with such molecules, it finds a fat cell in your body in which to store them. The more you eat anti foods, the more fat you will have and that fat becomes a literal waste dump for the body's unrecognizable chemicals. No wonder your long-term health is affected so negatively!

When you eat Clean foods, your body breaks down and uses every single molecule. Every one! Each one of those molecules makes it to some place in your body where it does something for your health. Protein molecules go to building and repairing tissue. Healthy fat molecules assist with lubricating cells and keeping hair, skin and other organs healthy. Molecules from complex carbohydrates provide usable energy. Fiber cleans out your system. Water carries the nutrients through your body. Mom was right – you really are what you eat!

If you want to live a long, healthy, vibrant life, then you will have to eat life-giving foods. That means foods as close to their natural state as possible … Clean foods.

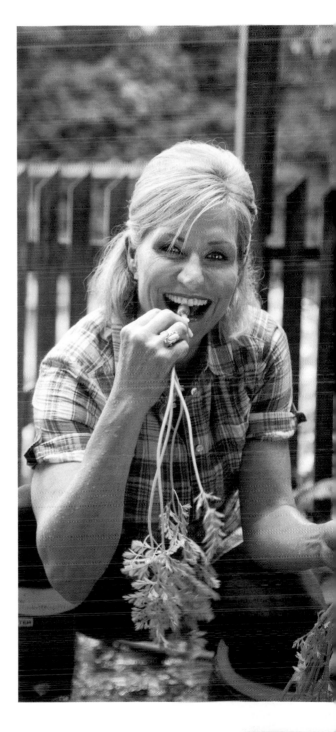

TOP CAUSES OF DEATH AND HOW TO PREVENT THEM

LEADING CAUSES OF NON-ACCIDENTAL DEATH*

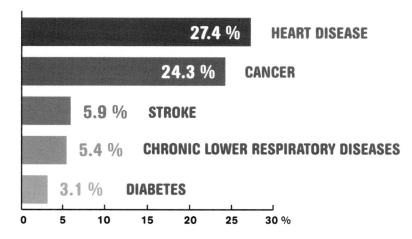

27.4 %   **HEART DISEASE**

24.3 %   **CANCER**

5.9 %   **STROKE**

5.4 %   **CHRONIC LOWER RESPIRATORY DISEASES**

3.1 %   **DIABETES**

0   5   10   15   20   25   30 %

*Statistics courtesy of the US Department of Health and Human Services, Centers for Disease Control and Prevention, 2006.

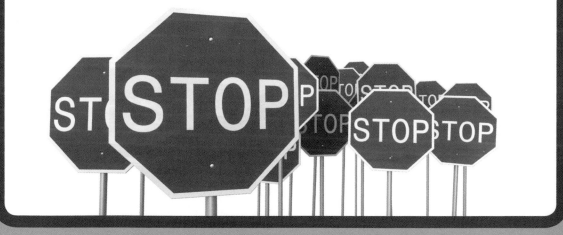

You can prevent disease and illness by following these preventative measures:

HEART DISEASE

(1) **DON'T SMOKE!** If you smoke, make it a priority to quit and if you don't smoke, don't start. Avoid smoke-filled areas, because ingesting second-hand smoke is just as dangerous to health.

(2) **EXERCISE REGULARLY.** Regular physical exercise strengthens the heart and lungs while controlling your weight and your stress – significant contributing factors in heart disease.

(3) **EAT CLEAN.** A diet rich in fresh fruits and vegetables, whole grains, legumes and lean proteins, and low in saturated and trans fats is the best diet for your heart. Make sure to consume enough omega-3 fatty acids and other healthy fats in balance. Minimize alcohol consumption.

(4) **STAY LEAN.** Even a weight gain of as little as five pounds means extra work for your heart. The extra weight further increases your chances of developing high blood pressure, high cholesterol and diabetes – all risk factors for developing heart disease.

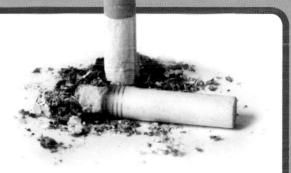

(5) **SCHEDULE A PHYSICAL.** It's easy to put off going to the doctor when you feel that nothing is wrong, but you may never know you have dangerous risk factors including high blood pressure or high cholesterol until it's too late. Scheduling an annual physical check up with your physician is a good investment in your health.

CANCER

(1) **GIVE UP THE CIGARETTE HABIT!** Quitting smoking reduces the risk of developing various cancers. Avoiding second-hand smoke is equally important in maintaining health.

(2) **EAT CLEAN.** Eat loads of fresh fruit and vegetables, plenty of whole grains and lean meats and drink enough water every day. Eat the correct balance of healthy fats but avoid trans and saturated fats.

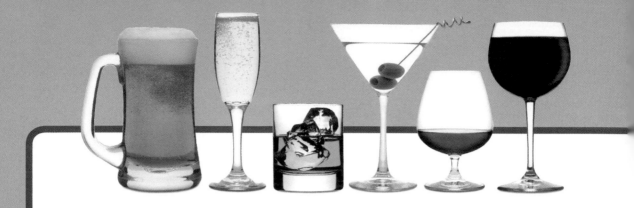

③ LIMIT ALCOHOL CONSUMPTION. The occasional glass of wine or alcoholic beverage – one or two glasses per week – is acceptable. Excessive alcohol consumption, however, is associated with an elevated risk of developing various types of cancer.

④ USE SUNSCREEN WITH A MINIMUM SPF OF 15. The powerful rays of the sun can break through even on a shady day. The sun is at its maximum strength between 10 am and 2 pm so try not to spend too much time unprotected and outdoors during these hours. Be vigilant about your moles – if you see any suspicious changes in your skin or your moles, please visit your doctor.

⑤ AVOID CARCINOGENS. Toxins are everywhere and difficult to avoid, but the more aware you are, the more readily you can avoid them. Common culprits include pesticides, car fumes, plastics, cleansers, preservatives and personal-care items from shampoo to soap to cosmetics. Avoid these cancer-contributing products when possible. Drink water from an inert metal water bottle and eat plenty of greens to fortify antioxidant levels in the body. Stay abreast of public health messages.

STROKE

① LIMIT ALCOHOL INTAKE. Alcohol consumption is a significant contributing risk factor for stroke. Consuming more than two alcoholic beverages each day significantly increases the risk of stroke. This is one instance where less is definitely more.

② QUIT SMOKING. Smoking doubles your risk of developing a stroke.

③ EXERCISE REGULARLY. Develop the habit of working out. Strive to perform 30 to 45 minutes of cardiovascular or resistance exercise at least three or four times per week.

④ CONTROL BLOOD SUGAR AND BLOOD PRESSURE. Eating Clean helps with both of these, especially if you consume a diet low in saturated and trans fats and limit your table salt intake. Switch to sea salt for a healthier salt option and follow the Eat-Clean Principles listed at the beginning of this book.

(5) SCHEDULE A REGULAR ANNUAL PHYSICAL. If you have a risky lifestyle or a family history of stroke, book a regular, yearly physical with your doctor. Doing so screens you for potential health issues and provides you with tools to offset illness. Home blood-pressure devices are available to help monitor blood pressure regularly.

CHRONIC LOWER RESPIRATORY DISEASES (BREATHING AND LUNGS)

(1) QUIT SMOKING. The number one way to avoid lung disease is not to smoke. Every cigarette package warns the public of this danger. Second-hand smoke should be avoided as well.

(2) EAT CLEAN. Your diet affects the potential of developing lung disease. Eating a diet rich in plants contributes to your body's ability to fight cancer and breathing/lung problems with the help of antioxidants.

(3) EXERCISE REGULARLY. Cardiovascular exercise strengthens the heart and lungs, making them less susceptible to disease.

(4) AVOID EXPOSURE TO ANTAGONIZING AGENTS: Radon is the second-leading cause of lung disease and cancer. Check your home and business for radon levels. Don't buy a home before checking radon levels. It is your right.

Asbestos is common in many households built before the 1970s. Asbestos is easily disturbed, especially during home renovations, creating toxic dust that seeps into the lungs. A work or home environment that has you breathing in small particles of asbestos may put you at risk for developing disease. Don't guess. Check asbestos levels in your home and office.

Farm workers often breathe in mold from various crops, and factory workers often breathe in fibers from cotton, jute, flax and hemp. Wear a particulate filter mask to avoid breathing in toxic particles.

(5) AVOID POLLUTION. Pay attention to the air quality each day and follow environmental warnings. If smog is high, don't go for a run outside. If possible, live in an area with cleaner air. Offset toxic accumulation by Eating Clean. Certain plant foods such as wheatgrass contain known anti-toxic agents that help to rid the body of pollutants.

DIABETES

(1) EAT CLEAN. The most powerful way to prevent type 2 diabetes is to control your blood sugar and body weight through diet. Avoid refined sugars and flours and foods made with these ingredients. Avoid or limit alcohol intake. Eat small, frequent meals consisting of lean protein and complex carbohydrates eaten together. Eat healthy fats to help slow digestion and also to nourish the brain.

(2) CONTROL YOUR WEIGHT. Nearly 90 percent of people who have diabetes are overweight! That is a staggering number. Weight control is the most powerful preventive medicine.

(3) BUILD MUSCLE. A body with less fat and more lean muscle tissue is less likely to develop diabetes. Body composition is more relevant than just body weight – where the fat collects is also significant. If your weight is predominantly around your middle,

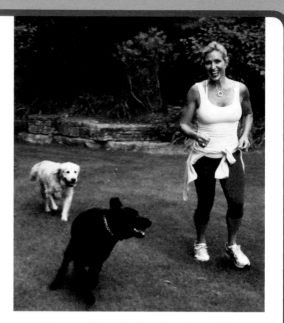

your chance of developing the disease is much greater. Work to build more lean muscle mass (while losing fat) to offset potential illness.

(4) EXERCISE REGULARLY. Both cardiovascular and resistance exercises are important to physical health. Cardiovascular exercise increases circulation, strengthens the heart and lungs, and promotes a lean physique. Include regular exercise in your health regimen.

(5) DON'T SMOKE. People who smoke are at a greater risk of developing diabetes. Live in a smoke-free environment.

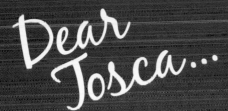

I'm a 29-year-old mother of twin boys (five months old) and I was looking in my local bookstore one day (the boys were actually cooperating with me!) and I came across your book, *The Eat-Clean Diet*. I skimmed through a few pages and thought that it sounded like good old-fashioned common sense so I purchased it and *The Eat-Clean Diet Cookbook*. (I love the recipes by the way.)

This letter is not about me though... it is about my 68-year-old father. I purchased a second copy of the book for my stepmother (who is really into health and fitness) and she subsequently purchased a copy of your cookbook for herself. She has been cooking from your book exclusively for the past two months and I would like to share a bit of news I got from my stepmother today about my father.

She said that when he had his three-month "check up" at the gym he goes to regularly (he likes to keep active but didn't always eat the best), the trainer was astonished to find that he had lost 7 percent body fat from the last time he was measured. She was very curious to find out what he was doing. He said that he'd just been eating different foods that his wife was making (from your cookbook) and that he'd changed nothing else. (My father has never been "fat" per se, but just not in the best shape.)

I am so proud that a man at 68 years of age (almost 69) is able to lose 7 percent body fat in a matter of a few months. He looks great, feels great and is leaner and more "cut." Obviously your strategies work very well for all.

Sincerely,

Stephanie Roch

London, Ontario

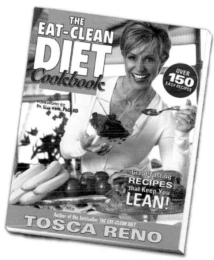

HOW TO LIVE A LONG LIFE

Many books and studies have been written on living a long life. While the media likes to pull out little sound bites such as "eat yogurt," there is a commonality to long-living societies. Here are the top five ways to live a long, active, vibrant, energetic life:

1 EAT CLEAN. I hope I've managed to convince you of this by now! Clean food nourishes, enriches and energizes. Dirty food destroys, diminishes and devastates.

2 GET ENOUGH REST AND SLEEP. If you can, follow your body's natural sleep rhythms. When you are tired, sleep. When your body has had enough sleep, you will awake naturally. Your body knows how much sleep it needs. Not giving it enough will negatively impact your health, your weight, your mood and ultimately your lifespan. You also need to take downtime. There is no such thing as a perpetual motion machine, so stop trying to be one. We all need time to sit and gaze at the stars, a beautiful sunset or nothing at all.

3 SPEND QUALITY TIME WITH THOSE YOU LOVE. By quality time I don't mean going to a Shakespearean play, although that's okay too. I mean real time. Cooking together time. Raking the yard together time. Walking together through the crunchy snow, talking about nothing time. It is these simple moments of life that make for the real, solid relationships that improve both the length and the quality of your life.

4 STAY ACTIVE. This means more than just going for your one-hour workout each day, though of course exercise such as this will benefit you immensely. In societies where people live a long time, they continue to labor right up till they die. That might mean farm work, preparing food, cleaning, walking, whatever they need to do … but they do not sit around on their rumps. This doesn't mean you have to go back to an agrarian way of life (although it's not a bad idea!) but whatever you do, make sure you keep doing it. And while you're at it, make sure to stay physically active too. As the saying goes, "Use it or lose it."

5 LIGHTEN UP! Enjoy yourself. Don't get angry over nothing – it's just not worth it. For the good of your happiness, for the happiness of those around you and for the good of your health, keep a sense of humor. Laughter is indeed the best medicine and no more so than when you can laugh at yourself, with true pleasure.

"Laughter is indeed the best medicine and no more so than when you can laugh at yourself, with true pleasure."

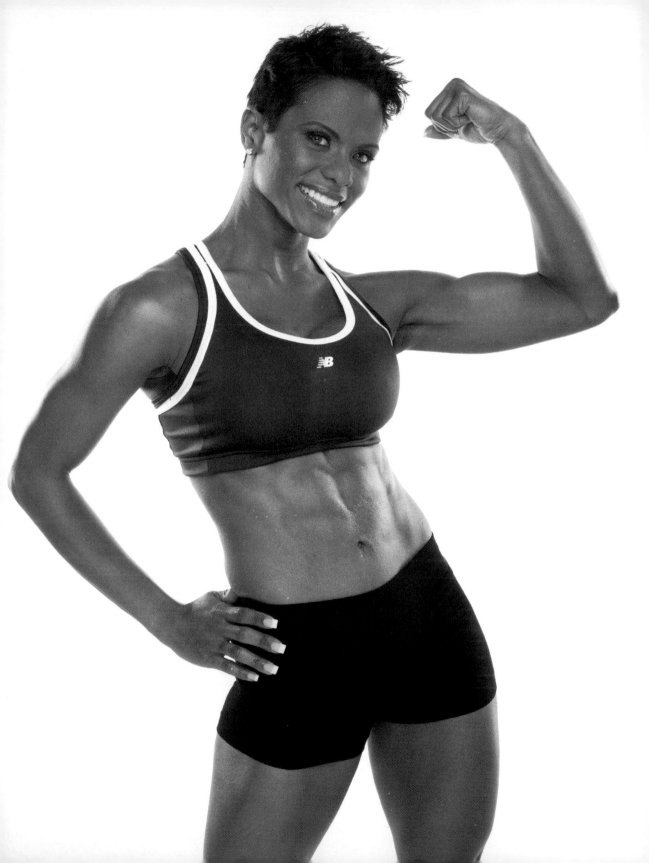

MAKING THE MOST OF SUPERFOODS

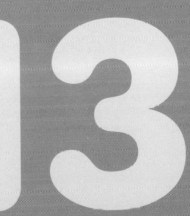

13

LET FOOD DO THE WORK

There is an innate sense of laziness, which I prefer to call efficiency, in all of us. Why do something the hard way when there is a more effective way to achieve similar results? Weight loss happens to be something many millions of us are very concerned with, yet we struggle with accomplishing this most difficult human task. We can accelerate weight loss in a natural, wholesome manner that does not feel like punishment at all. By now, you know the answer is Eating Clean, the backbone of which involves foods that are in the most natural state possible – I call this "eating close to the ground."

Some foods you will encounter while Eating Clean seem to possess Superhero powers. These foods, when consumed, make you feel like you have done something good for yourself. They are vastly different from the foods most North Americans eat of late. Compare the sense of satisfaction you feel after eating a quantity of steamed fresh vegetables – maybe a mixture of broccoli, asparagus and carrots – with the very empty sense you experience after consuming a greasy hot dog. Yet millions of us make such destructive foods our primary source of nutrition. It makes no sense.

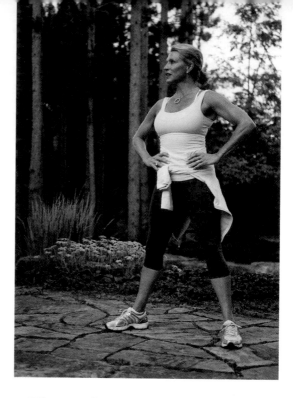

"Some foods you will encounter while Eating Clean seem to possess Superhero powers."

Since I have your attention I would now like to familiarize you with some foods that should start appearing on your plates with increased frequency from now on. Be careful! You will end up loving the results so much you probably will never eat another Twinkie again! I certainly hope so!

Why not get started right away? These powerful foods will make the job of looking and feeling better a thousand times easier. None of them are expensive nor are they dangerous to health — on the contrary, they are life giving!

FLAXSEED – GET HEALTHY FOR FIVE CENTS A DAY

There is nothing more powerful you can do for your health right away than add flaxseed to your diet. If you don't do anything else, you will still be coming out ahead. Flaxseed has been around for thousands of years. Cultivated in the Nile River Valley by the Egyptians, the flax plant yielded both valuable linen fibers from which to make cloth, and flaxseed. Nothing beats a stylish pair of linen pants, but flaxseed helps to create the healthy body that fills those pants out. Pharaohs valued the high nutritional content of ground flaxseed. They ate it ritually and Egyptians carried the seeds with them in case of emergency. Flaxseed was known to relieve abdominal pains and constipation. Roman soldiers carried flaxseed as food rations when they went to war.

King Charlemagne, ruler of the Franks, found flaxseed so nutritious and beneficial to health that he passed a law requiring the public to eat it daily during the eighth century. Europeans and Africans have embraced the tiny seed for its nutrition with far more interest than most North Americans, although that is beginning to change.

The health benefits of flaxseed are numerous. There is almost no aspect of human wellbeing that is not positively affected by this powerful little seed, which is no bigger than an ant. For a start, eating two tablespoons of ground flaxseed each day will improve digestion   flaxseed is known to have a mildly laxative effect sufficient to move lazy bowels, another condition afflicting many North Americans. It works! Imagine being able to shed those cloying last 10 pounds just by going to the bathroom more regularly! Studies show most of us carry an average of 5 to 25 pounds of waste in the colon, as a result of not eliminating properly. Whaaat?! Do you see what I mean by starting right now? You could be pounds lighter tomorrow by downing two tablespoons of very inexpensive but highly effective flaxseed right now!

The cardiovascular system improves when flaxseed is consumed, probably thanks to the healthy omega-3 fatty acids, Alpha-Linolenic acid (ALA), fiber and lignans present in flaxseed. Omega-3s also help reduce the risk of heart disease by lowering elevated blood fat (serum triglycerides) and reducing blood pressure.

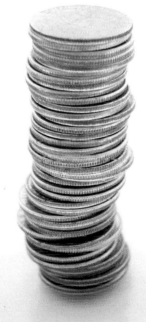

Most surprisingly, flaxseed has potent anti-cancer properties. Today's industrial diet is heavy in omega-6 fatty acids, skewing dangerously in the direction of actually causing cancer. When too many omega-6 fatty acids are consumed and not enough omega-3s, the body responds by creating an inflammatory environment ideal for developing cancer. Consuming more flaxseed and laying off of the industrial fats found mostly in packaged, refined foods helps to restore a healthy balance in the body. Those two tablespoons of flaxseed I recommend you take each day account for 140 percent of the body's daily requirement of omega-3 fatty acids, an amount that will cost you about five cents. Yes, a mere **five cents!**

Studies conducted in Toronto, Ontario, at the Women's College Hospital, show that some breast cancer tumors actually shrink in the presence of flaxseed. Similar results have been seen with prostate cancer. According to Doctors Richard Beliveau and Denis Gingras in their revealing book *Cooking with Foods that Fight Cancer,* "There is no doubt that flaxseed may have a highly positive and valuable impact on a diet designed to stave off cancer." The lignans or phytoestrogens in flaxseed are naturally occurring plant estrogens, which contribute to overall health by helping to prevent bone loss, reducing the risk of colon cancer and estrogen-related breast cancer, and mitigating the symptoms of menopause.

A LITTLE SEED, A LOT OF FAT!

Flaxseed may be tiny but it has an enormous beneficial impact when you are trying to lose weight. Part of the fear of dieting is the idea that you must go hungry. Our Superhero flaxseed steps in now to assist you once again. Full of healthy fats and fiber, flaxseed prolongs the sensation of fullness long after you eat it. Flaxseed fiber stays in your gut for an extended period, so you tend not to feel hungry soon after eating, the way you would if you ate a Cinnabon for breakfast. Empty calories, or anti-nutrient foods, never seem to satisfy in the same way as these natural foods do. Perpetual dieters who are unable to lose weight may know about this conundrum – the one where nutritionally lacking foods are eaten and hundreds of calories are consumed, but the dieter nonetheless remains unsatisfied and so the eating continues. Deprivation diets are never the answer to successful weight loss. Adding as little as two tablespoons of ground flaxseed daily to your diet can do the trick.

IMPORTANT FLAXSEED TIPS

✳ Use flaxseeds as opposed to flaxseed oil in order to get the full benefit of the lignans, which are present only in the seeds.

✳ Flaxseeds must be ground in order to release their full nutritional and health benefits, otherwise they will pass through you whole. Grind what you need for a week in a coffee grinder used solely for this purpose.

✳ An airtight opaque container will prevent volatile flaxseed oil from going off. Place the meal in the refrigerator to protect the fragile oils.

✳ I add two tablespoons of ground flaxseed to my cooked oatmeal every morning. I enjoy the pleasant, nutty taste.

✳ Find creative ways to enjoy flaxseed. I like to sprinkle the seeds over a leafy green salad for added texture. Another favorite way to enjoy flaxseed is to spread a whole-grain wrap with natural nut butter, place a peeled banana in the middle and sprinkle with flaxseed. Roll it up and enjoy!

✳ Use flaxseed as a garnish for home-baked goods such as breads, quick breads, meatloaf, muffins and fruit crumbles.

✳ The oils in flaxseed will go rancid if you mishandle the seeds. Always check to make sure the seeds don't smell foul before using. If they do, toss them. You aren't wasting much money and it isn't worth the health risk to consume them. Rancid oils contribute to disease.

MUSHROOMS - EAT MORE FUNGUS!

Don't be grossed out! Fungus is your friend, particularly if you are keen on shedding pounds. I have recently begun sampling the enormous variety of mushrooms out there by adding them to all things cooked at Chez Reno, partly because I am intrigued by the curious things I see every week at the produce counter and partly because I know how powerful they are, nutritionally speaking. It is a simple matter to sauté a small pan full of sliced mushrooms and serve them as a side dish to accompany virtually any entrée. Mushrooms are so meaty they can be used as a meat alternative, particularly the hefty portobello mushroom.

It's hard to believe a plant (which is not really a plant) that survives essentially on rotting organic material can be of nutritional significance for humans. They aren't green and they don't have fruit – the mushroom is actually the fruiting part of an enormous underground system of mycelium, or underground threads, which raid the soil for nutrients. That said,

their nutritional importance cannot be denied, either for health or weight-loss purposes. The Pharaohs once again knew the value of the fungus, reserving them for their own royal consumption. Beyond the frying pan, mushrooms have assumed a special place in the world of medicine, especially in Asia, where they are valued for their healing properties.

What do these spongy white forms have to do with weight loss? At the Johns Hopkins Bloomberg School of Public Health, fungi have been associated positively with weight loss. Researchers at the school pulled a fast one on participants. Taking advantage of the meatiness of certain mushrooms, meat was removed from the diet and replaced with mushrooms. The mushroom/meat switch proved successful. Over the four-day study the subjects ate fewer calories and shed weight. Another study conducted at San Diego State University found that people on a low-carbohydrate, mushroom-based diet were able to shed more pounds and have healthier blood-lipid profiles than those on a standard low-carb diet.

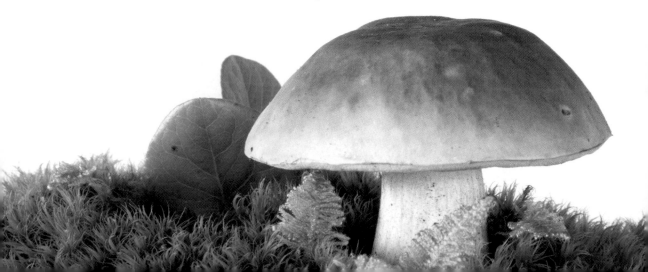

MUSHROOM FACTS

🍄 There are more than 100,000 known species of mushrooms, of which 2,000 are edible. Many are poisonous, so it pays to purchase or harvest mushrooms from a dependable source that can vouch for their origin.

🍄 Some mushrooms can be hallucinogenic. It is best to avoid these types, as they may store high concentrations of toxic chemicals including lead and mercury.

🍄 Mushrooms are implicated as powerful allies in the fight against cancer. Shiitake, enokitake, maitake and oyster mushrooms are loaded with anti-cancer agents that shrink the growth of tumors.

🍄 If you can't find fresh mushrooms, use dried. Many supermarkets carry dried mushrooms and it is a simple matter to reconstitute them. Place the mushrooms in a bowl. Cover with boiling water and soak for about 30 minutes. Drain the mushrooms and squeeze out any excess water.

🍄 Mushrooms are a rich source of nutrients. Vegetarians and vegans take note: mushrooms are rich in vitamin B12, a vitamin that is normally lacking or difficult to consume if you don't eat meat.

🍄 Mushrooms are rich in potassium, phosphorous, protein and fiber. In an Eat-Clean diet, mushrooms are valuable lean protein alternatives to meat.

🍄 Mushrooms are strong helpmates in the fight against disease, particularly heart disease.

🍄 You will be pleased to know that these funny fungi can facilitate your weight-loss efforts simply by eating them more often.

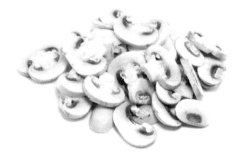

If you have been ignoring button mushrooms in favor of the more exotic ones such as shiitake, maitake, and reishi, consider this: research shows that the good old button mushroom contains just as much, if not more, antioxidant activity as its sexier-sounding counterparts.

The three most common button mushrooms are the ubiquitous white, the brown or tan-colored crimini or cremini and the portabella or portobello. The crimini and portobello are one and the same; in other words, crimini is an "immature" or "baby" portobello, while the portobello is sometimes called an overgrown crimini mushroom.

Although often found with vegetables in the grocery case, mushrooms actually belong to the kingdom Fungi — consisting of organisms without chlorophyll or vascular tissue, and including members as diverse as yeasts and molds. While most of the mushrooms consumed in this country are farmed or cultivated, many grow wild throughout the world. However, some mushrooms are poisonous, so avoid gathering and eating them in the wild without proper guidance.

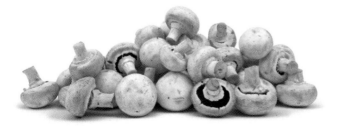

NUTRITION TIDBITS FOR PORTOBELLO MUSHROOMS

One cup of grilled portobello slices contains:

42 calories	5 g protein
0.9 g fat	2.7 g fiber
5.9 g carbohydrates	Low (below 55) Glycemic Index

In addition to being low in fat and high in fiber, portobello mushrooms pack a serious nutritional punch. For example, they are an excellent source of selenium (very important mineral for optimal antioxidant activity), many of the B vitamins and potassium. In addition, their polysaccharide and beta-glucan components exhibit anti-cancer properties.

When buying portobello mushrooms, look for smooth firm caps without wet slimy patches. Store them in the refrigerator inside a loosely closed paper bag or wrap them inside a damp cloth.

WAYS TO INCLUDE MORE MUSHROOMS IN YOUR DIET

- Add them to salads, pasta sauce, soups, stir-fries, casseroles or pizza.

- Use marinated and grilled portobello caps as flavorful burger "patties" — no need for meat here.

FERMENTED FOODS – YOGURT AND KEFIR

At this moment over 400 species of bacteria are living in your five-meter-long digestive tract, if you are healthy that is. Obviously such bacteria are of enormous benefit to humans, otherwise we would be in serious trouble. According to doctors Richard Beliveau and Denis Gingras, "The colon, for example, contains on average one thousand billion (one trillion) bacteria per milliliter, making it the planet's most densely populated microbial habitat!" Friendly bacteria ensure that healthy digestion is taking place at every moment of the day.

Certain foods contribute a positive effect to the already proficient inner workings of food processing. These are the fermented foods known as yogurt and kefir. Many variations of fermented foods can be considered important to your weight-loss efforts, but yogurt and kefir should be the focus right now. This is because they contain protein, which is important to consume at each of your six small Eat-Clean meals.

Yogurt products have taken the food industry by storm. If you are constipated or if you just need to increase your vitamin intake, there is a yogurt that claims to solve your problem. Forget the pseudo-yogurts that populate the shelves of your dairy case. Don't be lured by sugar, fruit and other so-called healthy ingredients. Yogurt is plenty healthy all by itself and you need to purchase a good-quality low-fat or nonfat plain yogurt.

I want you to consider real, healthy yogurt as the kind that contains only two ingredients – milk products and bacterial culture. This is what yogurt is supposed to be. If you want to add something sweet to it then do so with your own ingredients such as fruit or granola, other cereal grains or anything else you like, just not sugar! If you must sweeten yogurt, use natural honey, maple syrup, agave nectar or a bit of rapadura or Sucanat sugar. Use only a very small amount.

While we have known forever that dairy products, including yogurt and kefir, are essential for strengthening bones and teeth, we have recently learned the significance of these foods in managing weight. "Yogurt is the perfect food because it is high in calcium, [and] has carbs, protein and fat, which are what you need in every meal," claims Mireille Guiliano, author of the best selling *French Women Don't Get Fat*. She claims further that, "Yogurt is one of the French secrets to weight control." According to Guiliano, many French women eat yogurt at least twice a day, especially at breakfast. Yogurt contains lean protein, which is one half of the ideal weight-loss-fuel combo. If you add mixed berries you will get the other half of that equation, namely complex carbohydrates.

A study published in the *International Journal of Obesity* supports the notion that dairy products such as yogurt and kefir assist with weight loss. In the study published in April 2005, obese adults were asked to trim 500 calories a day from their diet. They did so while consuming three servings per day of low-fat yogurt. The study showed that the consumption of yogurt helped them shed significant amounts of fat, especially from around the waist.

Yogurt's lesser-known cousin, kefir, originates from Russia and Eastern European countries. It too is a fermented food made with only two ingredients: milk and live bacterial cultures. Stay away from kefir pimped out with sugar, chocolate chips or anything else that doesn't belong in your Eat-Clean food plan. Kefir is the Turkish word for "feel good" or "wellbeing," which is how you apparently feel after you eat this tangy fermented food. There is so much tryptophan in kefir that it imparts this natural "high" to those who eat it.

Kefir can be drinkable or thicker like yogurt. It has a similar taste to yogurt but is tangier and a bit effervescent thanks to the yeasts, which transform the lactose to carbon dioxide (that's the effervescence) and alcohol. Oh, now I know why they call it "feel good!" Kefir contains more bacteria than yogurt and for those who are lactose intolerant, fear not, the lactose sugars in kefir are pre-digested, so it is actually easier to digest and has no ill effects on the digestive tract. Many who cannot tolerate any other dairy products can tolerate kefir.

Along with healthy yeast and bacterial culture, kefir is also loaded with complete protein. Here then is another option for a lean protein source in your Eat-Clean food plan. The body more readily takes up the protein in kefir because the amino acids, much like the lactose, are partially pre-digested. The bacteria are doing all the work for you! Kefir also helps to fortify bones and teeth, since it is rife with calcium, magnesium and phosphorus. The latter is essential in helping to assimilate carbohydrates, fats and proteins as food passes through the digestive tract. The more plentiful this mineral, the healthier the cell and the more energy you have. As an added benefit, kefir fights cravings.

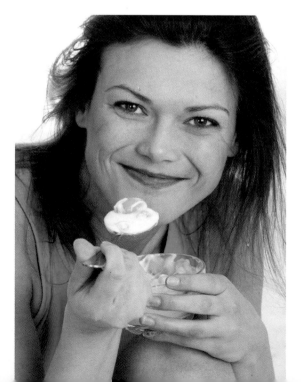

GET TO KNOW KEFIR

❖ If you are feeling really adventurous you can eat *koumiss*, a fermented food made from camel, mare or donkey milk.

❖ Kefir contains the B vitamins 1, 6 and 12, as well as vitamin K. The B vitamins are known to help fight depression.

❖ Many who eat kefir claim it is the fountain of youth, since kefir regulates the liver, kidneys and nervous system, chasing signs of old age and boosting energy levels.

❖ Russian biologist Elie Metchnikoff (1845-1916) is the founding father of immunology. The Nobel Prize winner is responsible for discovering the positive health attributes of lactic bacteria. He noticed that people living in the Bulgarian mountains enjoyed marked longevity and that they drank fermented milk called *yahourth*. Yahourth slowed premature aging by neutralizing toxicity in the gut.

❖ A probiotic is a beneficial bacteria usually from a plant source and found in the intestinal tract. Beware of what you are buying in the dairy case. Yogurt already has probiotics in it. Don't be duped by products that say they contain enhanced probiotic agents. They are all the same!

CHIA SEEDS

Centuries ago ancient Aztecs depended on chia as a valuable food source, believing it possessed mystical energy and supernatural powers. Mexicans and South Americans still incorporate it into their diet today. Chia is possibly better known as the cousin of the chia plant (think Chia pets). The plants produce tiny seeds, which may be black or grayish-white in color. The white seeds (marketed as Salba) have a slightly higher nutrition profile, but are more expensive than the black, which can usually be found in bulk food stores.

Chia is growing in popularity, as more and more North Americans are coming to know this tiny, grayish grain (that often gets stuck in your teeth) for its beneficial health qualities. Chia is important for its significant fiber content and hefty dose of healthy fatty acids. These are the omega-3 fatty acids, which are potent inflammation fighters, important for battling cancer. Omega-3s are effective in lowering LDL, or bad cholesterol levels, in the blood. The plentiful fiber in chia is the insoluble, or indigestible kind, which keeps your tummy full and your pipes cleaned out much the same as flaxseed. One serving of chia grains contains 4.2 grams of dietary fiber, mostly insoluble, which is responsible for stabilizing blood sugar levels. The white grains contain more protein than traditional grains including wheat, rice, corn or barley. In addition, chia has the highest fiber content of any food, including wheat bran. Chia can absorb many times its weight in water, which is one of the reasons it is so effective in a weight-loss program. It is this water-absorbing quality that slows digestion, promotes a feeling of fullness and moderates blood sugar levels. When you feel full you are not as likely to eat unnecessarily.

CHIA FACTS

➲ Chia has a neutral flavor so it can be readily used as a dietary supplement in smoothies, yogurt, kefir or cereal.

➲ Since chia is a seed it is gluten free and can be used in gluten-free diets. To make flour, mix one part ground chia with three parts flour made from gluten-free grains.

➲ Chia is rich with disease-fighting antioxidants and minerals.

➲ Two tablespoons of ground chia in half a cup of cold water can be used as an egg substitute for those who don't eat eggs.

TEMPEH, MISO AND MORE

Fermented soy products are part of a long Asian cultural history of health and wellness. Soy remains the outcast of a North American traditional diet and the butt of many jokes. "Are you really going to eat that rubber?" "Hmm, soy, tastes like cardboard," and more. Laugh all you like, you can't argue with its powerful health and weight-loss benefits.

Soy is an excellent source of non-animal, complete protein, which as you now know is essential to an Eat-Clean diet, especially when partnered with complex carbohydrates. Soy delivers more than just protein. It is chock full of nutrients including essential fatty acids, vitamins, minerals and disease-fighting phytochemicals, so it is a good idea to replace a few meals each week with dishes containing soy products. Miso, tempeh, edamame, tofu and soybean curd are all excellent options to consider.

Tempeh is a fermented (recall the benefits of eating fermented foods, namely yogurt, kefir, sauerkraut, some beer and wine) soy-based food made through a process where cooked soybeans are impregnated with a friendly mold. This *Rhizopus oligosporus* mold makes the soybeans stick together in a solid cake while the fermentation process occurs. The result is a meaty, mushroomy tasting food, densely packed with essential fatty acids (EFAs), vitamins, minerals and phytochemicals. Recall that EFAs keep the metabolism running at high speed while helping build lean muscle tissue. The prolific fiber in tempeh also keeps the tummy full.

Tempeh can be used in place of meat and is much like a portobello mushroom in flavor and texture. Slice it, season it, fry it or bake it and throw it into any dish you can conceive.

Miso is tempeh's stronger-tasting cousin. Soybeans are ground and injected with friendly bacteria called *Aspergillus orxyae.* The resulting fermented paste is mixed with other whole grains, including brown rice or barley, then placed in large holding vats where the mixture sits for as many as three years while fermenting. Miso is more of a condiment, like ketchup or mustard, and imparts a salty, tangy flavor to dishes. Miso soup is a dish enjoyed by many Asians, especially in Japan, where they eat it for breakfast.

Tempeh and miso are essentially pre-digested forms of soy, so they are easier to digest and assimilate into the body. Soy consumption must be done with a sense of balance, however, since there have been reports of health issues if soy is overconsumed or if women with a history of breast cancer eat it. If soy products are eaten within reason and with a clear idea of your own health (check with your doctor if you are in doubt), then soy can be a good source of nutrients. I eat it twice a week in the form of edamame or tempeh (that is how I like it best).

"Miso soup is a dish enjoyed by many Asians, especially in Japan, where they eat it for breakfast."

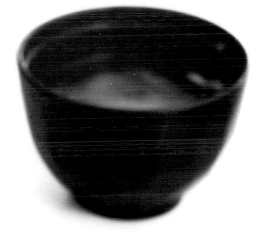

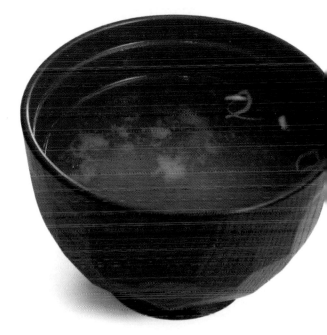

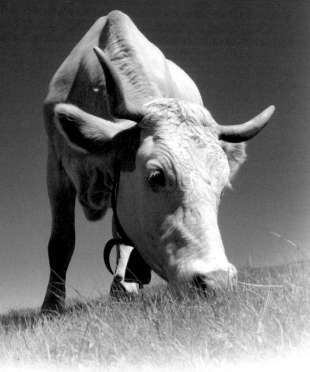

PASTURE-RAISED
MEATS AND POULTRY

It sounds odd to suggest that meat or poultry ought to be raised in pastures, but up until a few short decades ago that is where these animals roamed and ate. Now when you order a steak at a restaurant, you will read that the steak comes from "grain-fed animals," a fact that is obviously printed with some pride. But cattle are not meant to eat grain. Their digestive tracts are set up as ruminants with several stomachs to digest their preferred food – grass. When they eat grain, including corn and soy, their bellies become acidic and bloated, promoting disease, most predominantly *E. coli* (sound familiar?), which then contaminates anyone who eats the flesh of the diseased animal. Chickens love to scratch and roam, eating greens and bugs as they go. That is impossible to accomplish in the cages they are con-

fined to in most giant poultry operations. By definition, free-range implies that the animal probably has to search out his meal, rather than being confined to a concentrated feed lot, where conditions are inhumane and deplorable.

The meat of grass-fed animals – beef, venison, elk, bison and so on – is more nutrient dense, than is the meat of grain-fed animals. Grass-fed beef comes from cattle raised in open pastures, feeding on a steady diet of 100-percent organic grass. The flesh of grass-fed animals contains higher amounts of omega-3 fats, beta-carotene and as much as 400 percent more of vitamins A and E.

With respect to its role in an Eat-Clean lifestyle and in weight loss, the flesh of pasture-raised animals contains CLA (Conjugated Linoleic Acid), which is a powerful phytochemical shown to improve weight loss. Certain meats, including lamb, red meats and particularly thigh meat in poultry, already contain CLA, but animals that roam free concentrate it to higher degrees in their flesh. As Nina Planck states in her book *Real Food*, "CLA aids weight loss in several ways: by decreasing the amount of fat stored after eating, increasing the rate at which fat cells are broken down and reducing the number of fat cells." These are incredibly powerful reasons to make consuming grass-fed meats and free-range poultry a priority in your Eat-Clean lifestyle.

GAME MEATS

VENISON

This is the name commonly given to wild deer meat. Venison is nutritionally denser than beef, chicken or pork. It is a richly colored and flavorful meat that contains little fat, so it must be cooked with care.

BISON

One of my favorites, bison has a higher protein content and less fat than beef. Consuming sufficient EFAs is critical for a healthy diet and bison is an excellent source of these healthy fats.

ELK

Like venison, this richly colored meat is full of nutrients and little fat. Elk must be cooked with care as it contains little of its own fat. It is, however, a delicious meat.

ADZUKI AND MUNG BEANS

Beans have long been considered an excellent protein alternative to animal sources of meat for vegetarians. I love beans and I am not a full-fledged vegetarian, however I do call myself a "flexitarian," because at least twice, and sometimes three times a week, I make meatless dishes for dinner. I saw Michael Pollan, author of the *Omnivore's Dilemma* (one of my favorite eating-with-a-conscience books), on a recent *Oprah* show and he suggested the same, saying that, "Even one meatless day a week – a meatless Monday, which is what we do in our household – if everybody in America did that, it would be the equivalent of taking 20 million midsize sedans off the road." Now close your eyes and try to picture this. Realize that this is how much of a carbon footprint traditionally raised beef leaves behind. It's staggering! So I do my part and eat beans!

Beans come in handy on my meatless nights because I know if I partner them with rice, the result is a complete protein. Beans are also inexpensive, which again comes in handy during these times of economic difficulty. Beans, however, do not contain a complete array of proteins and this is why it is always suggested to partner them with rice. Adzuki and mung beans are ideal for an Eat-Clean lifestyle because they contain so much easily digested protein. They contain more protein per pound than a steak, yet they cost less and contain fewer unhealthy fats and calories.

How do beans help you lose weight? Beans have a low Glycemic Index (GI), which means they don't cause your blood sugar levels to sky-rocket after you eat them, since they provide slow-release energy. They are chock full of fiber, which also helps you feel full for longer, preventing possible bingeing. Some dieters make a tea with adzuki beans to accelerate weight loss, as these beans are known to promote weight loss and detoxify the body. Make your tea by simmering one cup of dried adzuki beans in five cups of water for one hour. Using a soup spoon, ladle out enough "tea" to fill a cup and drink it slowly. Drink half a cup of tea before meals. Both adzuki and mung beans help detoxify the body, which may assist you in jumpstarting your Eat-Clean lifestyle, particularly if you have had a long relationship with some detrimental foods, including sugar and other refined foods.

SPICES AND HERBS

The ever-inventive Romans were among the first to experiment with spices, but when Rome fell spices were nearly forgotten for some time. We think of spices as seasonings we can add to a dish to give it a signature flavor. What would chili con carne be without chili powder? However, a perhaps lesser-known fact is that spices can have a powerful effect on weight loss. It may be time to open your spice drawer and start shaking the goods onto your eats!

Brindell berry, or hila, is an herb that can promote weight loss as well as increase lean muscle mass. It works primarily by suppressing the appetite and blocking fat storage. The botanical name is *Garcinia cambogia.* Native to India and Asia, the plant produces small fruits that look like tiny pumpkins from which garcinia is harvested.

Psyllium. You may recognize this herb as the major ingredient in most products used to treat constipation. The fiber comes from the outer husk of the seeds of a plant whose botanical name is *Plantago ovata.* The husks are effective in weight loss, thanks to their effect of moderating blood sugar levels. It also promotes a sense of fullness when consumed, as many fibrous plants do, so you theoretically should not feel hungry after eating it. Psyllium also lowers blood serum cholesterol levels. This plant is most effective if you drink lots of water with it.

Capsicum, or hot pepper, is a fiery ingredient used to season many Mexican dishes. There are numerous varieties of peppers, each with its own intensity, including chili pepper, paprika and cayenne. Hidden in the brilliant flesh are plentiful antioxidants and the phytochemical capsaicin, which is capable of increasing body heat as it is digested. This metabolic event is called thermogenesis and stimulates your metabolism. When the metabolic rate is increased, more fuel is burned and capsaicin can help you maintain an elevated metabolic rate for as long as 70

"Greens, greens, greens! This is the battle cry of the Clean Eater. The more greens you pile into your diet, the better!"

to 90 minutes after ingestion. Capsaicin also boosts the mobilization of fat in the abdominal area.

Fennel is a beautiful plant with a mild licorice flavor. It's native to the Mediterranean, but the whole world has caught on to the wonderful flavor and usefulness of this bulbous plant. You will find it in teas, capsules, tinctures and lozenges. The fennel plant seems to help moderate the appetite, which is a valuable effect for those wishing to lose weight. Chewing the seeds also seems to suppress appetite. Fennel contains loads of fiber, which contributes to efficient elimination, again helpful when weight loss is the goal. Imagine your intestines as a series of pipes. Fennel is the brush that scrapes the colon walls clean of built-up waste products. Fennel stalks are commonly chewed after a large meal to relieve stomach discomfort.

Garlic is not only the world's most-loved cooking ingredient, it's also a natural diuretic. Garlic contains mustard oils, which cause peristalsis, powerful muscular contractions in the digestive tract. The contractions are so strong they help loosen and rid the body of unwanted fats. Garlic can also help to emulsify fatty clumps. Garlic is known to reduce blood-fat levels and this is currently being tested to evaluate its possible implications for weight loss.

Regardless, garlic is magnificent food, particularly when you roast it in a slow oven, bathed in a bit of olive oil for about 35 minutes. Heaven!

Quinoa. I think some of you may not purchase this wonder food simply because you are uncertain how to pronounce it. Say it like this: Keen-wah. Since quinoa is really the seed of the quinoa plant, those who are gluten intolerant can readily eat it. Even if you don't have digestive issues, quinoa is beneficial for an Eat-Clean lifestyle.

Quinoa is one of the few grains that contain protein — twice as much as any other cereal grain. It is ideal as a weight-loss and weight-management food because it is lower in carbohydrates than other cereal grains. It also contains plentiful healthy fats, iron, calcium, phosphorus, manganese and copper. The Aztecs and the Incas did not refer to it as the Mother Grain for nothing!

Quinoa is ideal for the Eat-Clean lifestyle because it sustains you while it satisfies you. The carbohydrates in this grain are released slowly, so when you have eaten quinoa it stays with you, releasing energy over time. This is beneficial for combating cravings and binges.

GREENS, GREENS, GREENS!

This is the battle cry of the Clean Eater. The more greens you pile into your diet, the better! I recently became aware that although I eat plenty of vegetables, I was developing a slight bias against the greens — literally the tops of plants — that I would see while in the produce section of the grocery store. I did not know how to cook them, so I decided I had better get smart and learn. I began to buy Swiss chard, kale, dandelion greens, and everything green and leafy I could think of. Soon a serving of lightly steamed greens began to accompany every meal. Greens are surprisingly easy to cook and are nature's nutritional gift to you.

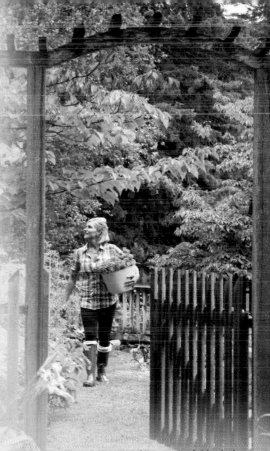

The Greeks know the power of greens! They make a practice of seeking out the *horta,* or wild greens, and even certain weeds. So this is what all those people are doing on the side of the roads in early spring and summer! In Greece, villagers gather greens from sites where no pesticides have been sprayed, then steam them and have them for dinner. They are best tossed with olive oil, a bit of sea salt and freshly ground black pepper, and given a spritz of lemon juice. Greeks value these plants because of their numerous health benefits. Many wild greens cure digestive ailments and cleanse the liver. Horta are also loaded with fiber and other nutrients essential to optimal health along with achieving and maintaining an optimal weight.

The most valuable wild greens (to your body) include dandelion, sow thistle, stinging nettles, purslane and mallow. However, it can be tricky to identify and harvest these greens before they are too tough and old to eat, or before they have bolted into maturity and are then also inedible. If you are gathering your own wild greens, you also need to worry about pesticide use, so check to make sure your horta patch is pristine first. Otherwise visit your produce section or farmers market and seek out other greens, already gathered for you. These include radicchio, chicory, dandelion, sorrel, arugula, endive, mustard and beet greens, as well as collard greens. I plan on planting several of these good greens in my next vegetable garden!

COCONUT BUTTER OR COCONUT OIL

You will find that I have included coconut oil and/or butter in many of the recipes in this book. I have done this with the intention of introducing you to a maligned yet incorrectly overlooked food – the coconut. For some time coconut oil has not been viewed in a favorable light. This is largely because it gets confused with palm oil, which is definitely not a good choice.

Coconut palms date back to prehistoric times, which means the plant is a survivor and has honed its evolutionary prowess over the millennia. Coconuts have been known to float in seas and oceans for months and still be viable afterwards. That may explain why the enormous "nut" has established itself in many tropical countries.

According to David Wolfe, author of *Eating For Beauty*, "Coconuts are one of the greatest gifts on this planet. No matter where you are, what you have done, how much you have mistreated your body, fresh young coconuts and coconut oil can save your life." I like the promise of this statement and have indeed found that when I have trained heavily or over-dieted during contest prep, drinking coconut water has a powerful energizing effect on me. It doesn't hurt that it also tastes delicious.

The coconut is a large nut, or seed, of the coconut palm. When you see coconuts hanging on trees they have a thick outer green layer. The nut itself is packaged cleverly with a dense fibrous outer layer, an inner white meaty layer (coconut meat), followed by a hollow space containing coconut water. Coconut water, which is sterile, contains a supply of electrolytes that is among the highest in nature. The reason for this high degree of purity is that it takes about nine months for the fibrous coconut to filter the water that eventually ends up inside the nut. The water from young coconuts can actually be used as intravenous fluid since it is identical to human blood plasma.

My favorite way to eat coconut is to find a young one that is still green outside and open it. Then, using a spoon, I scoop out the "jelly" or soft coconut meat. It is delicious and nothing like dried coconut at all. It is also highly nutritious, containing vitamins, minerals and healthy fats. This young coconut meat, or jelly, is known to contain high concentrations of plant nutrients that help fight free-radical damage.

COCONUT BUTTER AND OIL

Coconut oil is also called coconut butter. Don't confuse this with cocoa butter – they are not the same thing at all. Cocoa butter comes from the cocoa (think chocolate) plant. Coconut butter or oil comes from processing the meat from the mature brown coconut. The meat is removed from the ripe nut and shredded. Under specific pressing conditions, the oil filters out. Coconut oil and coconut butter *are* the same thing. The buttery form turns to a clear liquid when heated. Coconut oil is valued by chefs for its high smoke point, along with its delicious taste and pleasurable texture.

There are numerous health benefits to adding coconut oil to your diet. The medium-chain fatty acids in coconut oil are the healthy ones that are readily converted to energy by the body, so this is a much-needed healthy fat. Although coconut oil has been charged with increasing cholesterol, this is far from true. Coconut oil contains no cholesterol and better yet, has the ability to reduce serum cholesterol. For the sugar addicted among us, coconut oil is a must! By consuming the valuable oil regularly, you will shed the toxic addiction to sugar and its destructive effects on the body. Anyone with a big-time sugar habit knows what cravings are all about. Consuming coconut oil helps chase cravings away and goes one step further by stabilizing digestive hormones so you are not constantly hungry. Coconut oil even has a positive effect on metabolism, boosting a formerly sluggish rate to a more active one. I don't have to spell out what that means for those interested in weight loss.

STORAGE TIPS

Look for coconut oil that has been farmed and processed with you in mind. That is, look for fair-trade products not tainted with pesticides. You will need to keep it in a cool dark place to protect its healthful qualities. The best coconut oil comes in dark-colored or opaque containers. Coconut butter or oil is one of the most stable oil products, withstanding temperatures up to 170°C. This is important because most oils begin to form dangerous trans-fatty acids at high temperatures. Coconut oil and butter are a great addition to your Eat-Clean kitchen and diet.

FISH AND SEAFOOD

HEALTHY OR TOXIC?

Most nutritionists recommend that we eat fish at least twice a week for its healthful benefits, but seafood has its dark side. Some fish contain high levels of mercury and other poisons; others have been raised in questionable environments. This leaves us standing at the seafood counter scratching our heads. And as if that is not enough to worry about, now that over-fishing has depleted so many fish stocks to the point of near-extinction, we also have to think about whether we are contributing to that problem with our dinner selection.

It's worth putting in the effort to learn which are the best choices. Seafood is a wonderful source of protein and contains the very best fats, omega-3 fatty acids. A seafood-rich diet has been proven to improve the brain and visual development of babies and children, and helps to improve and maintain cardiovascular health. Evidence is beginning to mount that suggests eating seafood helps prevent or alleviate blood pressure, stroke, cancer, asthma, type 2 diabetes and Alzheimer's disease.

Seafood WATCH®, a program of the Monterey Bay Aquarium and a partner of SeaWeb's Seafood Choices Alliance, has come up with guidelines to help you figure out what the best choices of seafood are, bringing health and sustainability into consideration. They suggest that over 75 percent of the world's seafood is fished either right up to or beyond its sustainable limit. Fish farms seem like the logical answer, but some farms are run in a manner that produces fish inferior in taste and health benefits, and in a way that spreads disease both within the farm itself and then into the ocean at large.

BEST TO WORST
SEAFOOD CHOICES

Here, from the Environmental Defense Fund, are the best to worst seafood choices for your dinner table (avoiding mercury and PCBs).

NOTE: Young children are more at risk of mercury poisoning and PCBs than older children or adults. What may be a low or moderate risk for an adult could still be a high risk for young children.

LOW RISK (eat 2-4 times per month):

Sturgeon: Atlantic*	Snapper*
Tuna – albacore (canned, wild)*	Sole: English^
Tuna – yellowfin*	Trout: rainbow (farmed)^
Tilefish*	Monkfish*
Halibut*	Salmon (wild, Alaska)^
Mahi-mahi*	Sea bass – black*

MODERATE RISK (eat no more than twice per month):

Sea bass – Chilean*	Sea trout: spotted^*
Crab: blue^*	Grouper*
Lingcod*	Snapper – mutton*
Mackerel – Spanish*	Wahoo*
Rockfish^*	

HIGH RISK (eat no more than once per month):

Croaker – Atlantic^	Salmon – Atlantic^
Flounder^	Tuna – bigeye*
Opah*	Roughy – orange*

VERY HIGH RISK (women & kids should not eat at all):

Alewife^	Weakfish^*
Bass: striped (wild)^*	Mackerel – king*
Bluefish^*	Tuna – bluefin^*
Croaker – white^	Marlin*
Eel^*	Shark*
Shad^	Swordfish*
Sturgeon (wild, imported)^*	

> * Mercury is a main concern
>
> ^ PCBs is a main concern

Stay up to date! Go to www.montereybayaquarium.org/cr/cr_seafoodwatch/sfw_recommendations.aspx to download a pocket fish guide and an application for your phone (focus on environment and sustainability).

Go to www.edf.org to download a pocket guide with the focus on mercury and PCBs.

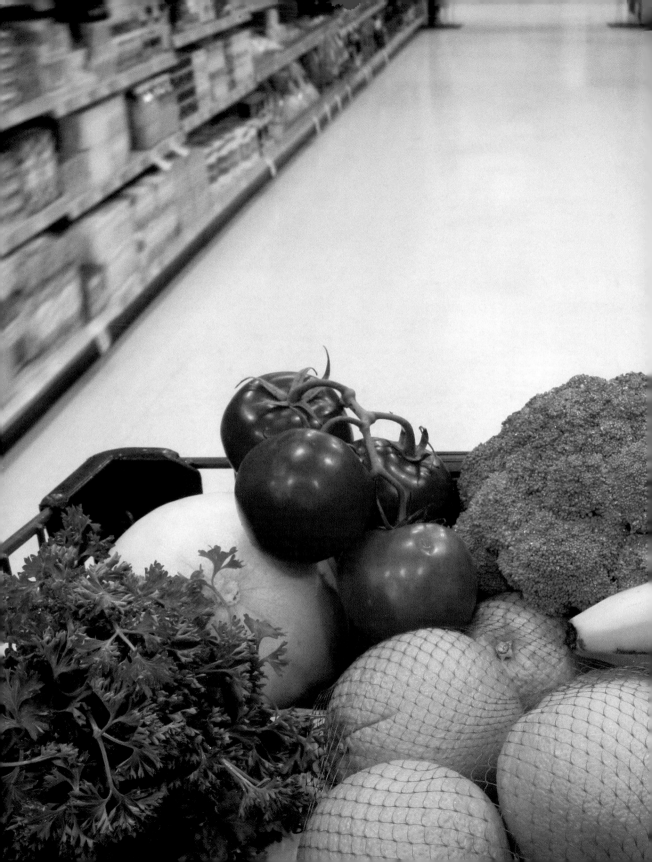

THE EAT-CLEAN DIET
RECHARGED

MEAL PLANS & GROCERY LISTS

14

COOLER PLANS

COOLER PLANS EXPLAINED

Each cooler plan is meant for a day's worth of food. Choose the cooler that is right for you at this time. Read over the Eat-Clean Principles on page 21 and refer to this checklist when packing your cooler:

◆ Eat more – eat six small meals each day.

◆ Eat breakfast every day, within an hour of rising.

◆ Eat a combination of lean protein and complex carbohydrates at each meal.

◆ Eat sufficient (two or three servings) healthy fats each day.

◆ Drink two to three liters of water each day.

◆ Carry a cooler packed with Clean foods each day.

◆ Depend on fresh fruits and vegetables for fiber, vitamins, nutrients and enzymes.

◆ Adhere to proper portion sizes.

If you are a vegetarian or vegan please refer to page 280 for lean protein options.

"Each cooler plan is meant for a day's worth of food. Choose the cooler that is right for you at this time."

COOLER PLAN #1   ➜ Hardcore eating for rapid results

WHAT IT'S FOR:

- ☑ Breaking plateaus
- ☑ Losing last 5 to 10 pounds
- ☑ Early contest preparation
- ☑ Photo shoots
- ☑ Showing increased muscular definition
- ☑ Quick weight loss
  - * Cooler one should be followed for a maximum of two weeks at a time.
  - * Eat your last meal at 6 PM, or four hours before bed.

WHAT IT IS:

Please note that this is the strictest of the cooler plans and will not be easy for some of you. There is very little room for indulgence and you may feel a little foggy due to lack of complex carbs. If it is too much, you can add more complex carbohydrates (yam, apple, or brown rice) to one of your early meals. But hardcore eating promises results, and that is what you will get!

HOW IT WORKS:

Follow the Eat-Clean Principles on page 21.
(for a menu-plan example, see page 268)

COMPLEX CARBOHYDRATES FROM FRUIT:

- ◆ 1 apple or pear per day (½ in the morning and ½ in the afternoon or evening)

COMPLEX CARBOHYDRATES FROM VEGETABLES (RAW OR STEAMED):

- ◆ 2 cupped handfuls eaten five times per day of cucumbers, radishes, tomatoes, leafy greens, broccoli, spinach, asparagus, green beans, sprouts, celery, bok choy or other high-water content, non-starchy, low-Glycemic Index vegetables

COMPLEX CARBOHYDRATES FROM WHOLE GRAINS AND STARCHY CARBOHYDRATES:

- ◆ 1 handful per day of cooked quinoa, brown rice, oatmeal, millet or Cream of Wheat

  Top this with:

  2 to 4 tablespoons of ground flaxseed

  2 to 4 tablespoons of bee pollen
- ◆ 1 hand-sized sweet potato or yam serving per day (½ in the morning and ½ in the afternoon or evening)

LEAN PROTEIN:

- ◆ 1 palm-sized portion eaten five times each day of chicken, tuna, egg whites, turkey, bison, elk or non-oily fish
- ◆ Good-quality, sugar- and chemical-free protein powder (hemp, soy, or whey) may be substituted for any protein serving

BEVERAGES:

- ◆ 1 gallon per day of distilled water, fresh water with no sodium or clear, unsweetened herbal tea

AVOID:

- ✗ Dairy products
- ✗ Juice
- ✗ Bread
- ✗ Salad dressings – except lemon juice and balsamic vinegar
- ✗ Spreads (margarine, butter, mayonnaise, etc.)
- ✗ High-sodium foods

COOLER PLAN #2

WHAT IT'S FOR:

☑ Steady weight loss

☑ Maintenance once your goal weight is reached

WHAT IT IS:

This IS Eating Clean. Do this year round for steady, healthy weight loss. But this plan can also be used for maintenance. Here's why: when your body begins approaching its set point (its genetically predetermined healthy weight) you will find weight loss will slow or stop.

The occasional treat (glass of wine, piece of chocolate, etc.) is permitted in limited amounts. Unhealthy sugars and fats are not recommended.

HOW IT WORKS:

Follow the Eat-Clean Principles on page 21.
(for a menu-plan example, see page 270)

COMPLEX CARBOHYDRATES FROM FRUIT AND VEGETABLES:

6 portions each day. A portion is:

* 1 cupped handful or piece of fruit, such as berries, grapefruit, melon, apples and mangoes
* 2 cupped handfuls of vegetables including broth-based/vegetable purée soups

COMPLEX CARBOHYDRATES FROM WHOLE GRAINS AND STARCHY CARBOHYDRATES:

2-4 portions each day. A portion is:

* 1 scant handful of high-protein, sugar-free cold cereals, such as Clean muesli or granola
* 1 handful of cooked cereal (see Cooler 1 for examples)
* 1 piece of whole-grain bread or wrap (seven-inch)
* 1 handful-sized serving of sweet potato, yam, banana, corn, carrots or squash

LEAN PROTEIN:

6 portions each day. A portion is:

* 1 cup / 1 handful of dairy products (low-fat soy, almond, hemp, rice or skim milk, cottage cheese, kefir, yogurt cheese or plain, fat-free, sugar-free yogurt)
* 1 scant handful of raw, unsalted nuts (also a healthy fat)
* 2 tablespoons of all-natural nut butters (also a healthy fat)
* 1 palm-sized portion of lean meats
* Good-quality, sugar- and chemical-free protein powder (hemp, soy or whey)
* For vegetarian options please see page 280

BEVERAGES:

* 2-3 liters per day of fresh water with no sodium
* Clear herbal tea (unsweetened)
* Black coffee (in moderation)
* Green / black tea

SWEETENERS: USE THESE IN MODERATION. AVOID ARTIFICIAL SWEETENERS.

✗ Agave nectar

✗ Maple sugar flakes

✗ Sucanat

✗ Rapadura sugar

COOLER PLAN #3

WHAT IT'S FOR:

☑ Getting used to the Eat-Clean lifestyle

WHAT IT IS:

This is Cooler #2 with more leniencies. If you are thinking about making changes to your current style of eating, you may be wondering where to begin. Make some of these changes to your current food habits to introduce your body to Eating Clean.

For many of you, especially newcomers, Eating Clean will be a departure from any diet or way of eating you have previously attempted. You will need to make some changes right away so you can begin to understand and experience the way Eating Clean can positively affect your health and body.

These are gentle changes, but still powerful enough to see some results. What may be the biggest surprise is how good natural foods will taste once you begin to toss out the junk.

HOW IT WORKS:

Follow the Eat-Clean Principles on page 21.

EAT:

- Oatmeal cooked with milk and sweetened with unsweetened applesauce or other fruits
- High-protein, sugar-free cereals
- Homemade soups and stews
- Plenty of fresh fruits and vegetables
- Leaner cuts of meats (grilled, broiled or baked) with no obvious fat
- Beverages: clear, herbal teas, green/black tea, black coffee, water or fruit juice cut with water

AVOID:

- ✗ Unhealthy fats, especially butter, margarine, lard, cream, ice cream, fatty dressings, sauces and meats
- ✗ Whole eggs (one may be eaten each day with egg whites)
- ✗ White table sugar
- ✗ Refined and processed foods
- ✗ Junk and fast foods
- ✗ Fried foods
- ✗ Excessive salt and sodium
- ✗ Excessive alcohol

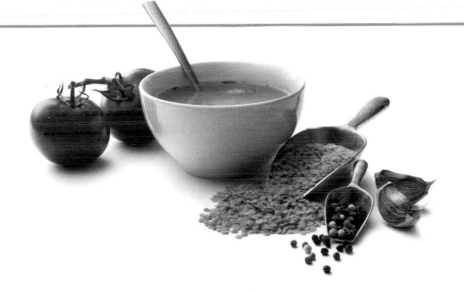

COOLER 1 MEAL PLAN

	BREAKFAST BOOSTER	MIDMORNING MUNCH	LUNCHTIME REFUEL
DAY 1	Oatmeal topped with flaxseed and bee pollen; scrambled egg whites; distilled water or herbal tea.	Grilled chicken breast; steamed green beans; distilled water.	½ sweet potato; romaine lettuce topped with grilled chicken breast, sprouts and squirt of lemon juice; distilled water.
DAY 2	Millet topped with flaxseed and bee pollen; scrambled egg whites; distilled water or herbal tea.	½ apple; water-packed canned tuna; distilled water.	½ sweet potato; spinach topped with grilled chicken breast, radishes, cucumbers and dash balsamic vinegar; distilled water.
DAY 3	Oatmeal topped with flaxseed and bee pollen; scrambled egg whites; distilled water or herbal tea.	1 pear; roasted turkey; distilled water.	Grilled chicken breast with ½ sweet potato; green beans; distilled water.
DAY 4	Cream of Wheat cereal topped with bee pollen and flaxseed; hardboiled egg whites; distilled water or herbal tea.	½ pear; protein shake made with water and 1 scoop protein powder; distilled water.	Bison tenderloin with ½ sweet potato; broccoli; distilled water.
DAY 5	Millet topped with flaxseed and bee pollen; scrambled egg whites; distilled water or herbal tea.	½ apple; water-packed canned tuna; distilled water.	Baked tilapia with ½ sweet potato; bok choy and steamed tomatoes; distilled water.
DAY 6	Quinoa topped with flaxseed and bee pollen; hardboiled egg whites; distilled water or herbal tea.	Grilled chicken breast; celery sticks; distilled water.	Spinach topped with water-packed canned tuna, sprouts; squeeze of lemon juice; distilled water.
DAY 7	Cream of Wheat cereal topped with bee pollen and flaxseed; hardboiled egg whites; distilled water or herbal tea.	½ apple; protein shake made with water and 1 scoop protein powder; distilled water.	Grilled tuna loin; ½ sweet potato; raw, sliced radishes; distilled water.

MID-AFTERNOON PICK-ME-UP

Protein shake made with water and 1 scoop protein powder; 1 pear; distilled water.

Water-packed canned tuna; cherry tomatoes; distilled water.

Roasted turkey breast; raw, sliced radishes; distilled water.

Grilled chicken breast; sliced cucumber, raw, sliced radishes; ½ pear, distilled water.

Water-packed canned tuna; celery sticks; distilled water. ½ apple.

1 pear; protein shake made with water and 1 scoop protein powder; distilled water.

Hardboiled egg whites; sliced tomatoes; ½ pear, distilled water.

DINNERTIME DELIGHT

Baked cod; ½ sweet potato; steamed bok choy; distilled water.

Roasted turkey breast; ½ sweet potato; steamed asparagus; distilled water.

Grilled bison tenderloin; ½ sweet potato; steamed, sliced zucchini; distilled water.

Baked tilapia; steamed spinach; steamed broccoli; ½ sweet potato; distilled water.

Roasted elk; ½ sweet potato; steamed asparagus; steamed green beans; distilled water.

Baked chicken breast; ½ sweet potato; steamed broccoli; distilled water.

Grilled chicken; ½ sweet potato; steamed, sliced zucchini; steamed asparagus; distilled water.

GROCERY LIST

WHOLE GRAINS
- ❏ Cream of Wheat
- ❏ Millet
- ❏ Oats

PRODUCE
- ❏ Apples
- ❏ Asparagus
- ❏ Bok choy
- ❏ Broccoli
- ❏ Celery
- ❏ Cherry tomatoes
- ❏ Cucumbers
- ❏ Green beans
- ❏ Kale
- ❏ Lemons
- ❏ Pears
- ❏ Radishes
- ❏ Romaine lettuce
- ❏ Spinach
- ❏ Sprouts
- ❏ Sweet potatoes
- ❏ Tomatoes
- ❏ Zucchini

PROTEINS
- ❏ Bison
- ❏ Chicken
- ❏ Cod
- ❏ Eggs
- ❏ Elk
- ❏ Protein powder
- ❏ Quinoa
- ❏ Tilapia
- ❏ Tuna loin
- ❏ Water-packed, canned tuna

MISC.
- ❏ Balsamic vinegar
- ❏ Herbal tea

FAMILY MEAL PLAN

	BREAKFAST BOOSTER	MIDMORNING MUNCH	LUNCHTIME REFUEL
DAY 1	Picante Frittata (pg 289); 1 slice whole-grain toast; water; black coffee or herbal tea.	1 cup vegetable crudités with lowfat hummus; hardboiled egg whites; water.	Water-packed canned tuna mixed with yogurt cheese on a whole-grain wrap with sprouts, shredded carrots and sliced apple; water.
DAY 2	Cookie cutter shaped whole-grain pancakes with unsweetened applesauce; scrambled egg whites; water; black coffee or herbal tea.	Lentil Spread (pg 306); cherry tomatoes and sliced cucumber; water.	Leftover Asian Noodle Bowls; 1 orange; water.
DAY 3	Whole-grain English muffin with almond butter, topped with sliced banana and flaxseed; water; black coffee or herbal tea	Nonfat plain yogurt; 1 banana; water.	Leftover Sloppy Joes; 1 banana; water.
DAY 4	Cream of Wheat cereal with 1 scoop protein powder, topped with sliced peaches, blueberries, flaxseed and bee pollen; water; black coffee or herbal tea.	1 Clean protein bar; 1 pear; water.	Salmon Salad (made with leftover salmon) on a whole-grain pita with celery, radishes and salad greens; a handful of grapes; water.
DAY 5	Ultimate Smoothie (pg 293); water; black coffee or herbal tea.	Hummus; cherry tomatoes, sliced cucumbers and radishes; water.	Leftover roast turkey dinner; water.
DAY 6	Granola with nonfat, plain yogurt, flaxseed, bee pollen and sliced strawberries; water; black coffee or herbal tea.	Nonfat cottage cheese with berries and flaxseed; water.	Leftover chicken bites; vegetable crudités with yogurt cheese; water.
DAY 7	Oatmeal with chopped apples, cinnamon, flaxseed and wheatgerm; scrambled egg whites; water; black coffee or herbal tea.	Smoothie: ice, 1 scoop protein powder, 1 banana, strawberries, nonfat milk (or other non-dairy beverage); water.	Whole-grain pita stuffed with leftover bison tenderloin, mixed greens and balsamic vinaigrette; water.

MID-AFTERNOON PICK-ME-UP	DINNERTIME DELIGHT	BEFORE BED (IF HUNGRY)
Protein shake with 1/4 cup oatmeal, 1 Tbsp flaxseed, 1 banana and 1 cup soymilk; water.	Asian Noodle Bowls (pg 374); water.	1 apple; 1 handful unsalted almonds; water; herbal tea.
Nonfat cottage cheese with cubed melon; water.	Sloppy Joes made with lean, ground turkey breast on multi-grain buns; steamed vegetables; water.	Nonfat plain yogurt topped with 1 sliced banana; water; herbal tea.
Hummus; carrot and celery sticks; water.	Grilled salmon; brown rice; steamed asparagus; water.	1 Honey Almond Cookie (pg 390); 1 cup nonfat milk (or other non-dairy beverage); water.
Apple slices dipped in nonfat plain yogurt with a dash of vanilla; water.	Roasted turkey breast with roasted beets, roasted sweet potatoes, roasted carrots and roasted fennel; water.	1 Chocolate Coated Frozen Banana (pg 394); water; herbal tea.
1/2 cup nonfat plain yogurt, 1/2 cup chopped apple, 1/2 cup muesli; water.	Chicken bites; oven fries; mixed vegetables; water.	Unbuttered air-popped popcorn, sprinkled with olive oil, paprika and toasted walnuts; water.
1 whole-grain wrap with 1 hardboiled egg white mashed with hummus, grated carrot, tomato and cucumber; water.	Bison tenderloin; mashed sweet potatoes; steamed kale; water.	Sliced apple with nut butter (of your choice), water, herbal tea.
Nonfat plain yogurt with blackberries and 1/2 cup Clean granola; water.	Whole-grain pasta with meat sauce made with lean, ground turkey, spinach and garlic; water.	Power Balls (pg 385); water; herbal tea.

*For some great family-friendly recipes, see the *Eat-Clean Diet for Family and Kids*

GLUTEN-FREE MEAL PLAN

	BREAKFAST BOOSTER	MIDMORNING MUNCH	LUNCHTIME REFUEL
DAY 1	Picante Frittata (page 289); 1 slice whole-grain GF toast or rice cake; water; black coffee or herbal tea.	1 sliced apple, topped with all-natural peanut butter; water.	Gazpacho (pg 329); grilled chicken breast; water.
DAY 2	Oatmeal* topped with unsalted walnuts, unsweetened applesauce, cinnamon, bee pollen, and flaxseed; scrambled egg whites; water; black coffee or herbal tea.	Ultimate Smoothie (pg 293); water.	Water-packed canned tuna over spinach leaves with diced radishes, carrots and a squeeze of fresh lemon juice; water.
DAY 3	Brown rice cake topped with almond butter, sliced banana and flaxseed; water; black coffee or herbal tea.	Trail mix; 1 pear; water.	Mango Salsa (pg 309); grilled tofu; water.
DAY 4	Egg white omelet with red bell peppers, tomato, fresh cilantro, and mushrooms; water; black coffee or herbal tea.	2 celery stalks, topped with all-natural peanut butter and raisins; water.	Grilled tilapia; roasted sweet potatoes steamed spinach; water.
DAY 5	Sweet Potato Oat Bars (pg 290)*; hardboiled egg whites; 1 plum; water; black coffee or herbal tea.	Nonfat cottage cheese; mango; water.	Mixed greens topped with grilled chicken, chickpeas, cucumbers, corn, cherry tomatoes and slivered almonds; water.
DAY 6	Ultimate Smoothie (page 293); water; black coffee or herbal tea.	Hummus; cherry tomatoes; sliced carrots and cucumbers; water.	Leftover bison with spinach leaves, sliced tomato and avocado on brown rice wrap; water.
DAY 7	Hot rice milk overtop hot rice cereal, pumpkin seeds, raisins, chopped almonds and walnuts, flaxseed, cinnamon and nutmeg; water; black coffee or herbal tea.	Nonfat cottage cheese; blueberries; water.	Salmon Miso Soup (pg 333); mixed greens with squeeze of fresh lemon juice; water.

MIDAFTERNOON PICK-ME-UP	DINNERTIME DELIGHT	BEFORE BED (IF HUNGRY)
Trail mix; 1 pear; water.	Grilled salmon; steamed bok choy; steamed asparagus; brown rice; water.	Scrambled egg whites; sliced tomatoes; water or herbal tea.
Mediterranean Olive Spread (pg 302); rice crackers; sliced green bell pepper; water.	Chicken Explosion (pg 381); water.	Blackberries, raspberries and kefir mixed with GF protein powder; water or herbal tea.
1 sliced apple topped with all-natural peanut butter; water.	Red Snapper with Vegetables (pg 370); water	Lemongrass Gingermint Tea Infusion (pg 389); nonfat plain yogurt; 1 handful unsalted almonds; water.
Unsweetened applesauce with flaxseed and 1 scoop GF protein powder; water.	Chicken stir-fried with onions, carrots and bok choy; brown rice; water.	Nonfat cottage cheese with orange segments; water or herbal tea.
Hummus; cherry tomatoes; sliced carrots and cucumbers; water.	Bison tenderloin; lentils; roasted carrots, beets and fennel; water.	Unbuttered air-popped popcorn; 1 handful unsalted pecans; water or herbal tea.
2 celery stalks, topped with all-natural peanut butter and raisins; water.	Thai Steak on pure buckwheat Soba Noodles (pg 373); water.	Nonfat plain yogurt mixed with ground almonds and raspberries; water.
1 banana spread with natural peanut butter; water.	Roasted turkey breast; Brazilian Style Pumpkin (pg 365); steamed broccoli and kale; water.	Power Balls (pg 385)*; water or herbal tea.

*Use uncontaminated oats

VEGAN MEAL PLAN

	BREAKFAST BOOSTER	MIDMORNING MUNCH	LUNCHTIME REFUEL
DAY 1	Black beans, mushrooms, green onions, avocado and tomatoes on a brown rice wrap; water; black coffee or herbal tea.	Trail mix; 1 orange; water.	Brown Rice and Lentil Salad (pg 321); water.
DAY 2	Ezekiel bread topped with almond butter, sliced apples and flaxseed; water; black coffee or herbal tea.	½ banana sliced on a brown rice cake spread with almond butter; water.	Mixed greens topped with chickpeas, black beans, tomatoes, celery, carrots, corn, slivered almonds and cucumbers; squeeze of lemon juice; water.
DAY 3	Quinoa; sliced strawberries; almond milk; water; black coffee or herbal tea.	Peanut butter with sliced banana on a brown rice wrap; water.	Black beans with brown rice, chopped red and yellow bell peppers, chopped green onions, fresh cilantro, dash of avocado oil and fresh lemon juice; water.
DAY 4	Smoothie: 1 scoop hemp or soy protein powder, almond milk, ice, mango, blueberries, kiwi and flaxseed; water; black coffee or herbal tea.	Lentil Bread Spread (pg 306); carrot and celery sticks; water.	Meal in a Bowl Soup (pg 330); water.
DAY 5	Oatmeal topped with applesauce, cinnamon, walnuts, flaxseed, and wheat germ; water; black coffee or herbal tea.	Soy yogurt; unsalted pecans; dried apricots; water.	Leftover dinner from Day 4; water.
DAY 6	Toasted Ezekiel bread topped with black beans and salsa; water; black coffee or herbal tea.	Bruschetta with Tomato and Avocado (pg 301)	Brown rice wrap filled with quinoa, black beans, avocado, spinach and salsa; water.
DAY 7	Scrambled Tofu with Spinach and Tomato (pg 297); water; black coffee or herbal tea.	1 pear; 1 handful unsalted almonds; water.	Sesame Noodles (pg 357); grilled tofu; steamed bok choy; water.

MIDAFTERNOON PICK-ME-UP	DINNERTIME DELIGHT	BEFORE BED (IF HUNGRY)
1 pear; 1 handful unsalted almonds; water.	Citrus Barbeque Tofu with Zesty BBQ Sauce (pg 339); steamed asparagus; ½ sweet potato; water.	Unbuttered air-popped popcorn; 1 handful of unsalted cashews; water or herbal tea.
Lentil Spread (pg 306); cherry tomatoes; yellow bell pepper slices; water.	Brown rice; steamed swiss chard; roasted beets; steamed edamame; water.	1 apple spread with almond butter; water or herbal tea.
Soy yogurt; 1 handful unsalted pecans; dried apricots; water.	Whole-wheat couscous with toasted pine nuts; grilled tempeh; steamed asparagus; water.	1 apple spread with almond butter; water or herbal tea.
1 celery stick topped with all-natural peanut butter and raisins; water.	Cooked lentils; cooked bulgur; ½ sweet potato; steamed broccoli and cauliflower; water.	Sliced strawberries; 1 handful unsalted pecans; water.
½ banana sliced on a brown rice cake spread with almond butter; water.	Quinoa; sautéed firm tofu; roasted Brussels sprouts; water.	Chocolate-Coated Frozen Bananas (pg 394); water or herbal tea.
Trail mix; ½ grapefruit; water.	Paradise Island Bean Burgers (pg 343); corn on the cob; water.	Smoothie: 1 scoop hemp or soy protein powder, ice, kiwi, strawberries and almond milk; water.
1 scoop hemp or soy protein powder mixed into unsweetened applesauce; water.	Mexican Pinto Beans and Brown Rice (pg 354), water.	1 apple spread with almond butter; water or herbal tea.

⬇ GROCERY LIST FOR FAMILY

WHOLE GRAINS

- ❑ Brown rice
- ❑ Brown rice cakes
- ❑ Cream of Wheat
- ❑ Granola
- ❑ Muesli
- ❑ Oats
- ❑ Popcorn kernels
- ❑ Soba noodles
- ❑ Whole-grain buns
- ❑ Whole-grain English muffin
- ❑ Whole-grain pasta
- ❑ Whole-grain wrap

PRODUCE

- ❑ Apples
- ❑ Arugula
- ❑ Bananas
- ❑ Beets
- ❑ Berries (blackberries, blueberries, strawberries)
- ❑ Broccoli
- ❑ Carrots
- ❑ Celery
- ❑ Cherry tomatoes
- ❑ Cipollito onion
- ❑ Cucumber
- ❑ Fennel
- ❑ Fresh basil
- ❑ Fresh chives
- ❑ Fresh ginger
- ❑ Garlic
- ❑ Grapes
- ❑ Grape tomatoes
- ❑ Green onions
- ❑ Kale
- ❑ Kiwi
- ❑ Leeks
- ❑ Lemons
- ❑ Melon
- ❑ Onion
- ❑ Oranges
- ❑ Peaches
- ❑ Pears
- ❑ Peas
- ❑ Radishes
- ❑ Red and yellow beets
- ❑ Red bell pepper
- ❑ Romaine lettuce
- ❑ Spinach
- ❑ Sprouts
- ❑ Sweet potatoes
- ❑ Tomatoes
- ❑ Zucchini

DAIRY

- ❑ Nonfat cottage cheese
- ❑ Nonfat milk
- ❑ Nonfat, plain yogurt
- ❑ Soy milk

PROTEINS

- ❑ Bison tenderloin
- ❑ Chicken breast
- ❑ Eggs
- ❑ Lean, ground turkey breast
- ❑ Turkey breast

MISCELLANEOUS

- ❑ Agave nectar
- ❑ All purpose flour, unbleached
- ❑ Almond butter
- ❑ Almonds, unsalted
- ❑ Avocado oil
- ❑ Balsamic vinegar
- ❑ Bee pollen
- ❑ Black pepper
- ❑ Cashews, unsalted
- ❑ Clean protein bars
- ❑ Coconut butter
- ❑ Coffee
- ❑ Dark chocolate
- ❑ Dijon mustard
- ❑ Dried apricots
- ❑ Dried mint
- ❑ Dried oregano
- ❑ Fig vinegar
- ❑ Flaxseed
- ❑ Green tea
- ❑ Ground cumin
- ❑ Ground Cinnamon
- ❑ Herbal tea
- ❑ Honey, liquid organic
- ❑ Hummus
- ❑ Low-sodium chicken broth
- ❑ Low-sodium soy sauce
- ❑ Olive oil
- ❑ Paprika
- ❑ Pecans
- ❑ Pitted dates
- ❑ Protein powder
- ❑ Pumpkin seeds
- ❑ Pumpkinseed oil
- ❑ Puy lentils
- ❑ Rice wine vinegar
- ❑ Salsa
- ❑ Sea salt
- ❑ Sesame seeds
- ❑ Sunflower seeds
- ❑ Toasted sesame oil
- ❑ Tomato paste
- ❑ Trail mix
- ❑ Unsweetened applesauce
- ❑ Unsweetened, dried cranberries
- ❑ Vanilla extract
- ❑ Walnuts
- ❑ Wheat germ
- ❑ Whole-wheat pastry flour, unbleached
- ❑ White pepper

GROCERY LIST FOR GLUTEN-FREE

WHOLE GRAINS

- ❏ Brown rice
- ❏ Brown rice cakes
- ❏ Brown rice wraps
- ❏ Buckwheat soba noodles
- ❏ Multi-grain, gluten-free flour
- ❏ Popcorn kernels
- ❏ Rice crackers
- ❏ Uncontaminated oats

PRODUCE

- ❏ Apples
- ❏ Asparagus
- ❏ Avocado
- ❏ Bananas
- ❏ Beets
- ❏ Berries (blackberries, blueberries, raspberries, strawberries)
- ❏ Bok choy
- ❏ Broccoli
- ❏ Carrots
- ❏ Celery
- ❏ Cherry tomatoes
- ❏ Corn
- ❏ Cucumbers
- ❏ Fennel
- ❏ Fresh basil
- ❏ Fresh cilantro
- ❏ Fresh ginger
- ❏ Garlic
- ❏ Green bell pepper
- ❏ Kale
- ❏ Kiwi
- ❏ Lemons
- ❏ Limes
- ❏ Mangos
- ❏ Mixed greens
- ❏ Mushrooms
- ❏ Onions (green, purple, red, spring)
- ❏ Pears
- ❏ Plums
- ❏ Pumpkin
- ❏ Radishes
- ❏ Red bell peppers
- ❏ Red cabbage
- ❏ Romaine lettuce
- ❏ Salad greens
- ❏ Scallions
- ❏ Spinach
- ❏ Sprouts
- ❏ Sweet potatoes
- ❏ Tomatoes
- ❏ Turnip
- ❏ Yukon gold potatoes
- ❏ Zucchini

DAIRY

- ❏ Feta cheese
- ❏ Kefir
- ❏ Nonfat cottage cheese
- ❏ Nonfat, plain yogurt
- ❏ Skim milk

PROTEINS

- ❏ Bison tenderloin
- ❏ Chicken breast
- ❏ Chickpeas
- ❏ Edamame
- ❏ Eggs
- ❏ Flank steak
- ❏ Lentils
- ❏ Salmon
- ❏ Tilapia
- ❏ Turkey breast
- ❏ Water-packed canned tuna

MISC.

- ❏ Agave nectar
- ❏ All-natural peanut butter
- ❏ Apple juice
- ❏ Applesauce
- ❏ Avocado oil
- ❏ Baking powder
- ❏ Baking soda
- ❏ Bay leaves
- ❏ Bee pollen
- ❏ Black pepper
- ❏ Celery seed
- ❏ GF chicken stock
- ❏ Chili oil
- ❏ Cinnamon
- ❏ Coconut butter
- ❏ Coffee
- ❏ Dark chocolate
- ❏ Dried currants
- ❏ Dried lemongrass
- ❏ Dried onion
- ❏ Dried mint
- ❏ Flaxseed
- ❏ Fruit sugar
- ❏ Ground cardamom
- ❏ Herbal tea
- ❏ Honey
- ❏ Hummus
- ❏ Kalamata olives
- ❏ GF vegetable stock
- ❏ Maple syrup
- ❏ Miso
- ❏ Nutmeg
- ❏ Olive oil
- ❏ Onion powder
- ❏ Paprika
- ❏ GF protein powder
- ❏ Pumpkin pie spice
- ❏ Pumpkin seeds
- ❏ Raisins
- ❏ Rice milk
- ❏ Rice wine vinegar
- ❏ Sea salt
- ❏ Sesame oil
- ❏ Sesame seeds
- ❏ Slivered almonds
- ❏ Soy milk, plain
- ❏ Sundried tomatoes
- ❏ Tabasco sauce
- ❏ Trail mix
- ❏ Unsalted almonds
- ❏ Unsalted pecans
- ❏ Unsalted walnuts
- ❏ Vanilla extract

GROCERY LIST FOR VEGAN

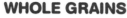

WHOLE GRAINS
- ❏ Brown rice
- ❏ Brown rice wrap
- ❏ Bulgur
- ❏ Couscous
- ❏ Ezekiel bread
- ❏ Ezekiel buns
- ❏ Oats
- ❏ Popcorn kernels
- ❏ Quinoa
- ❏ Sesame noodles
- ❏ Wheat germ
- ❏ Whole-grain bread

PRODUCE
- ❏ Apples
- ❏ Applesauce
- ❏ Avocado
- ❏ Asparagus
- ❏ Bananas
- ❏ Beets
- ❏ Blueberries
- ❏ Bok choy
- ❏ Broccoli
- ❏ Brussels sprouts
- ❏ Cabbage
- ❏ Carrots
- ❏ Cauliflower
- ❏ Celery
- ❏ Cherry tomatoes
- ❏ Chipotle peppers
- ❏ Corn
- ❏ Corn on the cob
- ❏ Cucumbers
- ❏ Fresh arugula
- ❏ Fresh basil
- ❏ Fresh cilantro
- ❏ Fresh parsley
- ❏ Fresh thyme
- ❏ Garlic
- ❏ Grapefruit

- ❏ Grapes
- ❏ Green onions
- ❏ Kiwi
- ❏ Leeks
- ❏ Lemons
- ❏ Limes
- ❏ Mango
- ❏ Mixed greens
- ❏ Mushrooms
- ❏ Onions
- ❏ Oranges
- ❏ Parsnips
- ❏ Pears
- ❏ Plum tomatoes
- ❏ Pumpkin
- ❏ Red bell peppers
- ❏ Shallots
- ❏ Spinach
- ❏ Sweet potatoes
- ❏ Swiss chard
- ❏ Tomatoes
- ❏ Yellow bell peppers
- ❏ Yellow potatoes
- ❏ Zucchini

PROTEINS
- ❏ Black beans
- ❏ Chickpeas
- ❏ Edamame
- ❏ Kidney beans
- ❏ Lentils
- ❏ Pinto beans
- ❏ Protein powder (hemp or soy)
- ❏ Puy lentils
- ❏ Tempeh
- ❏ Tofu (firm)

MISCELLANEOUS
- ❏ Agave nectar
- ❏ All-natural peanut butter
- ❏ Almond butter

- ❏ Almond milk
- ❏ Apple cider vinegar
- ❏ Avocado oil
- ❏ Balsamic vinegar
- ❏ Black pepper
- ❏ Chili powder
- ❏ Cinnamon
- ❏ Coconut butter
- ❏ Coffee
- ❏ Dark chocolate
- ❏ Dijon mustard
- ❏ Dried apricots
- ❏ Dried basil
- ❏ Dried oregano
- ❏ Flaxseed
- ❏ Ground coriander
- ❏ Ground cumin
- ❏ Herbal tea
- ❏ Molasses
- ❏ Olive oil
- ❏ Pine nuts
- ❏ Raisins
- ❏ Red wine vinegar
- ❏ Salsa
- ❏ Sea salt
- ❏ Sesame seeds
- ❏ Slivered almonds
- ❏ Soy yogurt
- ❏ Tahini
- ❏ Tamari
- ❏ Toasted sesame oil
- ❏ Tomato paste
- ❏ Tomato sauce
- ❏ Trail mix
- ❏ Unsalted almonds
- ❏ Unsalted pecans
- ❏ Walnuts

GROCERY LIST FOR COOLER 2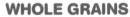

WHOLE GRAINS

- ❑ Bran
- ❑ Brown rice
- ❑ Brown rice cakes
- ❑ Couscous
- ❑ Ezekiel bread
- ❑ Ezekiel buns
- ❑ Granola
- ❑ Millet
- ❑ Multi-grain flour
- ❑ Oatmeal
- ❑ Popcorn kernels
- ❑ Wheat germ
- ❑ Whole-grain bread
- ❑ Whole-grain English muffins
- ❑ Whole-grain pasta
- ❑ Whole-grain wraps

PRODUCE

- ❑ Alfalfa sprouts
- ❑ Bananas
- ❑ Bay leaves
- ❑ Beets
- ❑ Blueberries
- ❑ Broccoli
- ❑ Brussels sprouts
- ❑ Carrots
- ❑ Celery
- ❑ Cilantro
- ❑ Corn
- ❑ Fresh basil
- ❑ Fresh chives
- ❑ Fresh rosemary
- ❑ Fresh thyme
- ❑ Garlic
- ❑ Grapes
- ❑ Green beans
- ❑ Green onions
- ❑ Heirloom tomatoes
- ❑ Kiwi
- ❑ Leeks

- ❑ Lemons
- ❑ Limes
- ❑ Mango
- ❑ Mixed greens
- ❑ Parsley
- ❑ Pears
- ❑ Peas
- ❑ Pineapple
- ❑ Purple onion
- ❑ Red bell pepper
- ❑ Shallots
- ❑ Spinach
- ❑ Sweet potatoes
- ❑ Tomatoes
- ❑ Watermelon
- ❑ Zucchini

DAIRY

- ❑ Bocconcini cheese
- ❑ Nonfat cottage cheese
- ❑ Nonfat milk
- ❑ Nonfat, plain yogurt
- ❑ Tzatziki

PROTEIN

- ❑ Bison tenderloin
- ❑ Black beans
- ❑ Chicken breast (boneless, skinless)
- ❑ Eggs
- ❑ Lamb chops (grass fed is best)
- ❑ Quinoa
- ❑ Rainbow trout
- ❑ Tofu
- ❑ Water-packed canned tuna

MISCELLANEOUS

- ❑ Agave nectar
- ❑ Almond butter
- ❑ Almonds, unsalted
- ❑ Apple cider
- ❑ Baking powder
- ❑ Baking soda

- ❑ Balsamic vinegar
- ❑ Bee pollen
- ❑ Black pepper
- ❑ Cashews, unsalted
- ❑ Cheesecloth
- ❑ Coconut butter
- ❑ Coffee
- ❑ Cumin
- ❑ Dijon mustard
- ❑ Dried mint
- ❑ Dried oregano
- ❑ Flaxseed
- ❑ Green tea
- ❑ Low-sodium chicken stock
- ❑ Low-sodium vegetable stock
- ❑ Olive oil
- ❑ Olives
- ❑ Protein powder
- ❑ Pumpkinseed oil
- ❑ Raisins
- ❑ Red pepper flakes
- ❑ Saffron
- ❑ Sea salt
- ❑ Unsweetened applesauce
- ❑ Unsweetened, dried cranberries
- ❑ Walnuts

SOLUTIONS FOR A BUSY LIFE

LIVING THE EAT-CLEAN LIFESTYLE DESPITE YOUR CALENDAR

Throughout human evolution, life has been primarily about gathering enough food to survive, and often that meant pursuing that food on foot. Our biology is largely unchanged, but life today is nothing like it was back then. The chore of finding food was a daily priority for our ancient ancestors, while we make little time for food — other than to grab it fast and gobble it down! Our hurry is often so great that we are blind to what we are actually eating. Eating is no longer a pleasure; it is just one more thing to mark off the "To-Do" list. We live among skyscrapers and jammed calendars in a jungle of our own making. And so we need answers not only to the perennial question: "What is there to eat?" but also the ubiquitous: "I only have five minutes, so I need something quick and easy!"

BREAKFAST – A PROBLEM OR A NECESSITY?

Despite the proven fact that breakfast is the most important meal of the day, many people struggle with squeezing it in. You already know how I feel about breakfast, so I won't allow you to skip it. The following are some creative ways to get this first meal into your stomach!

IT TAKES ONLY MINUTES TO:

- Mix 1/2 cup of low-fat kefir or plain yogurt with 1/2 cup of Clean granola and sliced berries. Top with ground flaxseed.
- Scramble one whole egg with four whites and place on toasted whole-grain bread.
- Throw 1/2 cup of low-fat kefir or plain yogurt into a blender with frozen fruit, skim milk, flaxseed and a dollop of natural nut butter. Make extra to take to work for another mini-meal.
- Spread a whole-grain wrap with natural nut butter, place a banana in the middle and sprinkle with flaxseed. Roll it up, cut it in half and eat it for breakfast or for a snack later.
- Place 1/2 cup of Ezekiel-grain cereal in a bowl. Cover with hot milk or water. Top with sliced fruit and flaxseed.
- Measure 1/2 cup of dry oatmeal into a bowl. Pour a cup of boiling water overtop and let stand, covered, for five minutes. Garnish with berries and a dollop of low-fat kefir or plain yogurt.
- Layer smoked salmon and sliced tomato on egg whites and place on top of a toasted whole-grain English muffin.
- Spread two slices of Ryvita with natural nut butter. Grab an apple or banana and you're done!

LUNCHTIME LUNACY

I consider lunch the perfect opportunity to make a green salad, dressed with loads of interesting toppings and drizzled with exotic oil. My current favorite is richly-colored, full-flavored pumpkinseed oil. I add some seeds to the mix to give it crunch then top it off with a tangy vinegar. Finally, I round out my meal with grilled fish or hardboiled egg whites.

If you get bored with lunch you will tend to give in to sugar and simple carbs. Boredom is a common reason for overeating or eating poorly. The following are just a few of literally millions of lunchtime ideas.

IT TAKES ONLY MINUTES TO:

- Spread hummus on Ryvita, then load anything else on top – sliced tomatoes, avocado, portobello mushrooms, pieces of grilled chicken, egg whites, turkey or fish.
- Slip portable packages of water-packed tuna into a cooler and add to a green salad.
- Fill your cooler with last night's leftovers (and save money!).
- Bring along dense, whole-grain breads, wraps, bagels and crackers, which make the perfect base for all kinds of fillings and toppings.
- Make a picnic-style lunch to take to work – pack cold chicken, hardboiled eggs, sliced cucumbers, cherry tomatoes, hummus, fruit and water.
- Take hardboiled eggs to work. Prepare several

in the morning and carry four to work along with a colorful salad. Eat one yolk and toss the rest! Use citrus juices and exotic oils for dressing rather than commercial products.

MORE LUNCH-IN-A-JIFFY IDEAS!

BAKED SWEET OR REGULAR POTATOES:

Baked sweet or regular potatoes are "vehicles" for carrying fillings, so consider them ideal lunch foods. Use a small baked sweet or russet potato as the base for any of the following fillings, or create your own.

- **Spicy Cancer-Fighting Lunch:** Halve a baked potato and scoop the flesh into a bowl. Add yogurt cheese, snipped chives, water-packed tuna or chopped cooked chicken. Sprinkle with curry powder, sea salt, black pepper and mix well. Stuff into potato skin
- **Beef and BBQ Lunch:** Cut leftover lean steak into small strips. Toss with a mixture of light soy sauce, tomato paste and Worcestershire sauce. Mix well and stuff into the hollowed out halves of a baked potato.
- **Smooth and Crunchy Lunch:** Place three tablespoons of hummus on top of a halved baked potato. Top with chopped red and green bell peppers, green onion and fresh cilantro.
- **Use-Up-the-Chili Lunch:** Spoon leftover chili on a split baked potato.

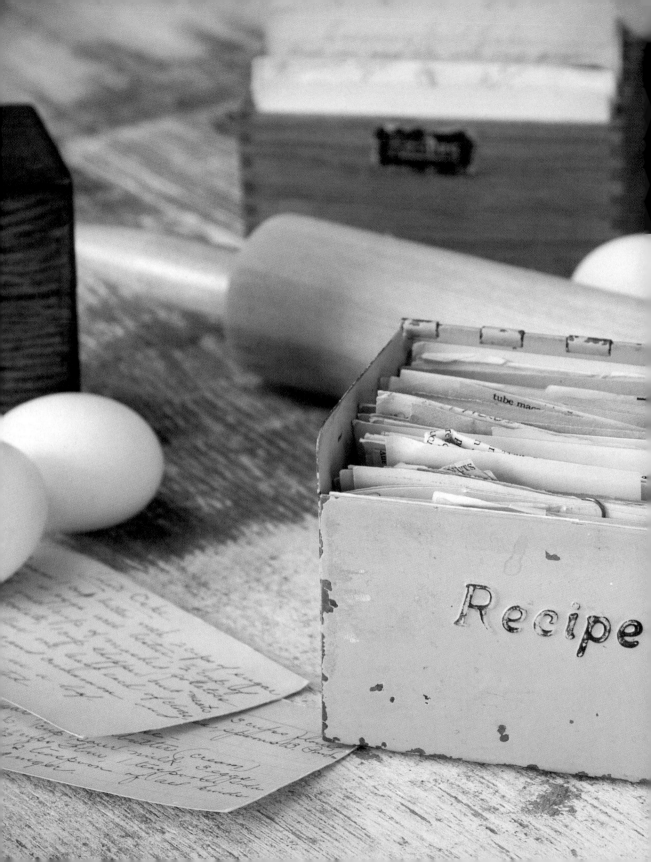

THE EAT-CLEAN DIET
RECHARGED

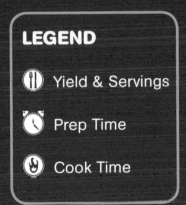

LEGEND

- Yield & Servings
- Prep Time
- Cook Time

RECIPES

15

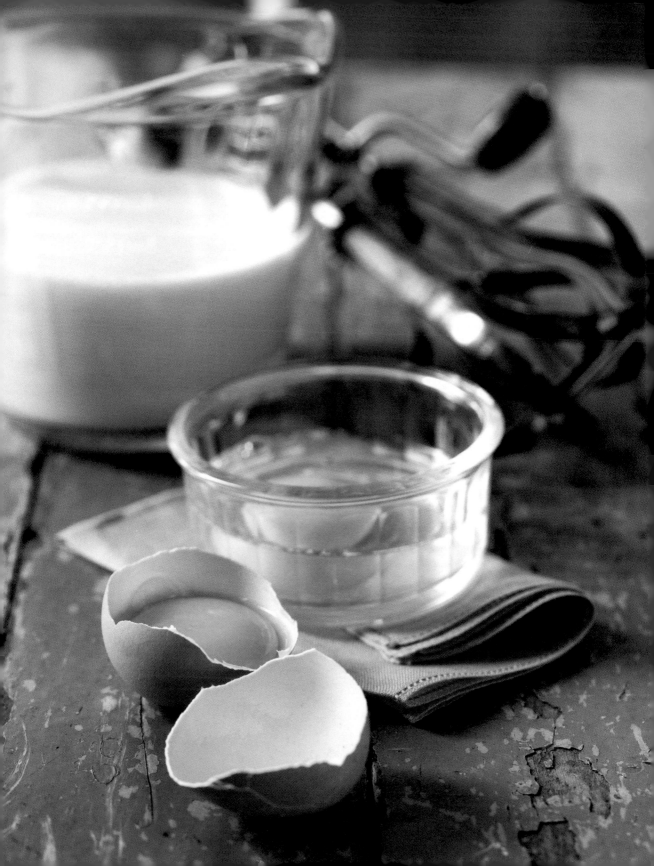

BREAKFAST

1

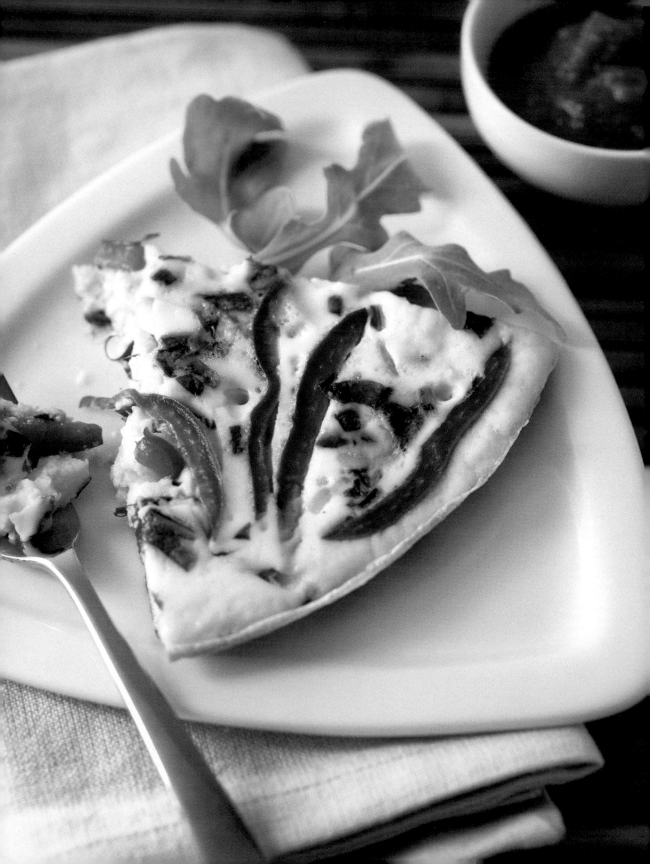

Picante Frittata

A frittata is an Italian omelet, which can be made simple or enriched with any ingredient from vegetables to meats, cheeses to spices or even pasta! (Your leftovers will never go to waste again!) Spice up your life with this peppery egg dish.

Ingredients

1 tsp / 5 ml extra virgin olive oil

1 Cipollino onion, peeled and minced

½ red bell pepper, seeded and deveined, cut into thin ribbons

1 cup / 240 ml baby spinach leaves, finely chopped

3 egg whites + 1 whole egg

¼ cup / 60 ml skim milk

¼ tsp / 1.25 ml sea salt

Pinch cumin

¼ tsp / 1.25 ml freshly ground black pepper

½ cup / 120 ml fresh salsa (homemade or commercial) as garnish (optional)

Method

1 Preheat oven to 350°F / 180°C. Make sure oven rack is in center of oven.

2 In a medium ovenproof skillet, heat olive oil over medium heat. Add vegetables to skillet and cook until soft, about five minutes.

3 While vegetables are cooking, combine eggs, milk, salt, cumin and pepper. Whisk well.

4 Pour egg mixture over cooking vegetables. Cook until edges are set and center is just beginning to set.

5 Transfer to heated oven and bake another five to eight minutes or until center is firm.

6 Transfer cooked frittata to heated plate and serve with salsa (optional).

Nutritional Value Per Serving:

Calories: 267 | Calories from Fat: 88 | Protein: 24g | Carbs: 24g | Total Fat: 10g | Saturated Fat: 2g | Trans Fat: 0g | Fiber: 5g | Sodium: 1459mg | Cholesterol: 211mg | Sugar: 14g

TIP Be sure to use an ovenproof skillet for the recipe, as it will end up in the oven. No plastic or wooden parts please!

Sweet Potato Oat Bars

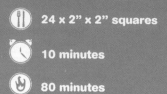

24 x 2" x 2" squares

10 minutes

80 minutes

The inspiration for this recipe came from a reader, Jeannie Sherin, who shared it with me wondering how it could be "Cleaned up." The original recipe had way too much sugar in it. Here it is in a slightly less sugar-overdosed form.

Ingredients

1 Tbsp / 15 ml olive oil

5 sweet potatoes, washed and trimmed of fibers (potatoes should be the same size)

4 cups / 960 ml oats (the 3 to 5 minute kind)

¾ cup / 180 ml skim milk soured with
    1 Tbsp / 15 ml lemon juice

¼ cup / 60 ml finely ground flaxseed

½ cup / 120 ml maple syrup (natural is best)

2 Tbsp / 30 ml pumpkin pie spice

2 Tbsp / 30 ml coconut butter

½ cup / 120 ml dried fruits (raisins, dates, cherries and/or blueberries), chopped

½ cup / 120 ml raw unsalted nuts (almonds, walnuts and/or pecans), chopped

Pinch sea salt

Method

1 Preheat oven to 350°F / 180°C. Prepare a 9" x 13" (1" deep) baking dish by coating lightly with olive oil.

2 Prick sweet potatoes all over. Place in oven and bake until tender. Remove from oven and let cool. When cool enough to handle, remove potato peels and place flesh in large mixing bowl. Leave oven on and set heat to 400°F / 200°C.

3 Add all remaining ingredients to sweet potato mixture. Mix well.

4 Press into prepared baking pan. Bake for 30 to 35 minutes or until golden on top.

5 Remove from heat and let cool. Cut into squares.

Nutritional Value Per Serving:
Calories: 189 | Calories from Fat: 43 | Protein: 6g | Carbs: 31g |
Total Fat: 5.5g | Saturated Fat: 1g | Trans Fat: 0g | Fiber: 4g |
Sodium: 20mg | Cholesterol: 0mg | Sugar: 8g

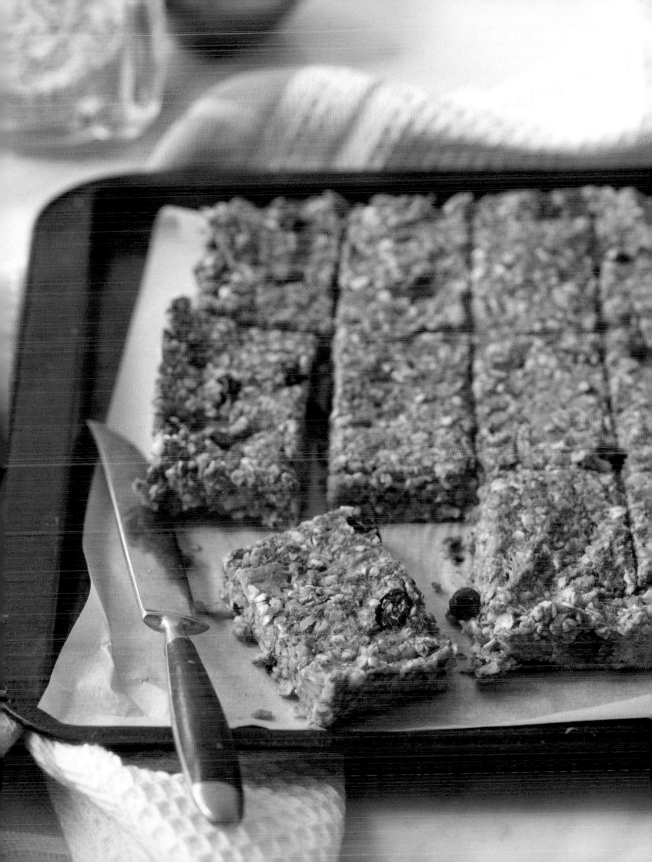

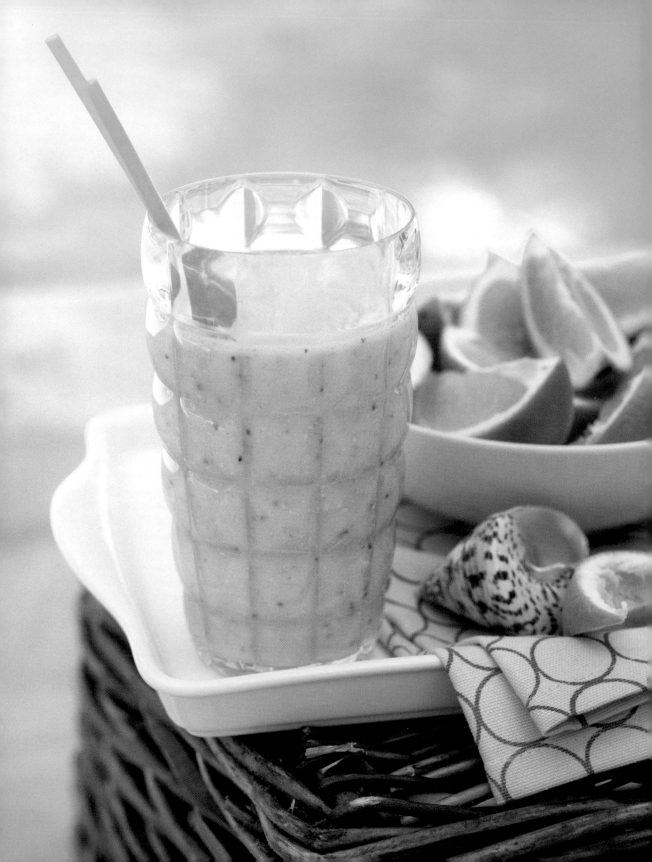

Ultimate Smoothie

There is something so refreshing about a cold smoothie on a hot summer morning. Cottage cheese gives this berrylicious beverage a protein punch – and makes it nice and thick. It's perfect for refueling after any workout!

Ingredients

1 cup / 240 ml ice cubes

1 cup / 240 ml skim, soy, rice or almond milk

¼ cup / 60 ml low-fat cottage cheese

½ cup / 120 ml fresh strawberries, sliced

1 kiwi, peeled and cut into chunks

½ cup / 120 ml green tea, chilled

Method

1 Toss all ingredients in blender and process until smooth.

Nutritional Value Per Serving:
Calories: 206 | Calories from Fat: 15 | Protein: 17g | Carbs: 33g |
Total Fat: 2g | Saturated Fat: 1g | Trans Fat: 0g | Fiber: 4g |
Sodium: 360mg | Cholesterol: 7mg | Sugar: 26g

Tam's Morning Constitutional Muffins

15 muffins

15 minutes

27 minutes

Start your morning on the path to regularity with these digestive delights. They work every time! I love them hot, right out of the oven for breakfast, but they also make an excellent addition to any midday meal.

Ingredients

½ cup / 120 ml multigrain flour
   (as natural as possible)

2 cups / 480 ml raw bran

1 cup / 240 ml ground flaxseed

1 cup / 240 ml raw wheat germ

4 tsp / 20 ml baking powder

2 tsp / 10 ml baking soda

8 egg whites

1 cup / 240 ml unsweetened applesauce

½ cup / 120 ml agave nectar

½ cup / 120 ml skim, butter, soy or almond milk

1½ cups / 360 ml water

1 cup / 240 ml raisins or pitted dates, chopped

Method

1 Preheat oven to 350°F / 180°C. Line muffin tin with unbleached paper liners or reusable silicon liners.

2 Combine all ingredients in large mixing bowl. Don't overmix or your muffins will be flat.

3 Bake for 25 to 30 minutes. Muffins are done when toothpick inserted in center comes out clean. Remove from heat and let cool. Serve or freeze individually.

Nutritional Value Per Serving:

Calories: 189 | Calories from Fat: 55 | Protein: 9g | Carbs: 31g |
Total Fat: 7g | Saturated Fat: 1g | Trans Fat: 0g | Fiber: 8g |
Sodium: 301mg | Cholesterol: 0mg | Sugar: 3.5g

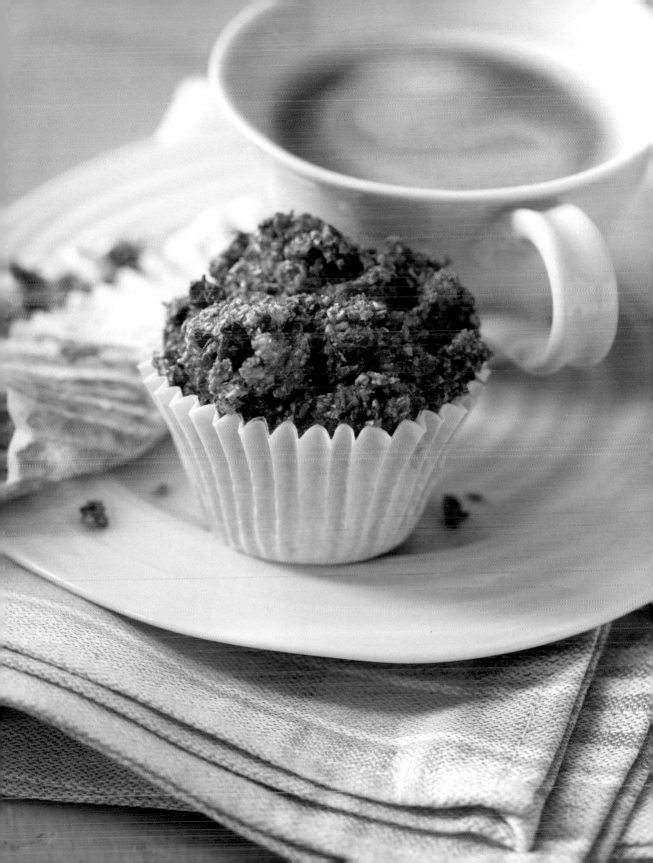

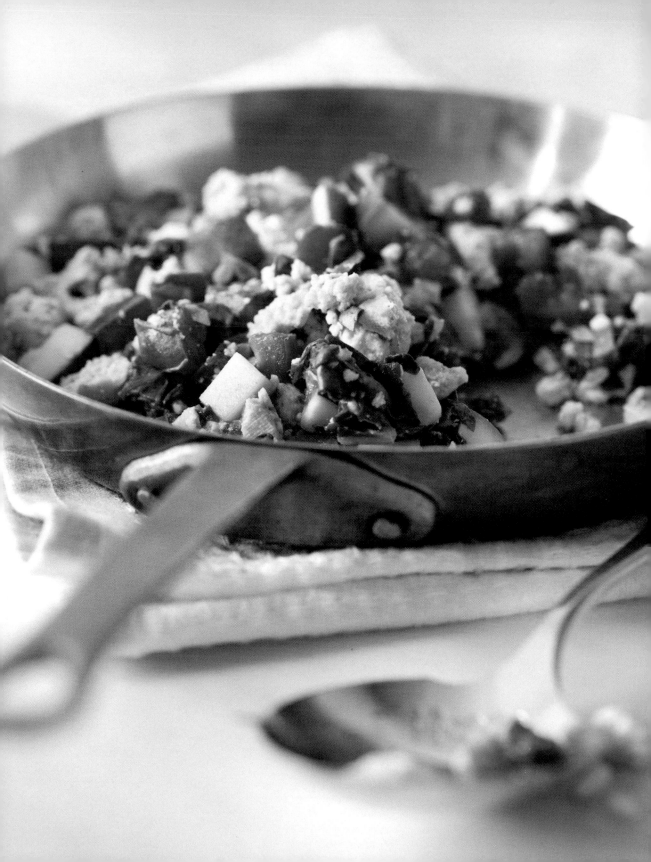

Scrambled Tofu with Spinach & Tomato

I don't mind eating a good scrambled egg dish but there are some of you who would like an alternative. Tofu springs to mind. It scrambles nicely and readily accepts any flavors you would like to add.

Ingredients

1 lb / 454 grams firm tofu, unflavored

3 Tbsp / 45 ml coconut butter, divided (if unavailable, use olive oil)

3 shallots, peeled and finely chopped

1 clove garlic, passed through a garlic press

1 small firm zucchini, finely chopped

4 plum tomatoes, chopped and set over a fine mesh sieve to drain

1 tsp / 5 ml ground cumin

4 cups / 960 ml spinach leaves, coarsely chopped

½ tsp / 2.5 ml sea salt

Freshly ground black pepper, to taste

Method

1 Press tofu (see recipe for Citrus Barbecued Tofu with Zesty BBQ Sauce on page 339 for pressing instructions).

2 Remove tofu from its press and break it up with your clean fingers. The pieces should look like scrambled eggs. Set aside.

3 In a medium skillet heat 1 Tbsp / 15 ml coconut butter. Add shallots and cook until fragrant.

4 Add garlic, zucchini and tomatoes. Cook until just soft. Remove from heat.

5 In another larger skillet, heat cumin gently over medium heat. Add remaining coconut butter and allow it to heat up a little.

6 Add crumbled tofu and cook through for several minutes. Add cooked vegetable mixture and chopped spinach. Heat through, stirring frequently.

7 Adjust flavor with salt and pepper. Serve hot.

Nutritional Value Per Serving:
Calories: 391 | Calories from Fat: 230 | Protein: 27g | Carbs: 19g |
Total Fat: 27g | Saturated Fat: 14g | Trans Fat: 0g | Fiber: 6g |
Sodium: 327mg | Cholesterol: 0mg | Sugar: 3g

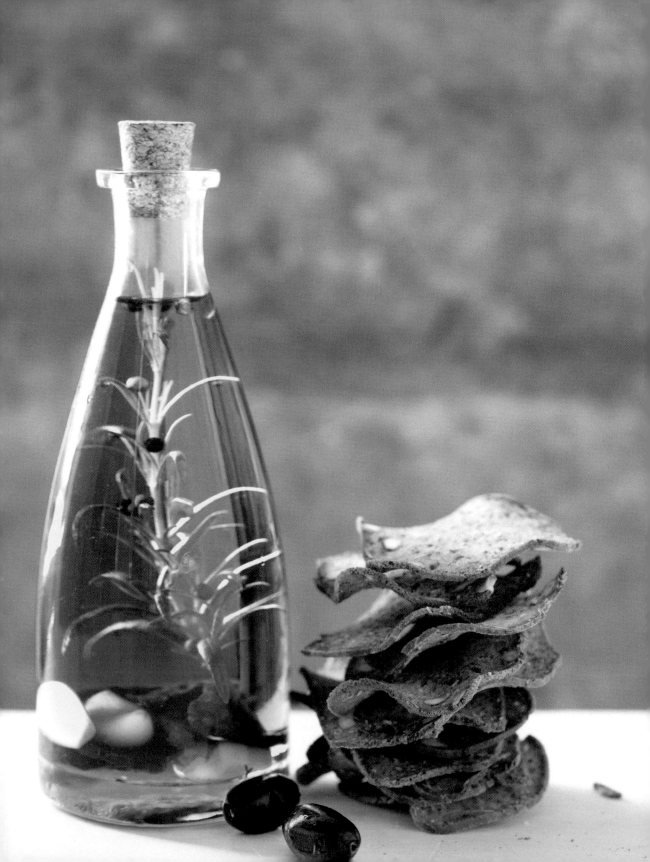

STARTERS

2

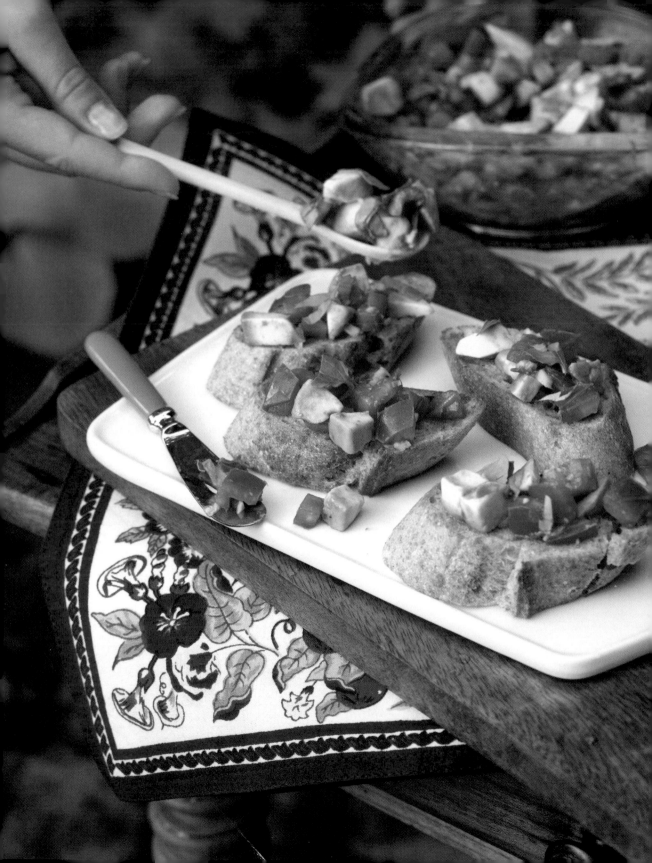

Bruschetta with Tomato & Avocado

12 slices

20 minutes

10 minutes

Commonly served as a snack or appetizer, bruschetta is an Italian-inspired dish dating back to at least the 15th century. The addition of avocado in this recipe bumps up the healthy-fat content and the taste factor. You can use the tomato mix in different ways – try it on whole-grain crisp breads, pita pizzas and more.

Ingredients

½ loaf whole-grain French, ciabatta or other thin loaf of bread

3 Tbsp / 45 ml extra virgin olive oil, divided

1 cup / 240 ml fresh chopped tomatoes

3 cloves garlic, passed through a garlic press

1 tsp / 5 ml sea salt

1 tsp / 5 ml freshly ground black pepper

1 handful fresh arugula leaves, finely chopped

1 handful fresh basil leaves, finely chopped

2 Tbsp / 30 ml best quality balsamic vinegar

2 fresh avocados

Juice of ½ fresh lemon

Method

1 Preheat oven to 375°F / 190°C. Line a baking sheet with parchment paper.

2 Slice bread into thin, ½-inch slices on the diagonal. Arrange slices on baking sheet. Don't overlap. Use another baking sheet if necessary.

3 Use a baking brush to lightly coat each piece of bread with olive oil. Bake for several minutes or until lightly toasted. Remove from oven. Set aside.

4 In a medium-sized oven-safe mixing bowl combine tomato, remaining olive oil, garlic, salt and pepper. Place in hot oven and bake for 10 minutes or until tomatoes are soft. Remove from heat.

5 Transfer cooked tomatoes to new mixing bowl. Add chopped arugula, basil and balsamic vinegar. Mix gently to combine. Set aside.

6 Peel avocados. Cut in half and remove pits. Dice avocado and toss with lemon juice.

7 Top each piece of bread with tomato mixture. Top with avocado. Serve.

Nutritional Value Per Slice with Topping:
Calories: 111 | Calories from Fat: 71 | Protein: 2g | Carbs: 9.5g |
Total Fat: 8g | Saturated Fat: 1g | Trans Fat: 0g | Fiber: 3.5g |
Sodium: 197mg | Cholesterol: 0mg | Sugar: 1g

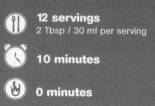

12 servings
2 Tbsp / 30 ml per serving

10 minutes

0 minutes

Mediterranean Olive Spread

This make-ahead spread is perfect for game day or any holiday at all! Use in place of butter for a taste that's rich, decadent and healthy. It's sure to become a favorite in your repertoire of recipes.

Ingredients

1½ cups / 360 ml Yogurt Cheese*

1 Tbsp / 15 ml Do-it-Yourself Onion Soup Mix (see below)

3 cloves garlic, peeled and passed through a garlic press

2 sundried tomatoes, finely chopped

12 pitted kalamata olives, finely chopped

¼ cup / 60 ml feta cheese, crumbled (purchase a good-quality cheese that isn't full of chemicals)

✳ See Yogurt Cheese recipe pg 334

Method

1 Combine all ingredients well in a medium-sized bowl. Spoon mixture into a Mason jar with a tight-fitting lid and store in the refrigerator.

Nutritional Value Per Serving:
Calories: 40 | Calories from Fat: 16 | Protein: 2g | Carbs: 3g | Total Fat: 2g | Saturated Fat: 1g | Trans Fat: 0g | Fiber: 0g | Sodium: 160mg | Cholesterol: 0mg | Sugar: 2g

8 servings
2 Tbsp / 30 ml per serving

5 minutes

0 minutes

Do-It-Yourself Onion Soup Mix

Ingredients

¾ cup / 180 ml dried onion flakes

¼ cup / 60 ml low-sodium chicken bouillon

¼ cup / 60 ml onion powder

¼ tsp / 1.25 ml sea salt

¼ tsp / 1.25 ml celery seed

Method

1 Mix all ingredients well and store in a small Mason jar with a tight-fitting lid.

2 To make soup if desired, add all ingredients to 6 cups / 1.5 L boiling water. Simmer for 10 minutes.

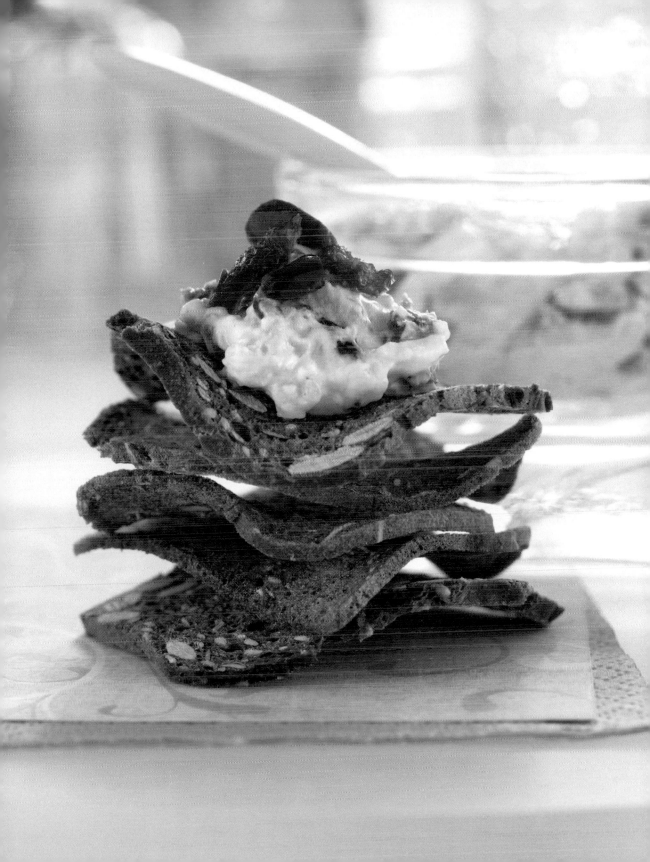

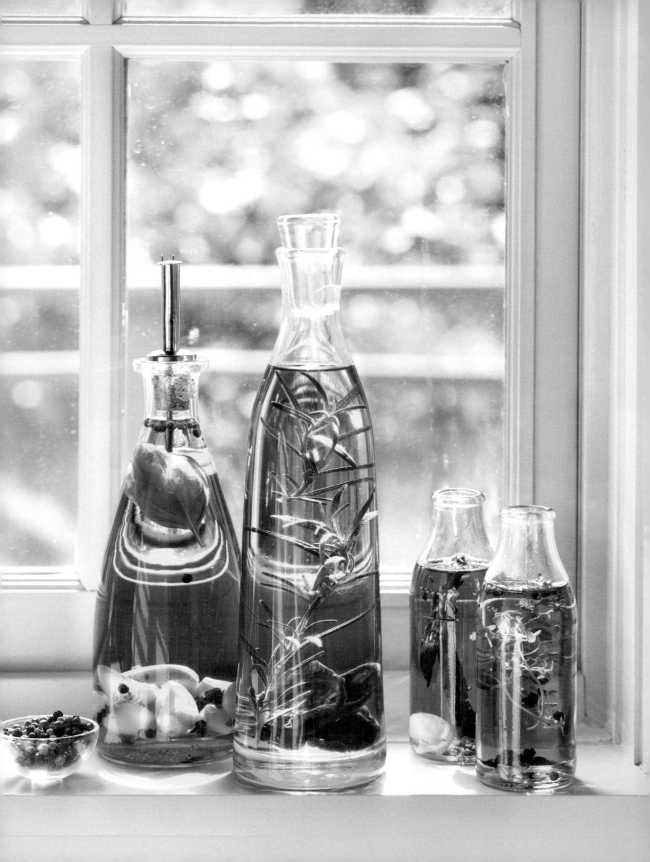

Spicy Herb & Garlic Infused Olive Oil

Olive oil is a delicious addition to so many recipes. I love cracking open a new bottle to sauté fresh veggies, drizzle on my salad, marinade meat, or use as a dip for hearty, crusty bread. Flavored olive oils make the meal that much better. This recipe teaches you how to prepare your own olive-oil creations at home. No more visits to the fancy culinary store required!

Note: This recipe takes one week to prepare.

Ingredients

1 x 32 oz / 1L bottle extra-virgin olive oil

1 bunch fresh herbs (basil, bay, chives, cilantro, dill, mint, oregano, parsley, rosemary, tarragon and/or thyme).

8 cloves garlic, peeled

4 long, dried chili peppers (optional for a spicy oil)

1 cup / 240 ml sundried tomatoes

Method

Day one:

1 Pour olive oil into a saucepan and heat over low heat. You want the oil to be warm.

2 Select a variety of fresh herbs to use for your infusion. You can use any combination you like. Trying out new flavors is half the fun. My favorite combination is rosemary and thyme. Wash and dry the herbs. Bruise them slightly to bring the flavors forward.

3 Stuff the herbs, garlic, chili peppers (if using) and sundried tomatoes into empty bottle. Use enough to fill the bottom quarter of the bottle.

4 Using a funnel, pour the warm oil into the bottle over your ingredients.

5 Store your olive oil in the refrigerator (since you are using perishable ingredients such as garlic).

Day Three:

1 Check on the flavor of the olive oil. Garlic can overpower the other ingredients. If it's just right you can remove the garlic cloves using a strainer. Be sure to put the other ingredients back in the bottle and store oil in the refrigerator.

Day Seven:

1 Strain the herbs, sundried tomatoes, chili peppers and garlic (if not previously removed) out of the olive oil. Store the oil creation in a cool, dark place.

2 If you choose to leave the ingredients in the oil you must keep it stored in the refrigerator. Use within a couple of months.

TIP Don't be concerned if the oil appears congealed. This happens because of the cool refrigerator temperatures. The oil will liquefy at room temperature.

Nutritional Value Per Serving:
Calories: 256 | Calories from Fat: 249 | Protein: 0g | Carbs: 2g | Total Fat: 28g | Saturated Fat: 4g | Trans Fat: 0g | Fiber: 0g | Sodium: 36mg | Cholesterol: 0mg | Sugar: 1g

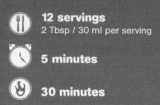

Lentil Spread

A hit at any party, this lentil spread makes butter obsolete! This protein-packed alternative tastes great on whole-grain breads, crackers, pitas and brown rice cakes. I like to use it as a dip for crudités.

Ingredients

2 Tbsp / 30 ml raw unsalted walnuts

1 cup / 240 ml Puy lentils, cooked

2 green onions, trimmed and coarsely chopped

2 cloves garlic

1 Tbsp / 15 ml grainy mustard

1-2 Tbsp / 15-30 ml avocado oil (or other
good-quality oil)

1 Tbsp / 15 ml low-sodium tamari or soy sauce

Sea salt to taste

Freshly ground black pepper

Method

1 Place all ingredients in food processor and process until smooth.

2 Adjust consistency by starting with 1 Tbsp / 15 ml oil and adding more if necessary.

3 Cover and refrigerate.

Nutritional Value Per Serving:
Calories: 86 | Calories from Fat: 29 | Protein: 4g | Carbs: 10g |
Total Fat: 3g | Saturated Fat: 0.5g | Trans Fat: 0g | Fiber: 5g |
Sodium: 46mg | Cholesterol: 0mg | Sugar: 0.5g

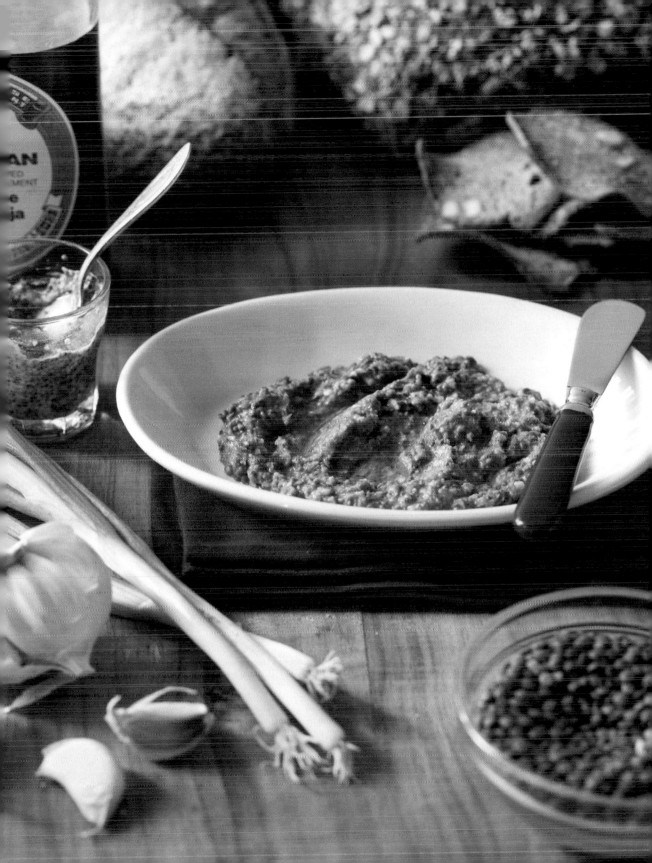

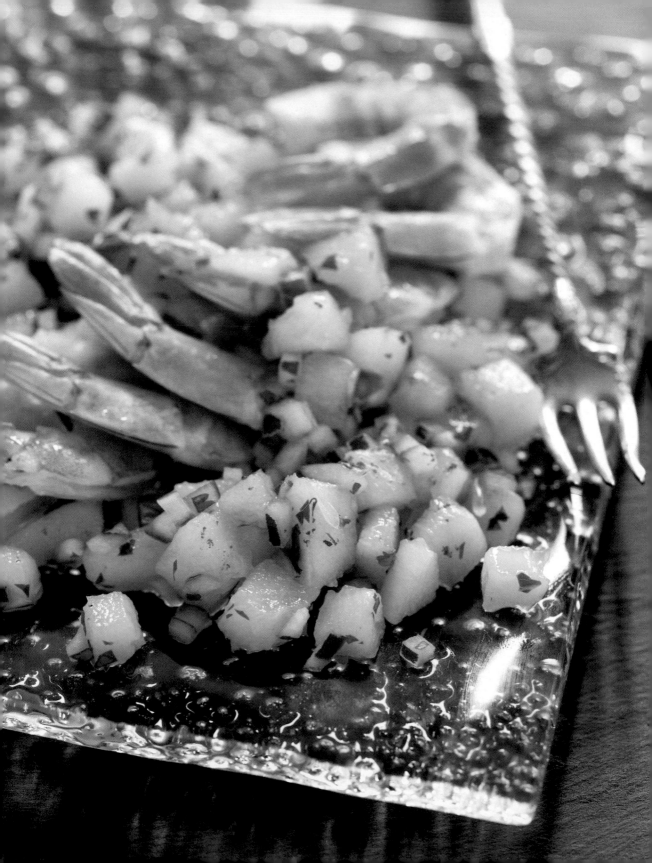

Mango Salsa

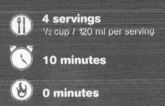

This refreshing salsa is perfect on a warm summer evening. The addition of cayenne or chili pepper offsets the sweetness of this fruity blend. It's excellent served on shrimp or white fish.

Ingredients

1 fresh near-ripe mango, peeled and finely chopped

½ small red onion, peeled and finely chopped

Juice of 1 fresh lime

3 Tbsp / 45 ml fresh cilantro, chopped

Pinch paprika

1 tsp / 5 ml sea salt

Freshly ground black pepper

Pinch cayenne or chili pepper (optional)

Method

1 Place all ingredients in a small mixing bowl. Mix well to combine.

2 Sprinkle with cayenne or chili pepper (if using).

3 Cover and refrigerate if not serving right away. Otherwise, serve at room temperature.

Nutritional Value Per Serving:
Calories: 42 | Calories from Fat: 2 | Protein: 0.5g | Carbs: 11g |
Total Fat: 0g | Saturated Fat: 0g | Trans Fat: 0g | Fiber: 1g |
Sodium: 394mg | Cholesterol: 0mg | Sugar: 8g

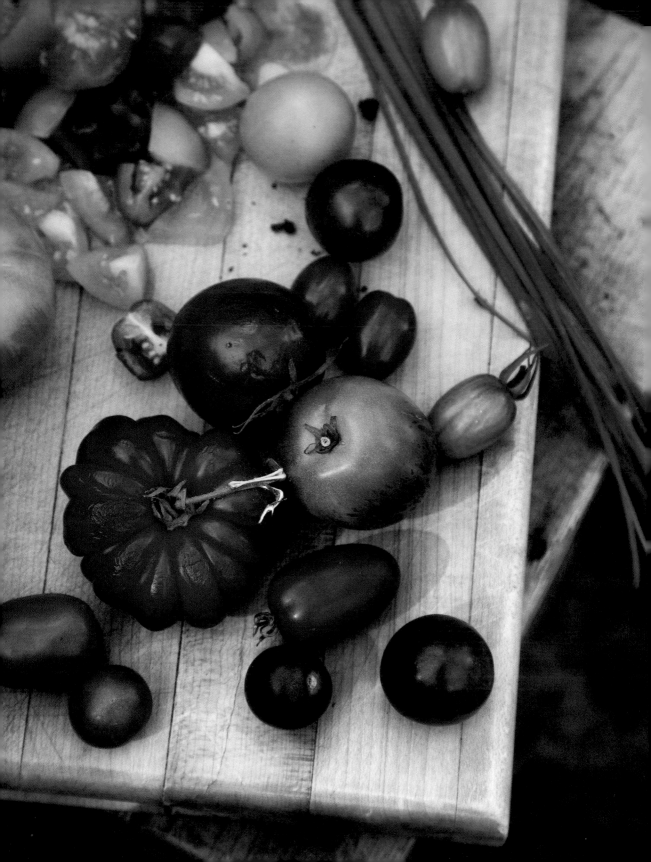

SALADS

3

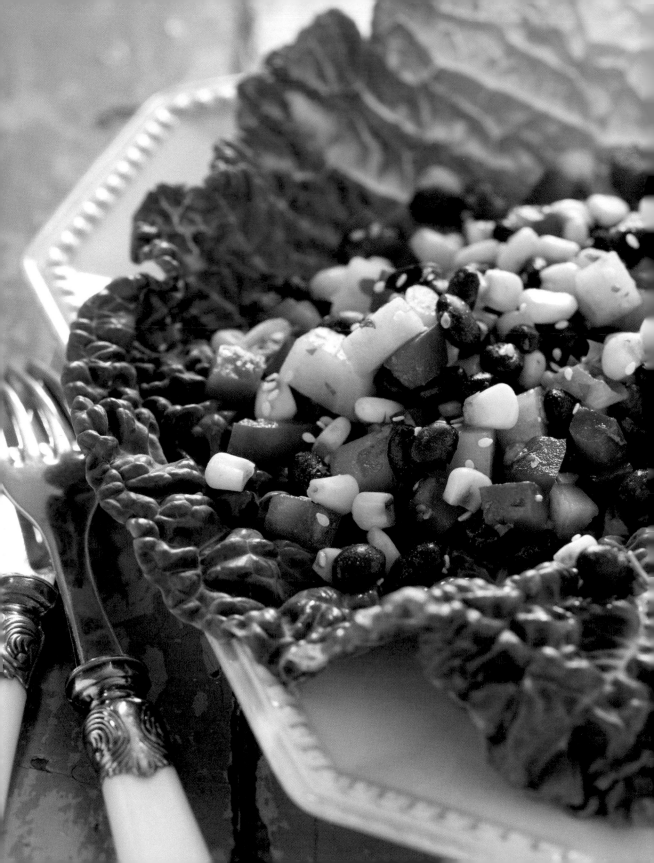

Black Bean & Corn Salad

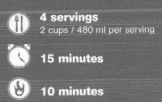

4 servings
2 cups / 480 ml per serving

15 minutes

10 minutes

Sesame adds a touch of nuttiness to this colorful salad with a tangy lemon dressing. Eat it on its own or use it as filling in a whole-grain wrap and give your lunch some life.

Salad Ingredients

1½ cups / 360 ml fresh cooked corn kernels

1 x 15 oz can black beans, rinsed and drained

2 yellow beets, cooked and chopped

1 red bell pepper, seeded, deveined and chopped

2 firm red tomatoes, chopped

4 green onions, sliced thin on the diagonal

1 Tbsp / 15 ml toasted sesame seeds

2 Tbsp / 30 ml fresh cilantro, chopped

Dressing Ingredients

Juice of 1 fresh lemon

1 Tbsp / 15 ml toasted sesame oil

1 Tbsp / 15 ml apple butter

1 Tbsp / 15 ml low-sodium tamari sauce

½ tsp / 2.5 ml sea salt

Method for Salad

1 Combine all ingredients in decorative salad bowl.

2 Pour dressing over salad and toss gently to coat. Serve immediately or cover and refrigerate.

Method for Dressing

1 Place all ingredients in glass Mason jar and seal. Shake well.

Nutritional Value Per Serving:

Calories: 261 | Calories from Fat: 24 | Protein: 14g | Carbs: 50g |
Total Fat: 3g | Saturated Fat: 0g | Trans Fat: 0g | Fiber: 14g |
Sodium: 39mg | Cholesterol: 0mg | Sugar: 8g

Beet & Arugula Salad

4 servings

20 minutes

60 minutes

Taste and texture come together exquisitely in this fresh, colorful salad. Sweet, earthy roasted beets, peppery arugula, crunchy sunflower seeds topped with the subtle tang of goat cheese … my mouth is watering already!

Ingredients

3 Tbsp / 45 ml extra virgin olive oil, divided

2 lbs / 908 g baby beets, washed and trimmed
   (all beets should be about the same size)

1 lb / 454 g Brussels sprouts, trimmed

2½ tsp / 12.5 ml sea salt, divided

Freshly ground black pepper, to taste

4 cups / 960 ml baby arugula

4 cups / 960 ml mesclun salad greens

¼ cup / 60 ml sunflower seeds, toasted

4 oz goat cheese, sliced into 8 pieces

2 Tbsp / 30 ml rice wine vinegar

Method

1 Preheat oven to 400°F / 200°C. Prepare baking dish by coating lightly with olive oil.

2 If beets are much bigger than Brussels sprouts, cut them in half; otherwise leave them whole. Toss beets and Brussels sprouts in 1½ Tbsp / 22.5 ml olive oil and season with 1 tsp / 5 ml salt and freshly ground black pepper.

3 Place vegetables in baking dish in single layer. Roast in hot oven for one hour. Remove from heat and let cool. Remove skins from beets when cool enough to handle.

4 Divide salad greens among four plates. Sprinkle with toasted sunflower seeds. Arrange beets and Brussels sprouts evenly between plates. Place two pieces of goat cheese on each plate. Drizzle each plate with vinegar and olive oil.

5 Season with a dusting of sea salt and black pepper.

6 Serve.

Nutritional Value Per Serving:
Calories: 426 | Calories from Fat: 224 | Protein: 18g | Carbs: 36g |
Total Fat: 26g | Saturated Fat: 9g | Trans Fat: 0g | Fiber: 13g |
Sodium: 1291mg | Cholesterol: 29.4mg | Sugar: 2g

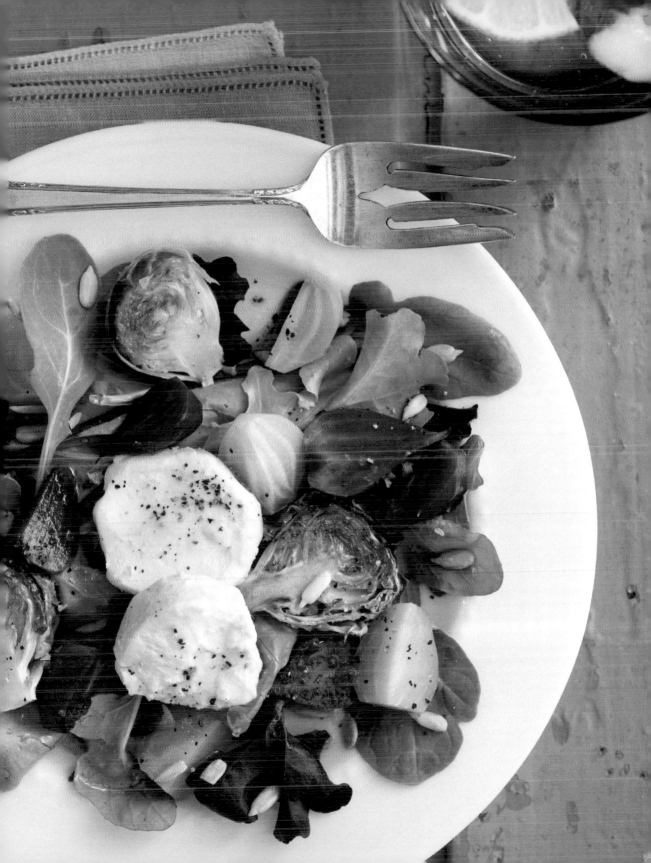

Balsamic vinegar is a lot like wine — the older the better. Make an effort to purchase the best quality you can find. This makes a huge difference!

Heirloom Tomato Salad

The joy of eating this salad is enhanced when the heirloom tomatoes come from your own garden. If you don't grow your own, make sure to purchase some the next time you hit a farmers market. Heirloom tomatoes are making a comeback thanks to their intense flavor. Although the ingredients are not many, the success of the salad lies in the quality of each. It is important to purchase the best you can manage to enjoy the most vibrant flavor. This happens to be one of my favorite salads, bar none!

Ingredients

2 lbs / 908 g heirloom tomatoes (go crazy and mix up the colors!)

1 cup / 240 ml bocconcini

2 generous handfuls fresh basil leaves

Several sprigs fresh chives

¼ cup / 60 ml best quality balsamic vinegar

¼ cup / 60 ml extra virgin olive oil

1 tsp / 5 ml sea salt

Freshly ground black pepper, to taste

Method

1 Wash the tomatoes well. Slice them into ¼- or ½-inch slices.

2 Divide the tomatoes among four plates.

3 Break up the bocconcini and divide the pieces among the plates.

4 Drop whole basil leaves on top of tomatoes and cheese.

5 Distribute the chives by snipping with scissors and letting pieces fall over salad.

6 Drizzle 1 Tbsp / 15 ml balsamic vinegar over each salad followed by 2 Tbsp / 30 ml olive oil.

7 Dust with sea salt and freshly ground black pepper.

Nutritional Value Per Serving:

Calories: 240 | Calories from Fat: 127 | Protein: 7g | Carbs: 8g | Total Fat: 20g | Saturated Fat: 6g | Trans Fat: 0g | Fiber: 1.5g | Sodium: 578mg | Cholesterol: 22mg | Sugar: 6g

Bocconcini is the Italian word for baby mozzarella. Do your best to get the freshest bocconcini possible. Again, this really makes a difference!

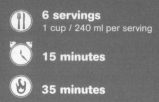
Brown Rice & Lentil Salad

Common in many diets around the world and a great way to use up pantry staples, this brown rice and lentil salad will please every palate. The pairing of rice and lentils makes a perfect protein, and it's hard to imagine a more healthy and delicious combination.

Ingredients

½ cup / 120 ml uncooked brown rice

½ cup / 120 ml dry Puy lentils

2 cups / 480 ml low-sodium chicken or vegetable stock (or water seasoned with 1 tsp / 5 ml bouillon)

1 Tbsp / 15 ml extra virgin olive oil

2 cloves garlic, passed through a garlic press

Juice of 1 fresh lime

2 Tbsp / 30 ml red wine vinegar (can use lemon juice or plain vinegar if that is what you have)

2 tsp / 10 ml Dijon mustard

½ tsp / 2.5 ml sea salt

Freshly ground black pepper

3 green onions, trimmed and chopped

1-2 tomatoes, chopped

1 Tbsp / 15 ml fresh parsley, finely chopped

Method

1 Combine rice and lentils along with stock or cooking liquid in medium saucepan and cook until all water is absorbed, about 40 minutes. You can use the oven method for cooking these too. Just place all ingredients in a covered casserole dish and bake at 350°F / 180°C for 40 minutes.

2 Remove cooked rice and lentils from heat. Place into decorative salad bowl and fluff with a fork. Let cool.

3 Prepare dressing by combining olive oil, garlic, lime juice, red wine vinegar, mustard, salt and pepper in small Mason jar. Put the lid on and shake well. Otherwise whisk well in small bowl.

4 Add chopped green onion, tomatoes and parsley to cooled rice and lentils.

5 Add dressing. Toss to combine. Serve chilled.

Nutritional Value Per Serving:
Calories: 177 | Calories from Fat: 34 | Protein: 8g | Carbs: 28g |
Total Fat: 4g | Saturated Fat: 1g | Trans Fat: 0g | Fiber: 6g |
Sodium: 269mg | Cholesterol: 0mg | Sugar: 3g

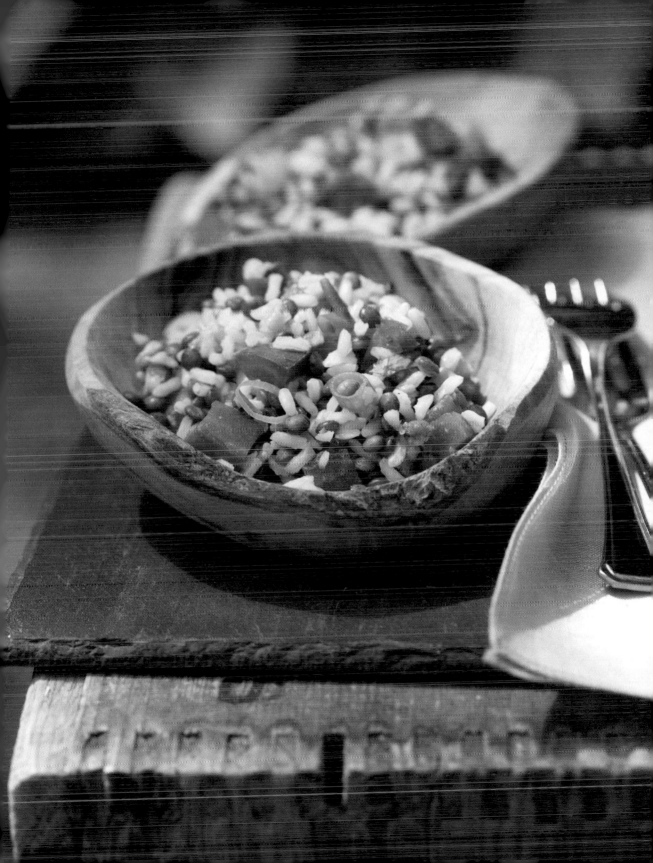

Leeks have to be washed and cooked before they can be eaten. To prepare leeks for washing, cut off the fibrous root, remove any tough or spotty leaves, trim the ends off the remaining leaves, cut the leek in half length-wise and then slice or chop. To wash, place your chopped leeks in a bowl of warm water and swirl them around to help loosen the dirt. Remove the leeks and place them in a colander, rinsing a second time.

Salad Greens with Spring Vegetables & Goat Cheese

4 Servings
2¹/₂ cups / 600 ml per serving

50 minutes

50 minutes

This colorful salad gives a new meaning to the phrase "restaurant quality." Serve it before dinner, or top with grilled chicken or fish for a lighter lunch.

Salad Ingredients

6 medium beets, washed and trimmed,
   leaving 2 inches of stems

4 leeks, whites only, cut in half lengthwise
   and rinsed

4 cups / 960 ml mixed greens (I like to mix up
   the colors for visual interest)

¼ cup / 60 ml soft goat cheese

¼ cup / 60 ml whole pecans, toasted

½ tsp / 2.5 ml sea salt

Freshly ground black pepper

1 tsp / 5 ml dried oregano

Vinaigrette Ingredients

Juice of 1 lemon

Juice of 1 orange

2 Tbsp / 30 ml agave nectar

¼ cup / 60 ml pumpkinseed oil

1 Tbsp / 15 ml rice wine vinegar

Method for Salad

1 Fill a medium saucepan with water, add beets and bring to a boil. Cook until tender. Remove from heat and drain. Rinse with cold water and let stand, changing the water frequently. When beets are cool enough to handle, slip skins off and trim stem ends. Cut into quarters or slice – however you like. Set aside.

2 Cut leek halves into quarters and place in a small saucepan. Bring to boil and cook until soft, about five minutes. Remove from heat and strain. Set aside.

3 Divide salad greens among four plates. Arrange cooked beets, leeks and goat cheese equally among the plates.

4 Garnish with toasted pecans.

5 Dust each plate with sea salt, black pepper and oregano.

6 Drizzle vinaigrette over each salad. Serve immediately.

Method for Dressing

1 Combine vinaigrette ingredients in glass jar with tight-fitting lid. Shake well.

Nutritional Value Per Serving:
Calories: 350 | Calories from Fat: 100 | Protein: 7g | Carbs: 35g |
Total Fat: 22g | Saturated Fat: 4g | Trans Fat: 0g | Fiber: 7g |
Sodium: 209mg | Cholesterol: 0mg | Sugar: 18g

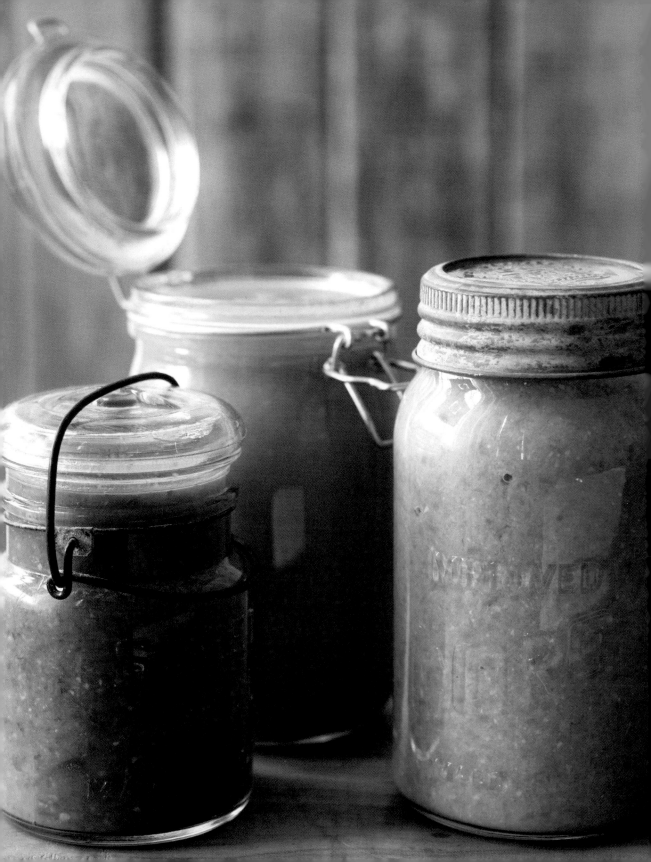

SOUPS & STEWS

4

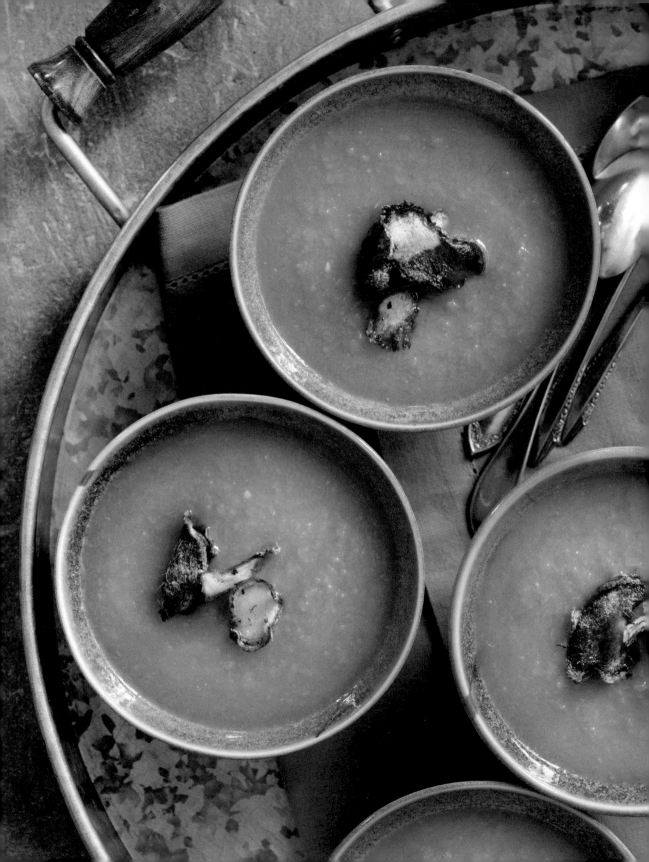

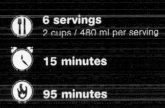

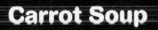

6 servings
2 cups / 480 ml per serving

15 minutes

95 minutes

Carrot Soup

There is nothing more satisfying than a hot bowl of soup on a brisk autumn or cold winter evening. You can easily turn this dish into a vegetarian or vegan meal, depending on your choice of cooking stock and garnishes. Enjoy!

Ingredients

½ cup / 120 ml melted coconut butter
 (if unavailable, use olive oil)

1 cup / 240 ml onion, peeled and chopped

6 cups / 1.5 L sweet carrots, peeled and
 coarsely chopped

1 large sweet potato, peeled and chopped

2 cloves garlic, passed through a garlic press

7 cups / 1.7 L low-sodium chicken stock

1 tsp / 5 ml freshly ground white pepper

1 Tbsp / 15 ml sea salt

Juice of 2 fresh oranges

2 Tbsp / 30 ml fresh ginger, grated

Optional

baked ginger and olive oil
Yogurt Cheese*
fresh chives

* See Yogurt Cheese recipe pg 334

Nutritional Value Per Serving:

Calories: 301 | Calories from Fat: 175 | Protein: 8g | Carbs: 27g |
Total Fat: 20g | Saturated Fat: 16g | Trans Fat: 0g | Fiber: 5g |
Sodium: 709mg | Cholesterol: 0mg | Sugar: 11g

Method

1 Place coconut butter in dutch oven. Heat over medium-high flame. Add onion and sauté until soft, about five minutes.

2 Add carrots, sweet potato and garlic. Cook until vegetables soften, about 15 minutes.

3 Remove from heat and add chicken stock, pepper and salt. Return to heat over medium-high flame.

4 When boiling, reduce heat and add orange juice and freshly grated ginger. Simmer for one hour.

5 Meanwhile, if garnishing with ginger, brush ginger with olive oil and bake at 400°F / 200°C until crisp.

6 Using an immersion blender, purée soup. Ladle into soup bowls and serve hot.

7 Garnish soup with a dollop of Yogurt Cheese, a few strands of fresh chives and baked ginger (if using).

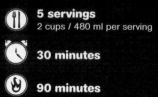
Lentil & Vegetable Stew

This vegetarian stew is hearty enough to convert any carnivore! Flavorful exotic spices are paired with Puy lentils (which conveniently don't break down or turn into mush during the cooking process like other kinds of lentils) and will warm your heart and soul on the coldest nights.

Ingredients

3 Tbsp / 45 ml olive oil

1 cup / 240 ml onion, chopped

3 cloves garlic, minced

3 carrots, peeled and chopped

3 parsnips, peeled and chopped

6-8 Brussels sprouts, tough ends removed,
   finely chopped

4 fist-sized potatoes, peeled and chopped

1 tsp / 5 ml ground cumin

Pinch cayenne pepper

1 tsp / 5 ml ground coriander

1 tsp / 5 ml turmeric

1 tsp / 5 ml ground ginger

½ tsp / 2.5 ml ground allspice

4 cups / 1 L low-sodium chicken or vegetable
   stock (or use water flavored with chicken
   or vegetable bouillon)

1 cup / 240 ml dry Puy lentils

2 tsp / 10 ml sea salt

3 bay leaves

Method

1 Heat oil in large Dutch oven over medium flame. Add all chopped vegetables and cook until soft.

2 Add all spices (except salt) and continue cooking until fragrant.

3 Reduce heat and add stock, Puy lentils, sea salt and bay leaves.

4 Cover and reduce heat to simmer. Cook for 45 to 60 minutes. Stew is done when lentils are cooked.

5 Serve hot over cooked brown rice or enjoy as is.

TIP This dish can be made in the slow cooker, but only needs about an hour or two to cook.

Nutritional Value Per Serving:
Calories: 218 | Calories from Fat: 46 | Protein: 10g | Carbs: 36g |
Total Fat: 5g | Saturated Fat: 1g | Trans Fat: 0g | Fiber: 10g |
Sodium: 133mg | Cholesterol: 0mg | Sugar: 4g

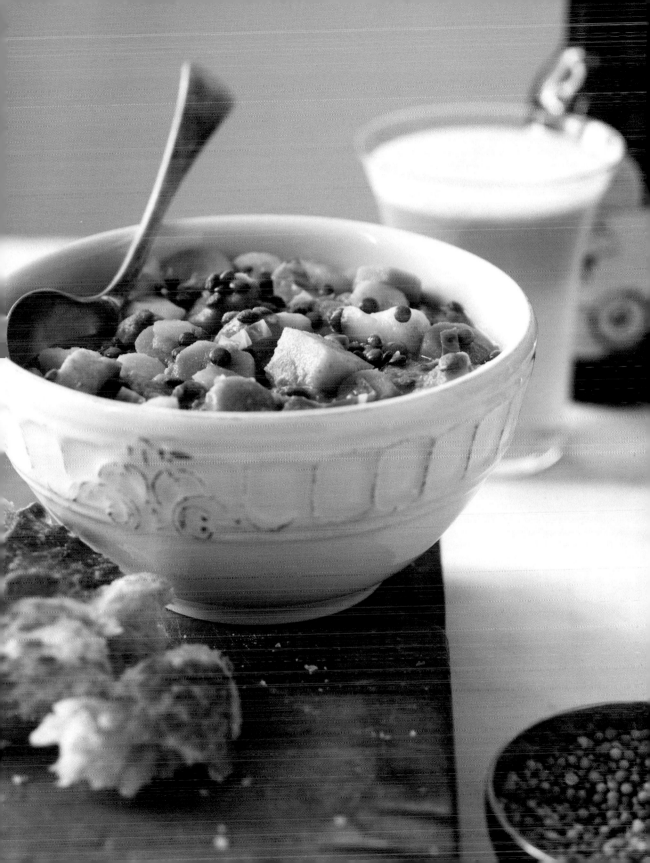

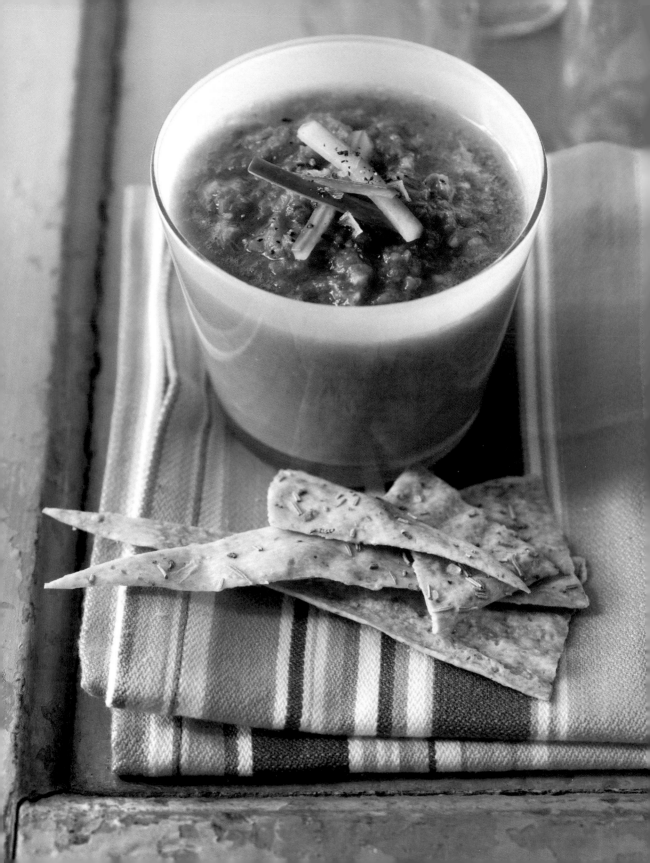

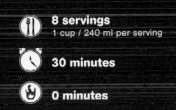
Gazpacho

There is nothing more nutritious and easy-to-make on a hot summer day than cool, refreshing gazpacho. This cold, tomato-based, raw vegetable soup is popular in Spain, Portugal and Latin America. You can experiment with the taste by throwing different vegetables into the mix.

Ingredients

4 lbs / 1.8 kg fresh ripe tomatoes, trimmed
    and cut into chunks

¼ cup / 60 ml extra virgin olive oil

¼ cup / 60 ml rice wine vinegar

1 cup / 240 ml juiced cucumbers

2 cloves garlic, peeled and trimmed

1 orange or red pepper, seeded and deveined,
    cut into chunks

1 Tbsp / 15 ml sea salt

½ cup / 120 ml fresh basil leaves, cut into ribbons
    (as garnish)

Freshly ground black pepper

Method

1 Place all ingredients in the bowl of a food processor. Process until smooth.

2 Transfer mixture to chilled serving bowls.

3 Garnish with chopped basil and freshly ground black pepper.

Nutritional Value Per Serving:
Calories: 109 | Calories from Fat: 64 | Protein: 2g | Carbs: 10g |
Total Fat: 7g | Saturated Fat: 1g | Trans Fat: 0g | Fiber: 3g |
Sodium: 405mg | Cholesterol: 0mg | Sugar: 7g

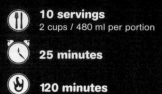

Meal-in-a-Bowl Soup

10 servings
2 cups / 480 ml per portion

25 minutes

120 minutes

Much can be made of a soup and this recipe puts emphasis on the word "much." It's got an intimidating looking ingredient list but don't let that get to you – the ingredients don't require much work. Just peel and chop then toss in the pan. Missing some of these ingredients? Don't worry. Use what you have and add something new. It will still taste fab!

Ingredients

¼ cup / 60 ml extra virgin olive oil

1 bunch celery, leaves included, trimmed
  and coarsely chopped

2 large onions, peeled and chopped

3 fat carrots, peeled and coarsely chopped

3 parsnips, peeled and coarsely chopped

1 head garlic, peeled and coarsely chopped

4 fist-sized yellow potatoes, peeled and
  coarsely chopped

1 head green cabbage (about the size of two
  hands cupped together), shredded

2 x 15 oz cans white kidney beans, rinsed and
  drained

8 plum tomatoes, coarsely chopped

12 cups / 3 L low-sodium chicken
  or vegetable stock

1 Tbsp / 15 ml sea salt

1 Tbsp / 15 ml freshly ground black pepper

2 Tbsp / 30 ml dried oregano

2 Tbsp / 30 ml dried basil

Method

1 In large Dutch oven or heavy-bottomed skillet, place olive oil and heat over medium-high flame.

2 Add celery, onions, carrots and parsnips. Sauté until onions are soft. Add garlic, potatoes, shredded cabbage and all remaining ingredients. Bring to a boil. Once boiling, reduce heat and let simmer for an hour or until vegetables are soft.

3 Serve hot.

Nutritional Value Per Serving:
Calories: 395 | Calories from Fat: 72 | Protein: 21g | Carbs: 66g |
Total Fat: 8g | Saturated Fat: 1g | Trans Fat: 0g | Fiber: 20g |
Sodium: 492mg | Cholesterol: 0mg | Sugar: 11g

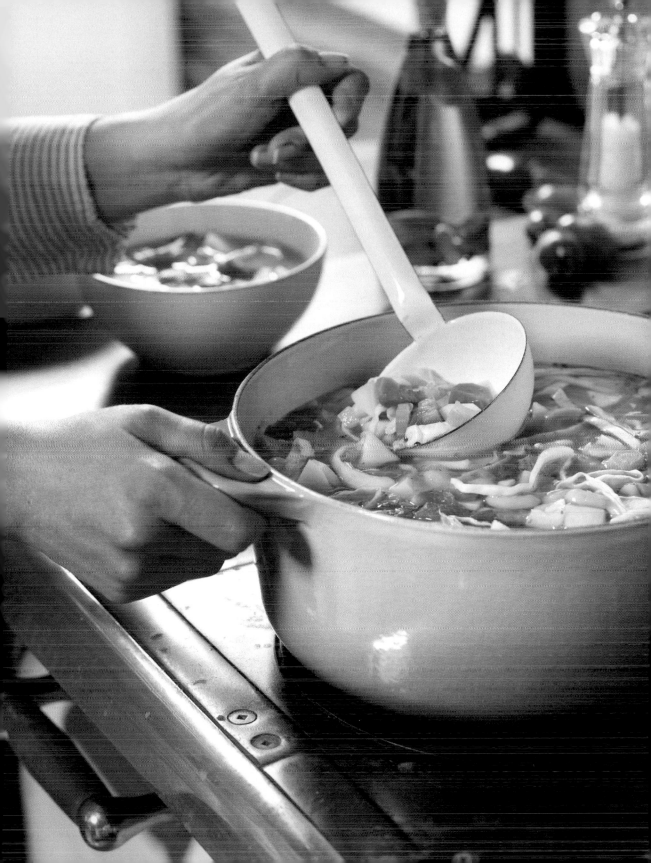

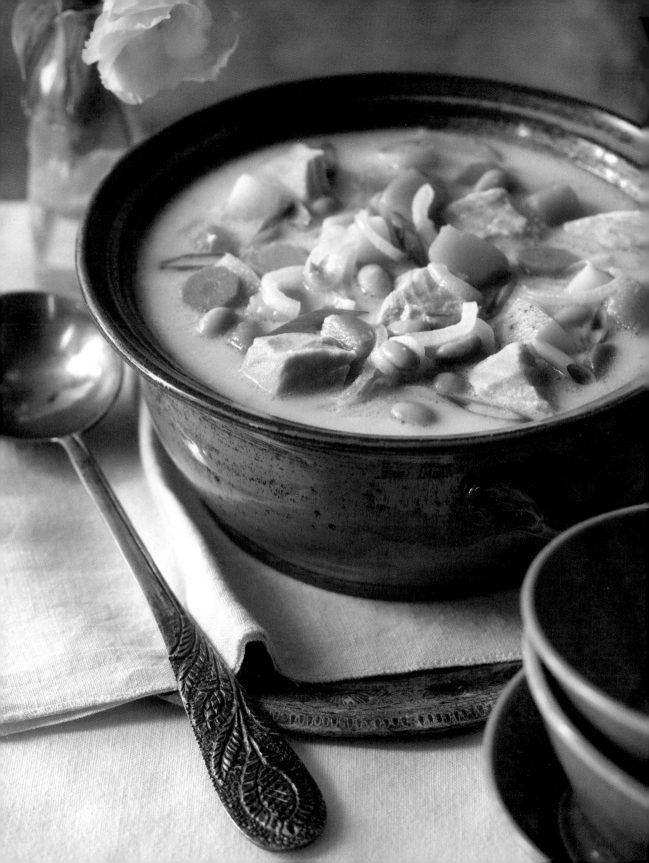

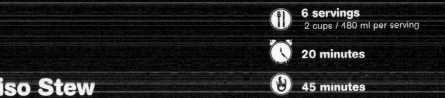

Salmon & Miso Stew

Seasoned by miso, which is the name for soybean paste, miso soup is the most popular soup in Japan – in fact, most Japanese meals include a small bowl of it. The salmon in this recipe adds a protein punch!

Ingredients

2 Tbsp / 30 ml coconut butter

2 cups / 480 ml thinly sliced onion

8 oz wild salmon, cut into 1-inch chunks

1 cup / 240 ml carrots, thinly sliced (like pennies)

3 cups / 720 ml low-sodium vegetable stock

2 bay leaves

2 cups / 480 ml chopped Yukon gold potatoes

1 cup / 240 ml 1-inch chunks pumpkin,
    skin removed

1½ cups / 360 ml plain soymilk

1 cup / 240 ml edamame

1½ Tbsp / 22.5 ml miso

3 scallions, trimmed and chopped on the diagonal

Method

1 In large Dutch oven heat coconut butter. Add onion and cook until soft, about five minutes.

2 Add salmon, carrots, vegetable stock and bay leaves. Bring mixture to a boil. Reduce heat to simmer and cover. Cook for 10 minutes.

3 Remove lid and bring mixture to a boil again. Add potatoes, pumpkin and soymilk. Cook over medium heat for five minutes. Don't let the soymilk come to a boil or it may curdle.

4 Add edamame. Simmer on very low heat for several minutes.

5 In small mixing bowl place miso. Using a soup ladle remove some of the broth and pour it over the miso. Mix broth and miso well. Transfer this mixture to the Dutch oven. Mix into soup and heat gently over very low heat.

6 Ladle into soup bowls and garnish with scallions. Serve hot.

Nutritional Value Per Serving:

Calories: 228 | Calories from Fat: 83 | Protein: 14g | Carbs: 24g |
Total Fat: 9g | Saturated Fat: 3g | Trans Fat: 0g | Fiber: 4g |
Sodium: 624mg | Cholesterol: 0mg | Sugar: 7g

Green Pea & Basil Soup

If anything says "spring," surely it must be fresh peas and fragrant basil. Put them together in a soup and you have heaven – exactly what you have been longing for after a dreary winter.

Ingredients

3 Tbsp / 45 ml extra virgin olive oil

1 small onion, chopped

3 stalks celery, leaves included, chopped

1 Tbsp / 15 ml dried basil leaves

1 tsp / 5 ml sea salt

Freshly ground white pepper, to taste

½ cup / 120 ml apple cider

3 cups + 1/3 cup / 800 ml fresh green peas, divided

4 cups / 960 ml low-sodium vegetable stock

1 generous handful basil, chopped

Optional

1 handful pea sprouts

1 cup / 240 ml Yogurt Cheese
   (see right for recipe)

Method

1 In large skillet heat oil for a few minutes. Add onion and celery. Sauté until onion is soft.

2 Add dried basil, sea salt and white pepper. Cook for three minutes, stirring constantly.

3 Add apple cider and let it come to a gentle boil. Add 3 cups / 720 ml peas and stock and bring to a gentle boil again. Cook for about 15 minutes.

4 Add chopped basil. Using an immersion blender, purée the mixture until smooth.

5 Ladle into soup bowls and garnish each with a handful of fresh peas and pea sprouts (if using). Each dish may also be garnished with a dollop of Yogurt Cheese if desired.

Yogurt Cheese

Ingredients

2 quarts / 1.9 L low-fat plain yogurt,
   dairy or soy based

Method

1 Place four layers of damp cheescloth in a fine mesh sieve or colander. Place the colander over a bowl.

2 Add yogurt and let it drain overnight in the refrigerator.

3 Discard the water from the bowl.

Nutritional Value Per Serving:

Calories: 127 | Calories from Fat: 54 | Protein: 6g | Carbs: 12g |
Total Fat: 6g | Saturated Fat: 1g | Trans Fat: 0g | Fiber: 4g |
Sodium: 210mg | Cholesterol: 0mg | Sugar: 6g

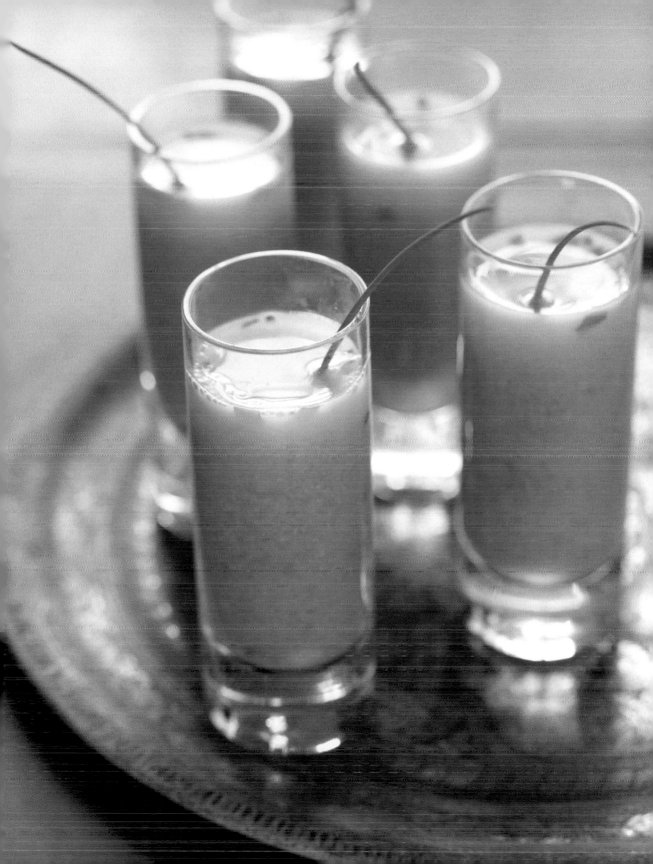

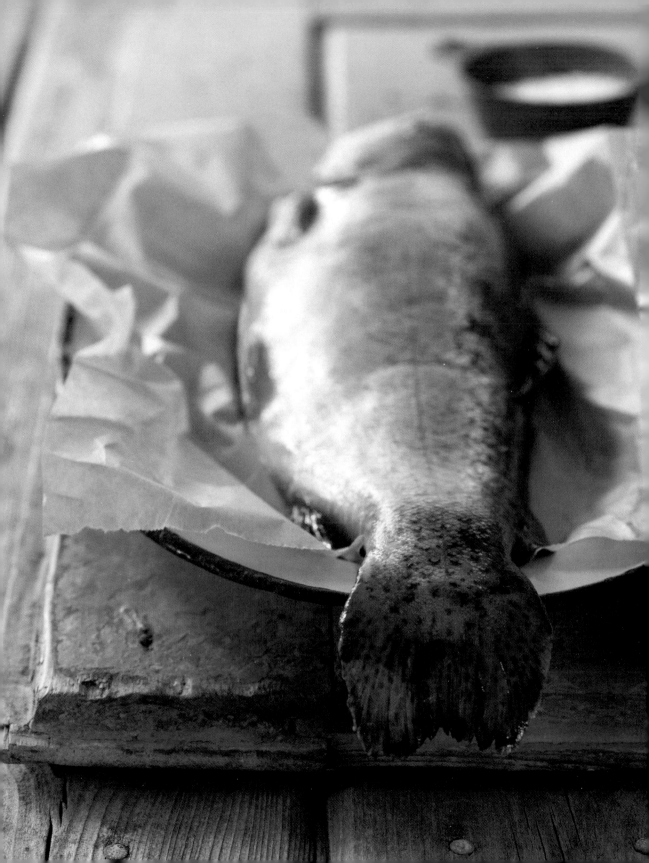

PROTEINS

5

Tofu. Just give it a chance! Tofu is for vegetarians what chicken is for meat eaters. It is the perfect canvas upon which to toss just about any flavor. Tofu soaks up and even requires an intensely flavored marinade in order to make it taste, well, better. Give it a good soaking for a few hours before cooking and see if you don't begin to like it too!

Citrus Barbecued Tofu with Zesty BBQ Sauce

🍴 6 servings

⏰ 20 minutes

🔥 15 minutes

Note: This recipe requires an overnight marinating. Plan ahead before making this dish.

Ingredients
1 lb / 454 g unflavored firm or extra firm tofu
1½ cups / 360 ml Zesty BBQ Sauce (recipe below)
Juice of 1 fresh lime
Juice of 1 fresh orange

Method
1 Tofu contains quite a bit of water, which must be removed before grilling for best results. This is easily accomplished by removing the tofu from its packaging and setting it on several layers of paper towel or a clean kitchen towel folded in four. Set toweling on a baking sheet and place tofu on top. Place a similar absorbent layer overtop of the tofu and another baking sheet on top of that. Weigh the whole arrangement down by placing a few heavy books on top. Let it sit this way for about an hour.

2 Meanwhile mix the citrus juice with the Zesty BBQ Sauce in a small bowl and set aside.

3 Extract the tofu from its press. Cut into ³/₄-inch squares for grilling.

4 Arrange tofu squares in a shallow glass baking dish or lasagna pan. Coat each piece well with marinade. Cover with plastic wrap and set in refrigerator overnight.

5 Put a light coating of cooking oil on clean BBQ racks. Preheat your grill to medium heat. When hot, place each tofu piece on grill and cook until grill marks appear. Turn and grill other side. Let tofu cook well on both sides, about 10 minutes each.

6 Use remaining marinade to baste tofu. Keep the grill on medium heat (not overly hot).

7 When tofu is properly grilled remove from heat and serve between toasted halves of a whole-grain bun, or as your protein to accompany an array of summer salads.

Zesty BBQ Sauce

🍴 1¹/₂ cups / 360 ml

⏰ 5 minutes

🔥 0 minutes

Ingredients
2 cups / 480 ml onions, sliced into rings
2 Tbsp / 30 ml extra virgin olive oil
3 whole cloves garlic
1 cup / 240 ml unsulfured organic molasses
½ cup / 120 ml organic apple cider vinegar
¼ cup / 60 ml tomato paste
¼ cup / 60 ml rice wine vinegar
1 tsp / 5 ml sea salt

Nutritional Value for ¹/₆ of Recipe Including Sauce:
Calories: 388 | Calories from Fat: 90 | Protein: 7g | Carbs: 75g | Total Fat: 10g | Saturated Fat: 1g | Trans Fat: 0g | Fiber: 11g | Sodium: 326mg | Cholesterol: 0mg | Sugar: 53g

Method
1 Place sliced onions and extra virgin olive oil in a medium saucepan. Slowly heat the mixture, letting onions caramelize for about 40 minutes. When the onions are perfectly caramelized they will be brown but not burnt.

2 Add the rest of the ingredients to the pan and let the mixture come to a gentle boil. Cook slowly for 15 minutes.

3 Remove from heat and cool for several minutes.

4 Puree in a blender or food processor until smooth. Pour into glass jar and store in refrigerator until ready to use.

Herb Marinated Grilled Lamb Chops

6 servings

10 minutes

10 minutes

I wasn't big on lamb until I practiced cooking it. What really sold me in the long run was getting the right combination of flavors with which to marinate the meat before cooking. In this recipe, a favorite of mine, the marinade boosts the Yum factor substantially. I think you'll like lamb after you try it this way.

Ingredients

6 lamb chops (grass fed is best, either cut from
    a rack of lamb or lollipop lamb chops)

2 Tbsp / 30 ml coconut butter, melted (if unavailable,
    use olive oil)

¼ cup / 60 ml balsamic vinegar

1 Tbsp / 15 ml agave nectar

1 tsp / 5 ml Dijon mustard

2 tsp / 10 ml dried mint

1 tsp / 5 ml freshly ground black pepper

½ tsp / 2.5 ml sea salt

2 cloves garlic, minced

1 Tbsp / 15 ml fresh rosemary, chopped

1 tsp / 5 ml dried oregano

Method

1 Marinate lamb chops before grilling. Prepare marinade by combining melted coconut butter or oil, balsamic vinegar, agave nectar, Dijon mustard, mint, pepper, sea salt, garlic, rosemary and oregano in small mixing bowl. Mix well to combine.

2 Place lamb chops in a shallow glass baking dish. Coat each chop with marinade. Cover and refrigerate for one hour.

3 When ready to cook preheat grill. Clean grill well and coat lightly with oil. Grill chops over a medium-high heat for about five minutes per side or until nicely browned. The trick is not to overdo the lamb as it gets tough fast.

Note: Nutritional value is for a 5-oz portion of lamb.

Nutritional Value Per Serving:
Calories: 388 | Calories from Fat: 90 | Protein: 7g | Carbs: 75g |
Total Fat: 10g | Saturated Fat: 1g | Trans Fat: 0g | Fiber: 11g |
Sodium: 326mg | Cholesterol: 0mg | Sugar: 53g

TIP Lamb chops should be grilled on a covered grill over a medium-high heat. Ideally, you should grill them to medium rare or medium. The trick is to keep a close eye on the chops, removing them from the grill when they are just done. Let the meat rest for a few minutes before you serve it.

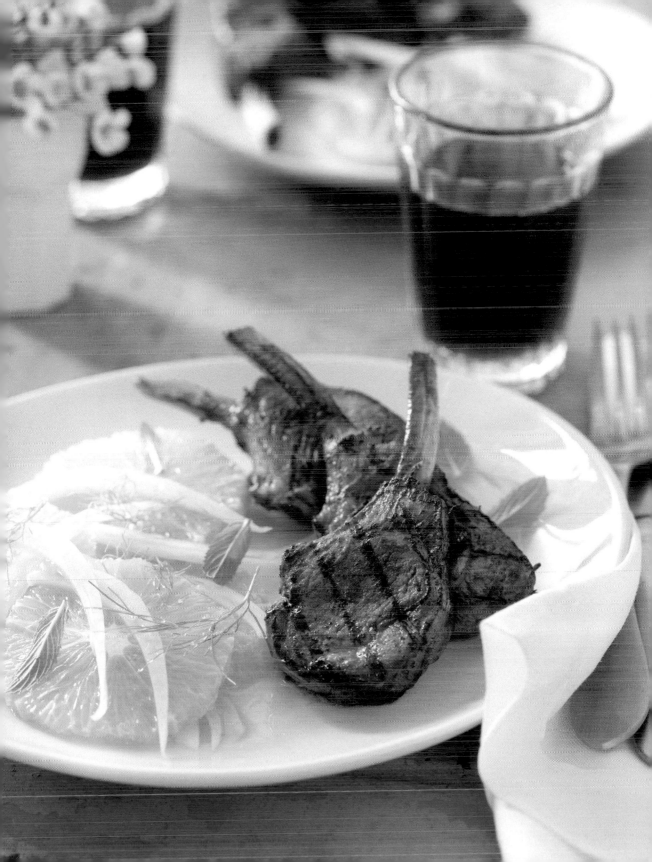

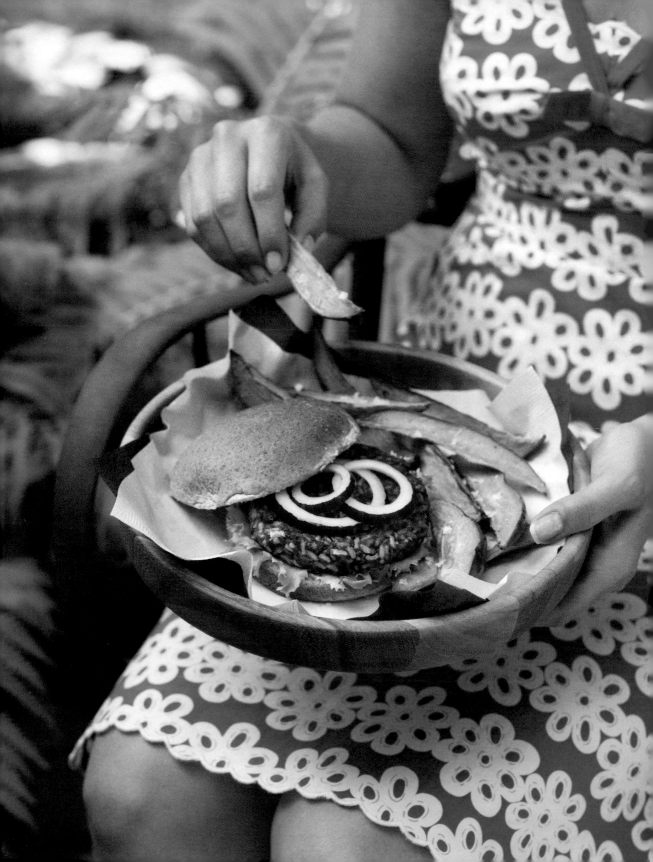

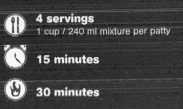

Paradise Island Bean Burgers

If you've never tried a bean burger before, you've been missing out! You can stay svelte in your swimsuit and enjoy a traditional meal, served hot right off the grill. Paradise is just around the corner.

Note: You'll need cooked rice for this recipe. I always make a big pot at the beginning of each week so I always have some ready for easy meals like this one.

Ingredients

1 cup / 240 ml black beans, rinsed,
    drained and mashed

1 cup / 240 ml cooked brown rice

1 clove garlic, passed through a garlic press

2 Tbsp / 30 ml leeks, whites only, finely chopped

2 Tbsp / 30 ml cooked and mashed sweet potato
    or pumpkin

1 tsp / 5 ml chili powder

½ tsp / 2.5 ml dried oregano

½ tsp / 2.5 ml dried basil

¼ tsp / 1.25 ml ground cumin

1 tsp / 5 ml sea salt

1 Tbsp / 15 ml extra virgin olive oil

4 Ezekiel buns, toasted

Method

1 Mix all ingredients except the olive oil and buns in a large bowl. Coat clean hands with olive oil to mix.

2 Divide mixture into equal fourths. Shape into patties.

3 Heat grill pan over medium flame and coat lightly with oil. Add patties and cook five minutes per side or until the patties are golden and crispy.

4 Serve on toasted burger buns.

5 Dress burgers with your favorite accoutrements.

Nutritional Value Per Serving:
Calories: 388 | Calories from Fat: 90 | Protein: 7g | Carbs: 75g |
Total Fat: 10g | Saturated Fat: 1g | Trans Fat: 0g | Fiber: 11g |
Sodium: 326mg | Cholesterol: 0mg | Sugar: 53g

Herbed Rainbow Trout

4 servings

25 minutes

30 minutes

Serving a whole fish is always a hit at dinner parties. The flavor of the fish comes from the poaching liquid – the flavors are infused into the fish while it simmers. How's that for table talk?

Ingredients

2 tsp / 10 ml extra virgin olive oil

1 yellow onion, peeled and chopped

2 cloves garlic, coarsely chopped

1 tsp / 5 ml sea salt

Freshly ground black pepper

8 cups / 2 L water

1 cup / 240 ml apple cider

4 bay leaves

5 whole fresh thyme sprigs

5 whole fresh rosemary sprigs

1 whole fresh rainbow trout

1 fresh lemon, sliced into ¼-inch thick rounds

5 green onions, trimmed, roots removed but
    otherwise left intact

Cheesecloth

Method

1 In a Dutch oven heat oil over medium heat. Add onion, garlic, salt and pepper and sauté until onion becomes soft, about five minutes.

2 Add water, cider and herbs and bring to soft boil. Reduce heat and simmer for 15 minutes.

3 Meanwhile, prepare your fish. Rinse well under cold running water, removing loose scales. Stuff lemon slices and green onion into fish. Wrap the fish in cheesecloth, making sure to leave a length of cheesecloth at either end. This will help you lower the fish into the boiling poaching liquid and remove it later.

4 Lower the fish into the hot poaching liquid, leaving the long ends of cheesecloth hanging over the side of the pan (not near the flame). Poach for 10 minutes.

5 Lift fish out by holding the long ends of cheesecloth. Place on flat surface and remove cheesecloth. Open the fish and remove the head, spine and tail, in one piece if possible.

6 Transfer remaining meat to a serving platter or plates and serve.

Nutritional Value Per Serving:

Calories: 388 | Calories from Fat: 90 | Protein: 7g | Carbs: 75g |
Total Fat: 10g | Saturated Fat: 1g | Trans Fat: 0g | Fiber: 11g |
Sodium: 326mg | Cholesterol: 0mg | Sugar: 53g

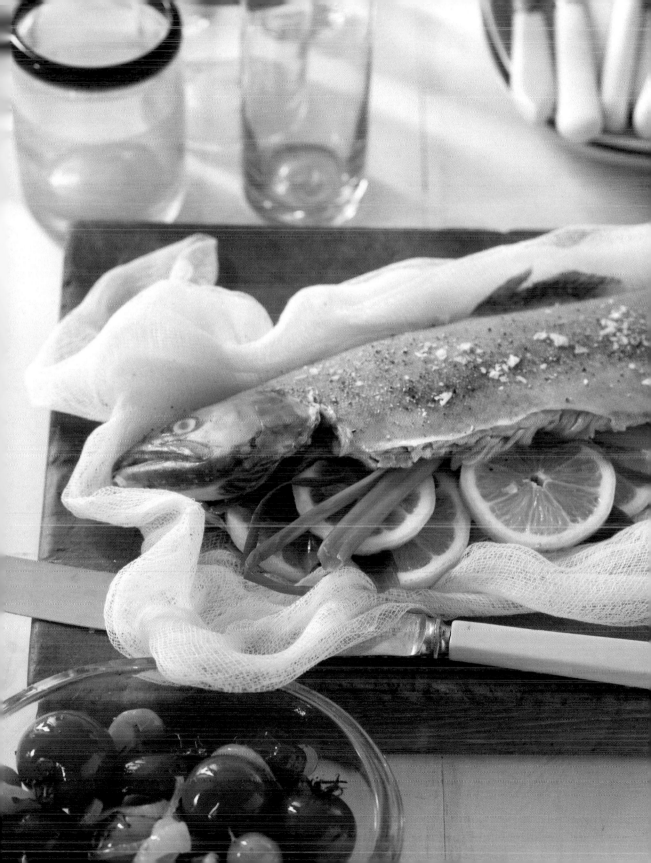

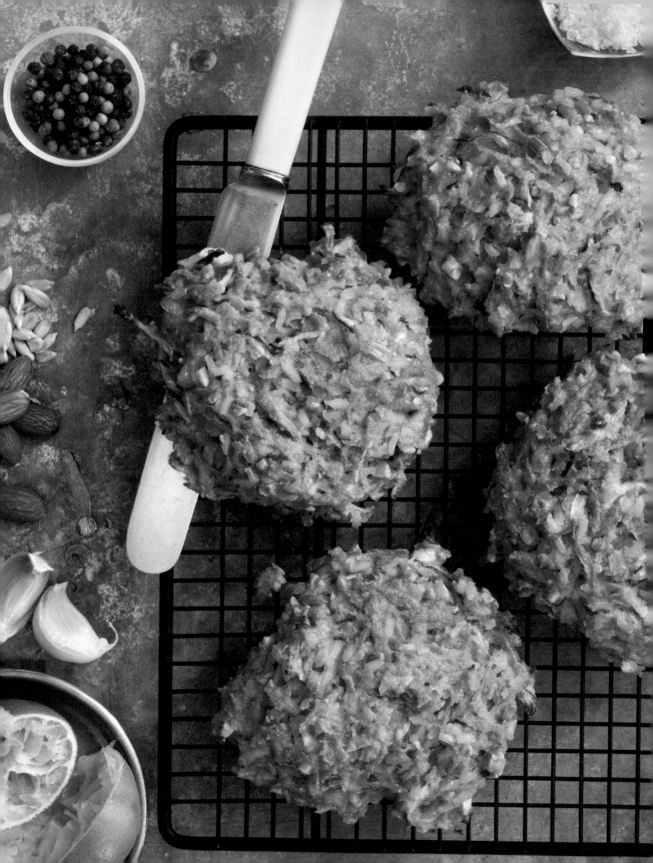

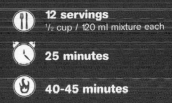
Brown Rice Patties

Perfect for a weeknight dinner, these nutty baked patties are not only nutritious and delicious, they're also economical and kid-friendly. It doesn't get any better than that! Toast Ezekiel buns and serve them burger-style, or for a lighter option, place atop a bed of fresh greens.

Note: You'll also need cooked rice for this recipe.

Ingredients

1 sweet potato, peeled and grated

1 firm green zucchini, washed, trimmed and grated

3 similarly sized carrots, peeled, trimmed and grated

1½ cups / 260 ml cooked brown rice

½ cup Power Flour (see recipe on page 385)

Juice of 1 fresh lime

Juice of 1 fresh lemon

1 Tbsp / 15 ml sesame oil

¼ cup / 60 ml raw unsalted almonds, coarsely chopped in food processor

¼ cup / 60 ml raw unsalted sunflower seeds, coarsely chopped in food processor

1 tsp / 5 ml sea salt

2 cloves garlic, passed through a garlic press

Freshly ground black pepper

1 egg

1 egg white

Method

1 Preheat oven to 375°F / 190°C. Line a large baking sheet with parchment paper.

2 Using a clean dishtowel, press any extra water out of grated vegetables.

3 Process almonds and sunflower seeds in food processor.

4 Combine all ingredients in large mixing bowl. Mix very well. Mixture should be fairly stiff.

5 Using a ½-cup scoop or measuring cup, scoop out mixture and shape into flat patties. Place on baking sheet.

6 Bake for 40 to 45 minutes or until lightly golden on top.

Nutritional Value Per Serving:

Calories: 388 | Calories from Fat: 90 | Protein: 7g | Carbs: 75g | Total Fat: 10g | Saturated Fat: 1g | Trans Fat: 0g | Fiber: 11g | Sodium: 326mg | Cholesterol: 0mg | Sugar: 53g

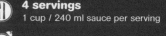

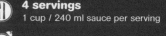**4 servings**
1 cup / 240 ml sauce per serving

25 minutes

45 minutes

Caribbean Chicken

The Caribbean is well known for its lively music, relaxed lifestyle and delicious food. With this perfect blend of sweet and spicy, you can pretend you're in the tropics … without leaving your own kitchen!

Ingredients

Juice and zest of 1 fresh lime, separated

Juice and zest of 1 fresh orange, separated

1 Tbsp / 15 ml agave nectar

1 Tbsp / 15 ml molasses

1 Tbsp / 15 ml fresh ginger, minced

4 cloves garlic, passed through a garlic press

½ tsp / 2.5 ml ground cinnamon

1/8 tsp / 0.6 ml ground nutmeg

1/8 tsp / 0.6 ml ground mace

1 tsp / 5 ml hot sauce (Tabasco or as hot as you like)

4 x 5 oz / 142 g boneless, skinless chicken breasts

1 Tbsp / 15 ml coconut butter

1 x 8-oz / 240 ml can crushed tomatoes

1 tsp / 5 ml sea salt

1 tsp / 5 ml freshly ground black pepper

TIP Use tuna or swordfish steaks instead of chicken to mix it up!

Method

1 Make a marinade in a small bowl or Mason jar by combining citrus juices (reserve the zest), agave nectar, molasses, ginger, garlic, cinnamon, nutmeg, mace and hot sauce. Shake or mix well.

2 Pour marinade over chicken breasts and let stand for at least an hour. The longer the chicken marinates, the stronger the flavor.

3 Heat coconut butter in large skillet over medium-high heat. Remove chicken breasts from marinade and place in skillet. Keep the marinade. Brown chicken on both sides.

4 Reduce heat and add reserved marinade, tomatoes and citrus zest. Add salt and pepper.

5 Cover and cook for 35 minutes. Check occasionally to make sure chicken does not stick to pan.

6 Remove chicken from pan and transfer to heated serving plate. Increase heat of skillet to reduce sauce. When it thickens, remove from heat and pour over chicken.

Nutritional Value Per Serving:

Calories: 388 | Calories from Fat: 90 | Protein: 7g | Carbs: 75g |
Total Fat: 10g | Saturated Fat: 1g | Trans Fat: 0g | Fiber: 11g |
Sodium: 326mg | Cholesterol: 0mg | Sugar: 53g

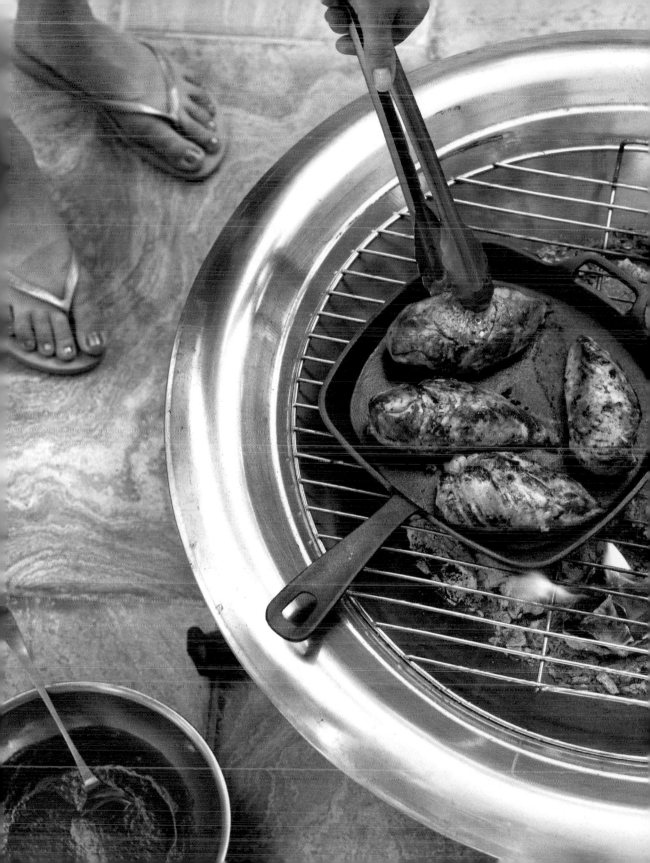

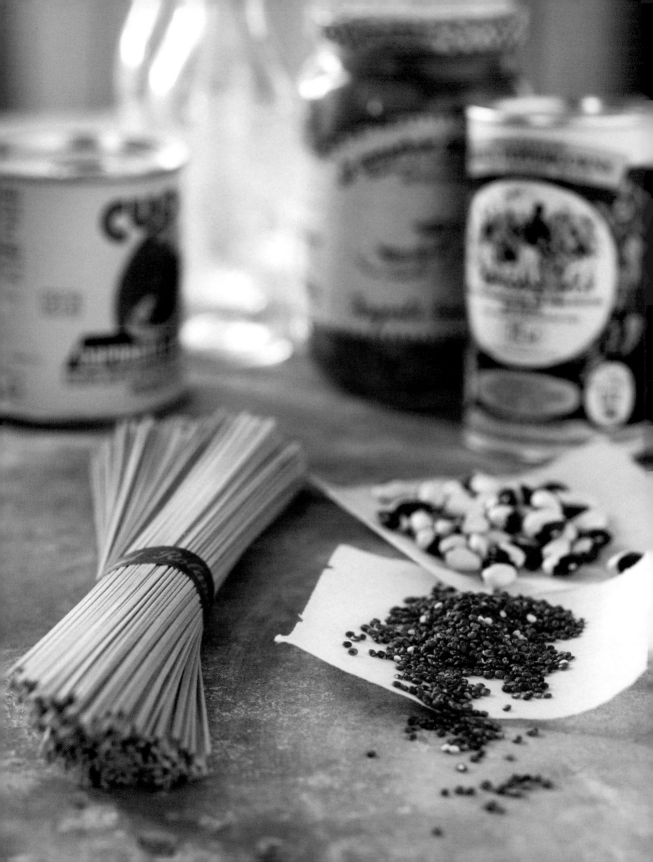

SIDES

6

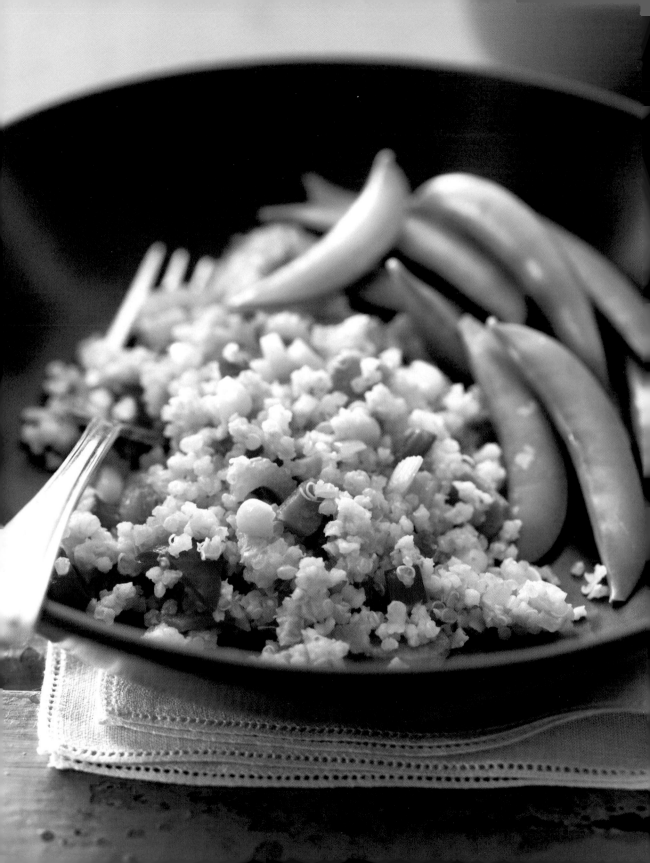

Baked Grains Pilaf

7 servings
1 cup / 240 ml per serving

20 minutes

40 minutes

I have long known that when I bake rice in the oven rather than boil it on the stove, the grains tend to remain firm and chewy. I like that and have learned to bake all my grains in the same way. If baked grains are on the menu, I will create my entire meal around "baking." That is, I will bake the grains alongside the fish and veggies. That way I am reducing the energy load and doing my bit for the Green Movement. This dish combines two of my favorite high-power grains, millet and quinoa.

Ingredients

1 Tbsp / 15 ml extra virgin olive oil, divided

1 onion, peeled and finely chopped

1 small carrot, peeled and finely chopped

3 stalks celery, leaves included, finely chopped

½ cup / 120 ml finely chopped bell pepper
(any color, although red looks nice)

½ cup / 120 ml corn kernels

¾ cup / 180 ml millet, rinsed well

¾ cup / 180 ml quinoa, rinsed well

3 cups / 720 ml low-sodium chicken
or vegetable stock

1 tsp / 2.5 ml sea salt

TIP Remember to wash millet and quinoa grains well before use by placing them in a fine mesh sieve and rinsing under running water until the water runs clear.

Method

1 Preheat oven to 350°F / 180°C. Prepare casserole dish by coating lightly with olive oil.

2 Place remaining olive oil in a medium skillet and heat gently. Add onion, carrot, celery, pepper and corn. Cook until onion is soft and translucent. Remove from heat.

3 Place washed grains in prepared casserole dish. Add cooked vegetables and mix to combine. Add chicken or vegetable stock and salt. Cover casserole dish with lid. Place in oven and bake for 30 minutes. Grains are cooked when all water has been absorbed. They will look slightly golden on the edges of the casserole dish.

4 Remove from heat and serve hot with any meal.

Nutritional Value Per Serving:
Calories: 205 | Calories from Fat: 42 | Protein: 8g | Carbs: 34g |
Total Fat: 0g | Saturated Fat: 1g | Trans Fat: 0g | Fiber: 4g |
Sodium: 278mg | Cholesterol: 0mg | Sugar: 2g

Mexican Pinto Beans & Brown Rice

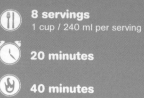
When you combine beans with rice you get a fast and easy, low-fat, high-quality protein meal. The creamy pinto beans paired with the spicy flavors from Mexico tastes even better after a day or two in the fridge, so be sure to make enough for lunch leftovers!

Note: You'll need cooked rice for this recipe.

Ingredients

3 Tbsp / 45 ml extra virgin olive oil

1 tsp / 5 ml ground cumin

1 tsp / 5 ml ground coriander

1 tsp / 5 ml ground cinnamon

1 Tbsp / 15 ml chili powder

1 medium onion, peeled and chopped

3 cloves garlic, chopped

2 cups / 480 ml cooked brown rice

4 cups / 960 ml canned pinto beans (or cooked
   from dried), drained and well rinsed

1½ to 2 cups / 360 ml – 480 ml low-sodium chicken
   or vegetable stock

3 Tbsp / 45 ml chipotle peppers, chopped,
   plus sauce

2 Tbsp / 30 ml tomato paste

1 tsp / 5 ml sea salt

Nutritional Value Per Serving:

Calories: 230 | Calories from Fat: 62 | Protein: 9g | Carbs: 34g |
Total Fat: 0g | Saturated Fat: 1g | Trans Fat: 0g | Fiber: 7g |
Sodium: 602mg | Cholesterol: 0mg | Sugar: 2g

Method

1 Heat oil in Dutch oven over medium heat. Add cumin, coriander, cinnamon and chili powder. Heat until fragrant.

2 Add chopped onion and cook until soft. Add garlic and cook a few minutes more.

3 Add cooked rice and rinsed beans, stock, chipotles, tomato paste and salt. Reduce heat and simmer for 20 minutes. Serve hot.

TIP 1 Add diced chicken or turkey breast to the dish to boost up the protein intake.

TIP 2 Serve with crisp tortillas and salsa.

TIP 3 If you are using canned beans, be sure to rinse well. This helps reduce the sodium.

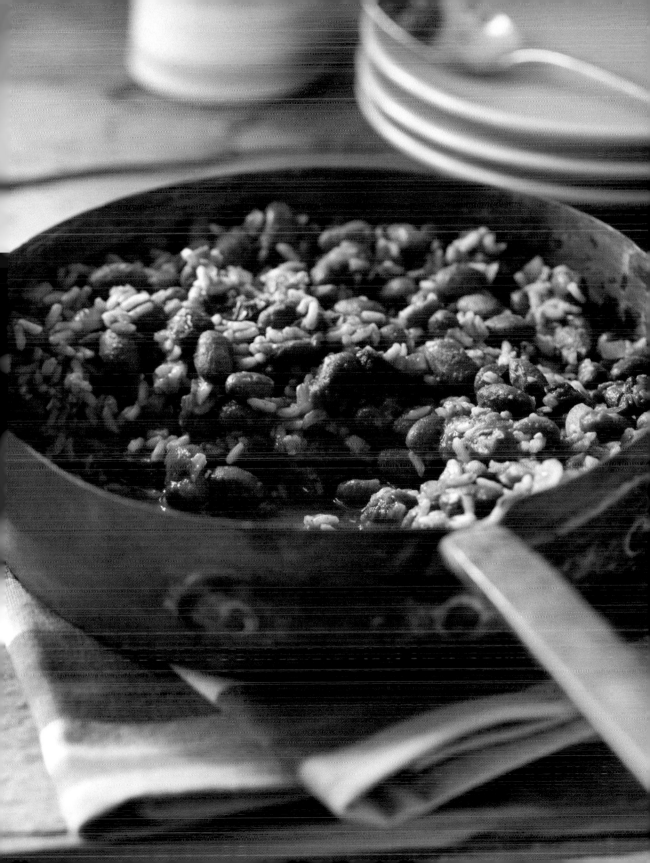

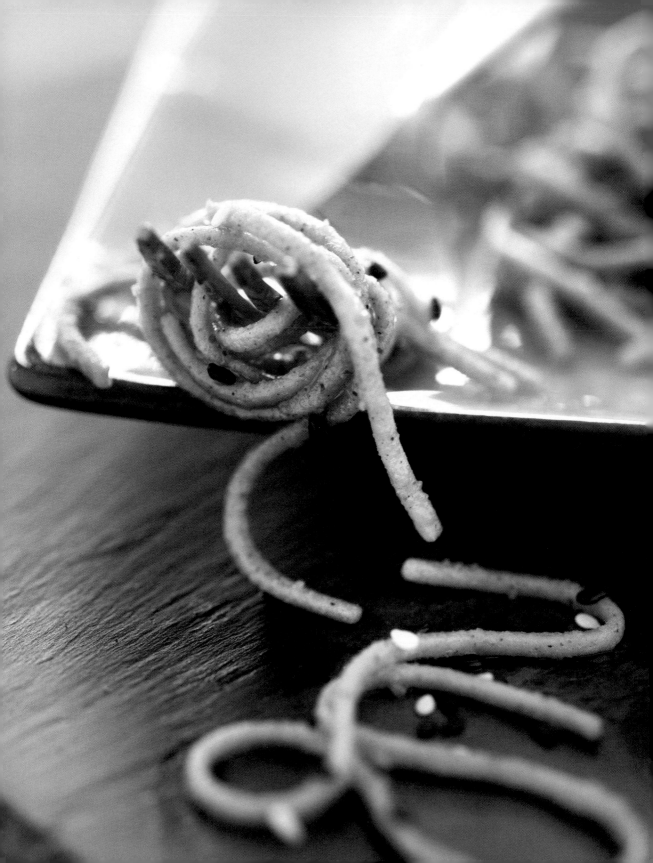

Sesame Noodles

Any recipe with nut sauce tastes decadent to me. Substituting peanut butter for almond gives this easy-to-prepare classic Asian noodle dish a rich, nutty twist. Try it with cashew butter for even more variety, and pair it with leftover veggies and chicken or shrimp to round out your Eat-Clean meal.

Ingredients

2 Tbsp / 30 ml tahini

2 Tbsp / 30 ml almond butter (or other natural nut butter of choice)

2 Tbsp / 30 ml brown rice vinegar

1 Tbsp / 15 ml agave nectar

2 Tbsp / 30 ml low-sodium tamari

1 tsp / 5 ml roasted sesame seed oil

1 x 8 oz package soba noodles cooked according to package instructions

2 Tbsp / 30 ml sesame seeds, toasted (black or white or combination of both)

Sea salt, to taste

Method

1 In medium saucepan combine tahini, almond butter, brown rice vinegar, agave nectar, tamari and sesame seed oil. Whisk mixture over gentle heat until well combined and a smooth sauce results.

2 Add cooked soba noodles to sauce and toss to coat. Sprinkle noodles with toasted sesame seeds and season with sea salt.

3 Serve hot.

Nutritional Value Per Serving:
Calories: 194 | Calories from Fat: 102 | Protein: 7g | Carbs: 17g |
Total Fat: 0g | Saturated Fat: 1.5g | Trans Fat: 0g | Fiber: 2g |
Sodium: 490mg | Cholesterol: 0mg | Sugar: 0g

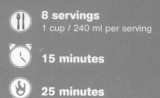

8 servings
1 cup / 240 ml per serving

15 minutes

25 minutes

African Potatoes & Beans

I've listed this recipe as a side, but it's definitely hearty enough to stand as a meal by itself. This dish is subtly seasoned and is perfect for any palate. The more adventurous can zest it up with a dash or two (or three!) of hot sauce.

Ingredients

2 Tbsp / 30 ml coconut butter (if unavailable, use olive oil)

1 red onion, peeled and sliced thin

2 stalks celery, leaves included, chopped

2 cloves garlic, passed through a garlic press

2 cups / 480 ml low-sodium chicken or vegetable stock

½ lb / 227 g red potatoes, coarsely chopped

½ lb / 227 g sweet potatoes, peeled and coarsely chopped

½ tsp / 2.5 ml sea salt

Freshly ground black pepper, to taste

1 x 15 oz can beans (any kind you like), rinsed and drained

1 x 15 oz can chickpeas, rinsed and drained

2 Tbsp / 30 ml tomato paste

1 Tbsp / 15 ml unsulfured molasses

Dash hot pepper sauce

¼ cup / 60 ml pumpkin seeds, toasted (optional)

Method

1 In Dutch oven or heavy-bottomed fry pan, heat coconut butter over medium-high heat. Add onion and celery and sauté until soft, about five minutes. Add garlic and heat through.

2 Add stock, both kinds of potatoes, salt and pepper. Boil mixture until potatoes are semi-soft, about 10 minutes.

3 Add beans, chickpeas, tomato paste, and molasses, and let simmer for 5 to 10 minutes or until heated through. Keep an eye on the pot, stirring once in a while so nothing sticks to the bottom.

4 Adjust flavor with salt, pepper and a dash of hot sauce.

5 Serve hot with grilled chicken or turkey. Garnish each dish with pumpkin seeds (if desired).

Nutritional Value Per Serving:
Calories: 221 | Calories from Fat: 38 | Protein: 8g | Carbs: 40g |
Total Fat: 4g | Saturated Fat: 2g | Trans Fat: 0g | Fiber: 6.5g |
Sodium: 231mg | Cholesterol: 0mg | Sugar: 6g

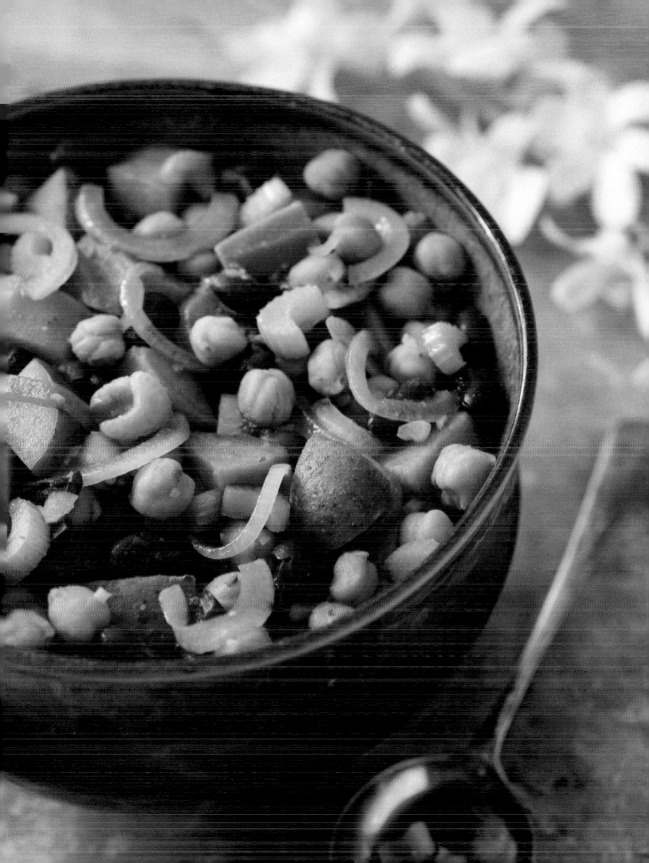

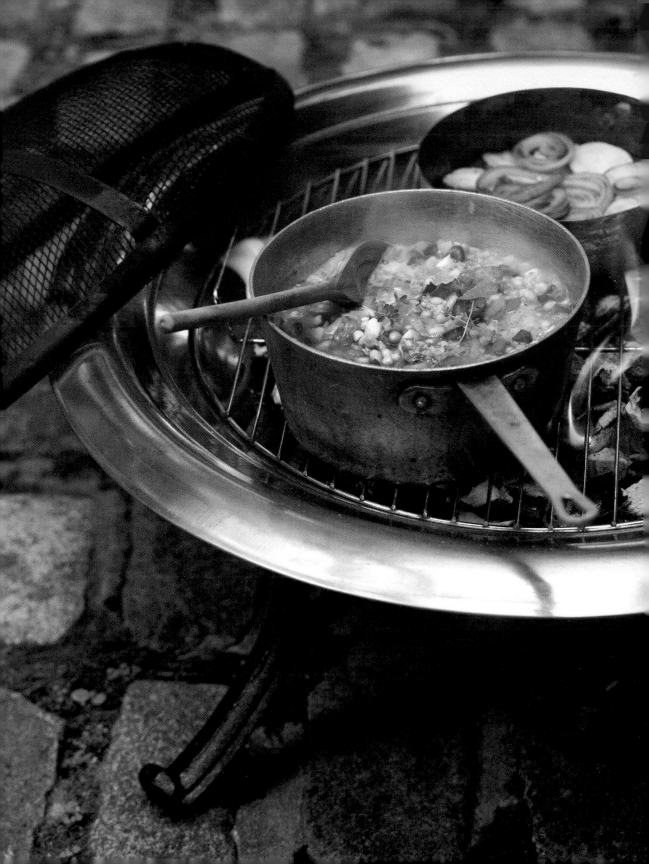

Braised Beans

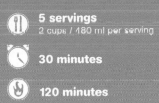

5 servings
2 cups / 480 ml per serving

30 minutes

120 minutes

Traditionally, braising means to cook something slowly in fat, in a closed pot with little moisture. In this recipe, I've removed the fat but kept the flavor … you can thank me later! Beans, beans – really are good for your heart!

Ingredients

1 cup / 240 ml dried beans of your choice, soaked overnight

5 bay leaves

1 small onion, left whole

4 sprigs fresh thyme, left whole, divided

2 sprigs fresh rosemary, left whole, divided

2 Tbsp / 30 ml coconut butter (if unavailable, use olive oil)

2 small yellow onions, peeled and chopped

3 cloves garlic, passed through a garlic press

5 Brussels sprouts, tough ends removed and finely chopped

1 small turnip or ½ regular sized turnip, peeled and finely chopped

2 stalks celery, leaves included, trimmed and finely chopped

1 large carrot, peeled, trimmed and finely chopped

1 tsp / 5 ml sea salt

½ tsp / 2.5 ml freshly ground black pepper

1 tsp / 5 ml finely chopped fresh thyme

1 cup / 240 ml low-sodium vegetable stock

4 fresh tomatoes, chopped (enough to make one heaping cup)

Note: On the night before you plan to make this dish, soak 1 cup / 240 ml dried beans of your choice – navy, Great Northern, broad, Lima etc. – in plenty of water and let sit overnight. Plenty of water means at least 5 cups / 1.2 L.

Method

1 After soaking beans overnight, drain and place in large soup pan or Dutch oven. Cover with about 6 cups / 1.5 L ml water and add bay leaves, whole onion, 2 sprigs thyme and 1 sprig rosemary. Bring to a boil over high heat. Reduce and let cook for an hour or until beans begin to split. Remove from heat. Drain and rinse. Set aside.

2 Meanwhile, heat coconut butter in Dutch oven over medium-high heat. Sauté onion, garlic, Brussels sprouts, turnip, celery and carrot until vegetables become soft.

3 Add sea salt, pepper, fresh thyme, remaining sprigs of thyme and rosemary, stock and tomatoes. Add beans. Let simmer over low heat for about 35 minutes. Serve hot.

Nutritional Value Per Serving:
Calories: 219 | Calories from Fat: 55 | Protein: 10g | Carbs: 33g | Total Fat: 6g | Saturated Fat: 3g | Trans Fat: 0g | Fiber: 8g | Sodium: 454mg | Cholesterol: 0mg | Sugar: 4g

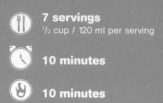
Golden Couscous

Couscous should be a staple in every pantry. This version is seasoned with saffron, a spice popular in Persian, Asian, European and Indian cuisines that is well known for its healing properties. Pigments of saffron have been found in 50,000-year-old paintings of prehistoric beasts. Sounds tested and true to me!

Ingredients

1 small leek, whites and light green only,
   finely chopped (about ⅓ cup / 80 ml)
1 clove garlic, passed through a garlic press
2 Tbsp / 30 ml finely chopped fresh parsley
1½ cups / 360 ml low-sodium chicken or
   vegetable stock
Pinch ground cumin
Several saffron threads, crumbled (you can use
   turmeric instead for a slightly different flavor)
1 cup / 240 ml couscous

Method

1 Place chopped leek, garlic and parsley in a medium saucepan with the stock, cumin and saffron. Bring to a boil.

2 Add couscous and cover tightly. Remove from heat immediately and let sit for several minutes to allow grains to absorb stock and flavorings.

3 Fluff with a fork before serving.

TIP An adult serving of cooked couscous is approximately ½ cup / 120 ml. Keep your portions in check!

Nutritional Value Per Serving:
Calories: 51 | Calories from Fat: 2 | Protein: 2g | Carbs: 10g |
Total Fat: 0g | Saturated Fat: 0g | Trans Fat: 0g | Fiber: 1g |
Sodium: 0mg | Cholesterol: 0mg | Sugar: 0.5g

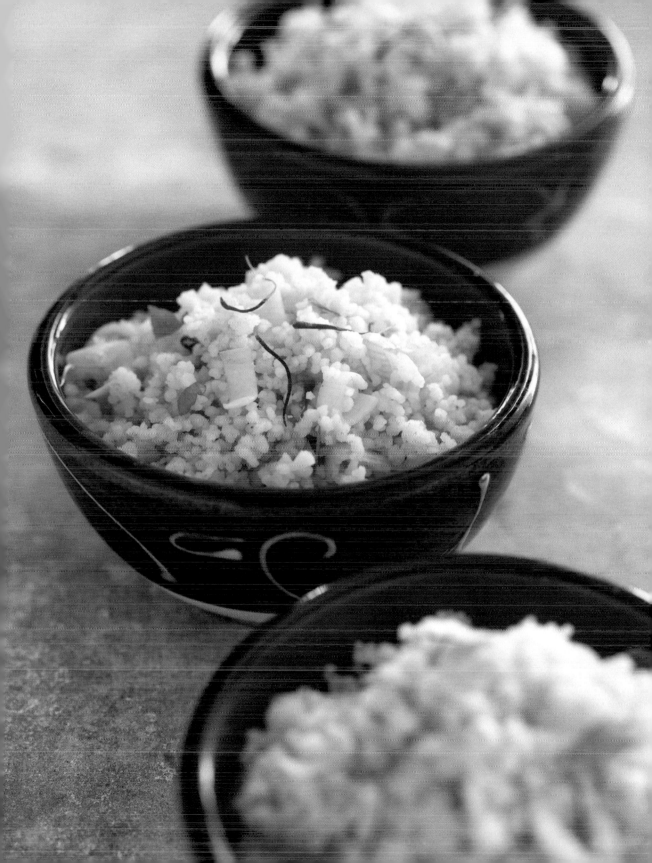

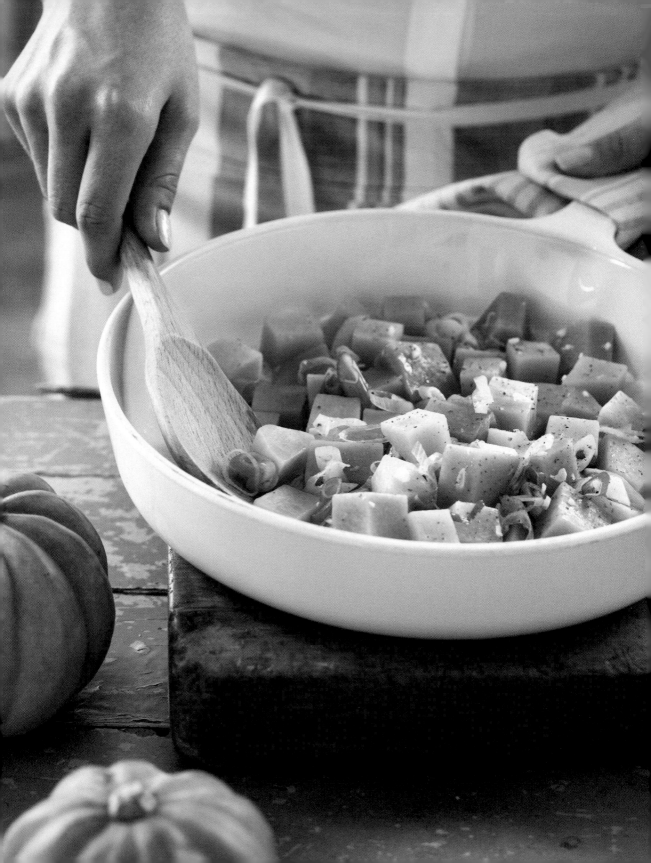

Brazilian Style Pumpkin

I believe that pumpkin is the new up-and-coming superfood, because it is dense with healthful nutrients and fiber. This recipe makes the very best of pumpkin by highlighting its rich flavor and wonderful texture.

Ingredients

2 Tbsp / 30 ml extra virgin olive oil

1 bunch scallions, trimmed and chopped into small pieces on the diagonal

2 cloves garlic, passed through a garlic press

3 cups / 720 ml pumpkin cubes (if you don't have pumpkin use a winter squash)

½ tsp / 2.5 ml sea salt

¼-½ cup / 60 ml-120 ml natural apple juice

Pinch cinnamon

Method

1 In Dutch oven heat olive oil over medium heat. Add scallions and cook briefly.

2 Add garlic, pumpkin, salt, apple juice and cinnamon. Cover and cook on low heat for 15 minutes or until pumpkin is soft. You may have to add more apple juice or water to keep the pumpkin from sticking to the bottom of the pan.

3 Serve hot as a side dish to any meat.

Nutritional Value Per Serving:
Calories: 107 | Calories from Fat: 61 | Protein: 1.5g | Carbs: 12g |
Total Fat: 7g | Saturated Fat: 1g | Trans Fat: 0g | Fiber: 1.5g |
Sodium: 202mg | Cholesterol: 0mg | Sugar: 5g

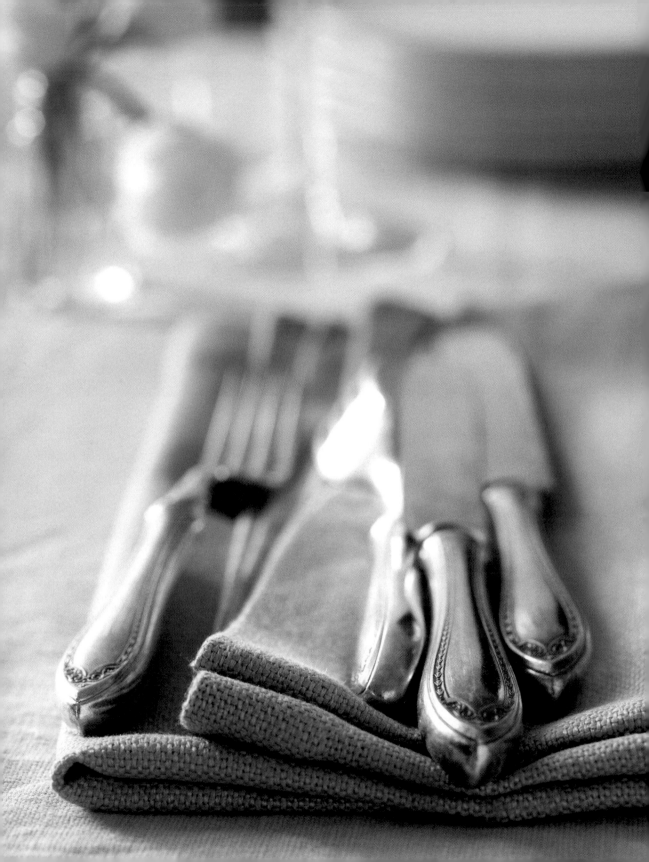

COMPLETE MEALS

7

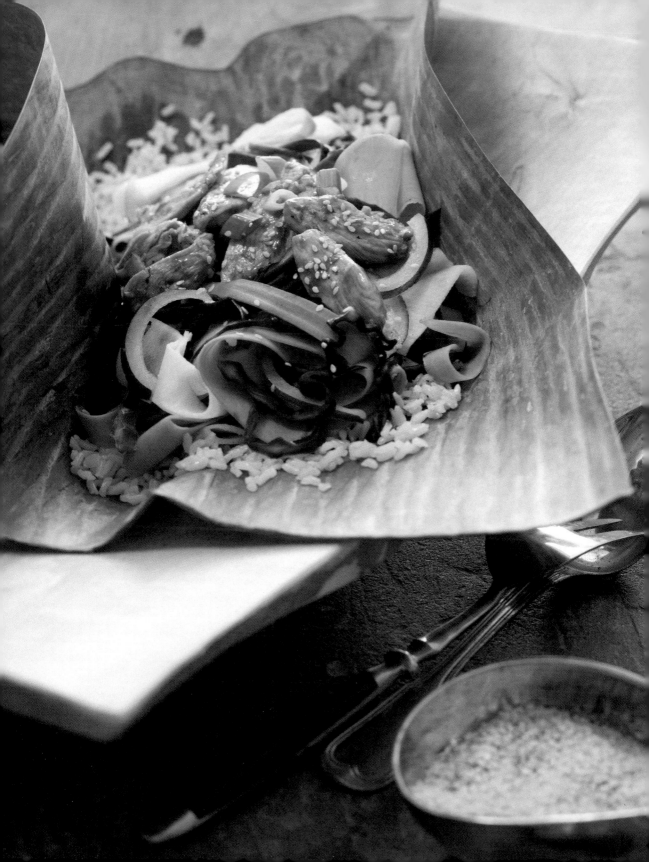

Colorful Chicken Stir-fry with Sweet Potatoes & Hoisin

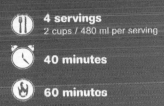

4 servings
2 cups / 480 ml per serving

40 minutes

60 minutes

Although hoisin is traditionally made from sweet potatoes, this Chinese dipping sauce is also referred to as "suckling pig sauce!" The name itself means "seafood," although there are no pigs or fish in the ingredients list. Thankfully, there is nothing confusing about the taste of this savory stir-fry.

Ingredients

2 Tbsp / 30 ml roasted sesame oil, divided

2 boneless, skinless chicken breasts,
    cut into ¼-inch strips

2 sweet potatoes, peeled and cut into ribbons

1 large purple onion, peeled and cut into ribbons

1 turnip, peeled and cut into ribbons

1 carrot, peeled and cut into ribbons

1 Tbsp / 15 ml fresh ginger, minced

3 cloves garlic, passed through a garlic press

4 - 5 cups / 960 - 1200 ml red cabbage, sliced

3 Tbsp / 45 ml Hoisin sauce

4 Tbsp / 60 ml sesame seeds, toasted

4 scallions, trimmed and chopped on the diagonal

Method

1 Heat 1 Tbsp / 15 ml oil over medium-high heat. Stir-fry chicken strips until cooked.

2 Add more oil if necessary and stir-fry potatoes, onion, turnip and carrot until tender-crisp. Add ginger and garlic. Cook two minutes more.

3 Add red cabbage and stir-fry until soft, adding more oil if needed.

4 Add hoisin sauce and reduce heat. Toss to coat.

5 Divide mixture among four heated serving bowls. Garnish with sesame seeds and scallions.

Nutritional Value Per Serving:
Calories: 246 | Calories from Fat: 73 | Protein: 28g | Carbs: 13g |
Total Fat: 8g | Saturated Fat: 1g | Trans Fat: 0g | Fiber: 2g |
Sodium: 112mg | Cholesterol: 69mg | Sugar: 3g

TIP You can serve this over cooked brown rice to make a complete meal.

Red Snapper with Vegetables

4 servings

40 minutes

50 minutes

Red snapper is a delicate-tasting fish that is very versatile in recipes. The simple baking method in this recipe allows the natural flavor of the fish to shine through. Paired with vegetables, this delectable dish is a light meal that doesn't scrimp on taste.

Note: This recipe requires that you prepare Fig Vinegar in advance (see below).

Ingredients

1 cup / 240 ml grape tomatoes

1 Tbsp / 15 ml olive oil, divided

¼ cup / 60 ml Fig Vinegar* (or red wine vinegar)

4 tsp / 20 ml fresh basil, coarsely chopped

1 tsp / 5 ml dried oregano

1 bunch spinach, trimmed, tough stems removed, coarsely chopped

1 Tbsp / 15 ml coconut butter (if unavailable, use olive oil)

1 clove garlic, passed through a garlic press

2 small firm zucchini, trimmed and sliced into ¼-inch slices lengthwise

8 small, thin carrots, peeled and left whole

4 x 4 oz / 113 g fresh red snapper filets

1 tsp / 5 ml sea salt

Freshly ground black pepper

1 x 8½ oz / 250 ml can artichokes, drained and sliced thin

✳You can find the recipe for Fig Vinegar at www.eatcleandiet.com/figvinegar

Method

1 Preheat oven to 425°F / 220°C.

2 Slice tomatoes in half and place in skillet with olive oil and Fig Vinegar. Cook until tomatoes break down. Add fresh basil and oregano. Heat through.

3 Sauté spinach in new skillet with coconut butter and garlic until wilted.

4 Grill zucchini until soft but not mushy. It should remain intact.

5 Boil carrots until tender.

6 Prepare baking dish by coating with oil. Season fish with salt and pepper. Place fish skin side down in baking dish. Place in hot oven and bake until nicely done, about 10 minutes. If you wish to warm your artichokes, add them to oven in a separate dish.

7 Divide steamed spinach among four plates. Set one piece of fish on each pile of spinach. Divide remaining vegetables (including artichokes) among plates. Serve hot.

Nutritional Value Per Serving:

Calories: 243 | Calories from Fat: 71 | Protein: 12g | Carbs: 32g | Total Fat: 8g | Saturated Fat: 3g | Trans Fat: 0g | Fiber: 11g | Sodium: 609mg | Cholesterol: 10.5mg | Sugar: 14g

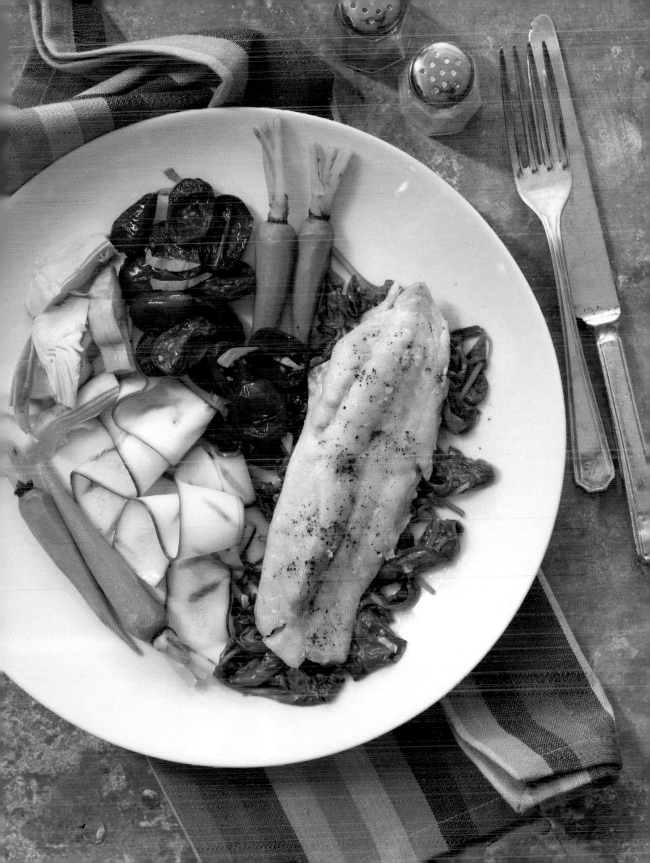

East meets West with this hearty steak served atop Japanese soba noodles, which are made from buckwheat and taste wonderful in both cold and hot dishes. Marinating the steak in Thai-style ingredients is the key to keeping it flavorful and tender, and serving this dish is a perfect way to get your meat lovers eating more greens!

TIP Make sure your pan has no plastic or wood on it or it will catch on fire in the oven!

Thai Steak on Soba Noodles

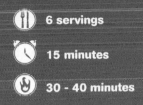

6 servings

15 minutes

30 - 40 minutes

Note: This recipe requires at least serveral hours' marinating time.

Ingredients

1½ lbs / 681 g flank steak, flattened to 1-inch
   thickness with a meat tenderizer

Juice of half fresh lemon

¼ cup / 60 ml + 1 tsp / 5 ml avocado oil, divided
   (if unavailable, use olive oil)

¼ cup / 60 ml chopped fresh cilantro

2 cloves garlic, passed through a garlic press

Dash Tabasco sauce (or other hot sauce of
   your liking)

3 tsp / 15 ml agave nectar

1 tsp / 5 ml sea salt, divided

1 tsp / 5 ml freshly ground black pepper, divided

½ cucumber, chopped

1 x 8 oz / 225 g package soba noodles

6 cups / 1.5 L salad greens (the darker green the
leaf,
   the better)

1 cup / 240 ml sprouts (broccoli, alfalfa or bean)

¼ cup / 60 ml sesame seeds, toasted

1 bunch green onions, trimmed and chopped
   coarsely on the diagonal

Method

1 Prepare marinade for steak by combining lemon
   juice, avocado oil, cilantro, garlic, Tabasco, agave nectar, salt and pepper in small bowl or Mason
   jar. Mix well. Set aside.

2 Place meat in lasagna pan or other shallow dish.
   Pour half marinade mixture over steak. Cover and let
   marinate for several hours in the refrigerator.

3 Preheat oven to 400°F / 200°C.

4 When ready to cook, remove meat from refrigerator.
   Using tongs remove meat from marinade and let it
   drip off a little before cooking. Discard this marinade.

5 Place chopped cucumber in small bowl and toss with
   three quarters of remaining marinade. Set aside.

6 Place 1 tsp / 5 ml of oil in large ovenproof skillet. Heat
   over medium-high heat. When hot, place marinated
   meat in skillet and brown on both sides, seasoning
   with salt and pepper while cooking.

7 Place skillet in oven and let meat cook for 10 minutes
   or to desired redness.

8 Meanwhile cook soba noodles according to direc-
   tions on package.

9 Remove meat from oven and place on cutting board.
   Let it cool while the soba noodles are cooking. After several minutes, cut meat on the diagonal in thin
   slices using a sharp knife.

10 Divide soba noodles on six plates. Place salad
   greens atop noodles. Divide sprouts among the six
   plates and arrange over greens. Drizzle remaining
   quarter of marinade overtop greens and sprouts.

11 Arrange marinade-tossed cucumber over the greens.

12 Divide cooked sliced beef equally on each
   plate. Sprinkle with sesame seeds and chopped
   green onions.

Nutritional Value Per Serving:
Calories: 764 | Calories from Fat: 246 | Protein: 54g | Carbs: 77g |
Total Fat: 38g | Saturated Fat: 8g | Trans Fat: 0g | Fiber: 5g |
Sodium: 1017mg | Cholesterol: 120mg | Sugar: 4g

Asian Noodle Bowls

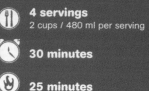

4 servings
2 cups / 480 ml per serving

30 minutes

25 minutes

On an evening when I am drawing a blank as to what to serve for dinner, I often turn to Asian noodle bowls because I can throw just about anything into the bowl and I can get it done fast. My favorite addition is greens. Anything from spinach to bok choy or nappa cabbage, rapini and even broccoli gets a turn swimming in the sesame-flavored broth. Make this your next "go-to" dish. It is so easy and so good you will surprise yourself.

Ingredients

2 large boneless, skinless chicken breasts, sliced into ¼-inch strips

2 Tbsp / 30 ml low-sodium soy sauce

1 tsp / 5 ml fresh ginger, minced

1 clove garlic, passed through a garlic press

2 Tbsp / 30 ml rice wine vinegar

2 Tbsp / 30 ml toasted sesame oil

4 cups / 960 ml low-sodium chicken or vegetable broth

1 package / 8 oz dry soba noodles or Asian noodles

½ cup / 120 ml frozen peas

2 cups / 480 ml broccoli spears

¼ cup / 60 ml thinly sliced sweet red pepper

1 small carrot, peeled and grated

4 green onions, thinly sliced on the diagonal

4 generous handfuls spinach

Method

1 Combine chicken, soy sauce, ginger, garlic, rice wine vinegar and toasted sesame oil in small saucepan. Over medium heat begin to heat mixture.

2 Add broth and bring to a gentle boil. Continue cooking until chicken is no longer pink – at least 10 minutes.

3 Add noodles, peas, broccoli and red pepper. Cook until broccoli turns bright green and is tender-crisp. Reduce heat and let sit, covered.

4 Stir in carrot and green onion.

5 When ready to serve, divide spinach leaves among four bowls at the bottom of each bowl. Ladle soup into each bowl, making sure to divide ingredients as evenly as possible. Garnish with peanuts (if using).

Optional

¼ cup / 60 ml roasted peanuts, chopped

Nutritional Value Per Serving:
Calories: 459 | Calories from Fat: 65 | Protein: 46g | Carbs: 56g | Total Fat: 6g | Saturated Fat: 1g | Trans Fat: 0g | Fiber: 5g | Sodium: 937mg | Cholesterol: 69mg | Sugar: 4g

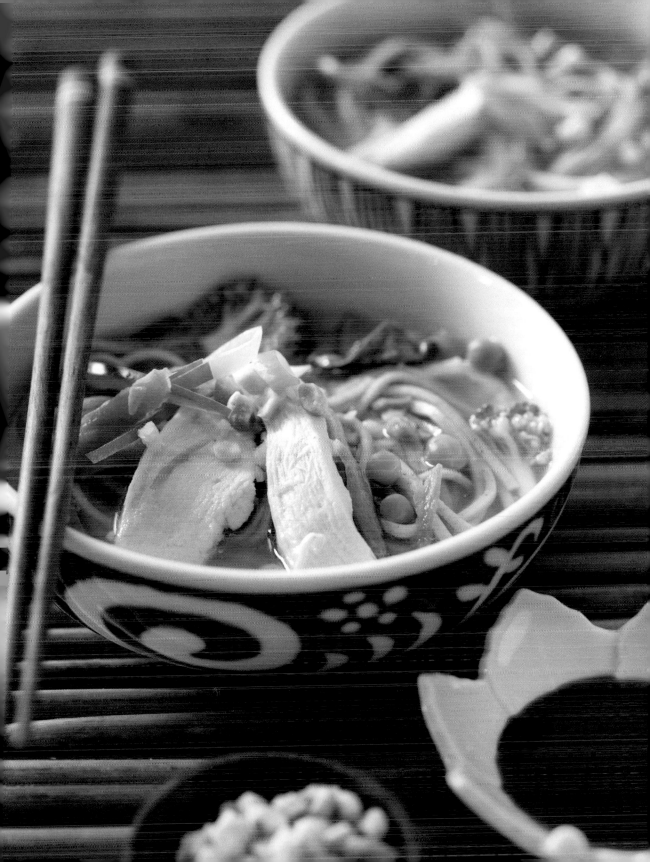

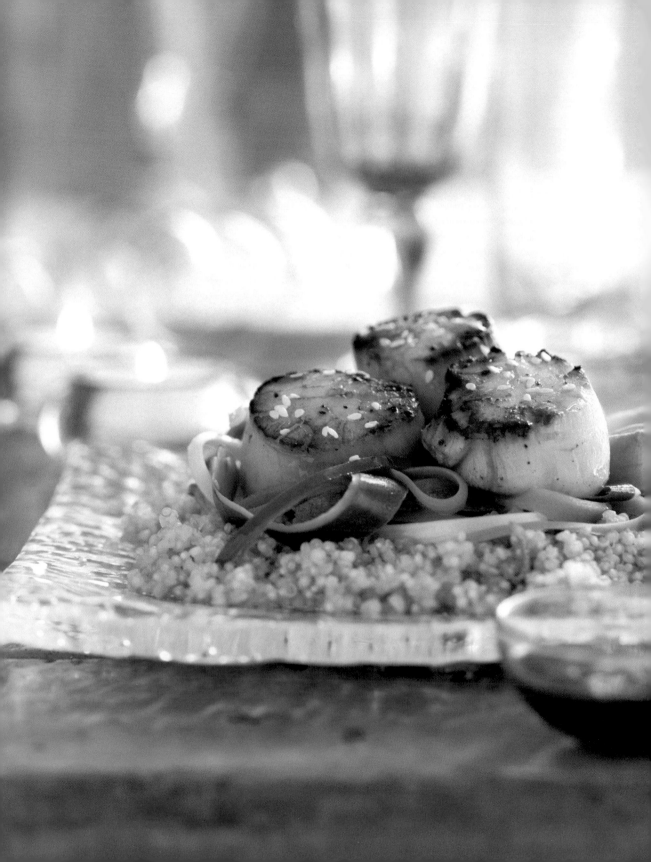

Scallops with Vegetables & Quinoa

4 servings

20 minutes

30 minutes

These scallops are crisp on the outside, and tender and moist on the inside – perfect for a family meal or a romantic dinner for two. Paired with vegetables with a hint of nutty flavor and served over a bed of fluffy citrus quinoa, this dish is packed with character and is guaranteed to impress.

Ingredients

1 lb / 454 g scallops or 3-4 scallops per person

3 Tbsp / 45 ml olive oil, divided

1 cup / 240 ml uncooked quinoa, well rinsed

2 cups / 480 ml low-sodium vegetable stock

6 small zucchini

4 similarly sized carrots, trimmed and peeled

1 red bell pepper, seeded and deveined,
     cut into long strips

5 scallions, trimmed, cut lengthwise into fours

Juice and zest of 1 fresh lime, divided

2 Tbsp / 30 ml white sesame seeds

2 tsp / 10 ml roasted sesame seed oil

½ tsp / 2.5 ml ground ginger

2 Tbsp / 30 ml low-sodium tamari sauce

Method for Scallops

1 Heat 2 Tbsp / 30 ml olive oil in skillet. Add scallops and pan sear over medium heat, two minutes per side. Remove from heat.

Method for Quinoa

1 Rinse quinoa grains well – this removes the bitter coating, so it's essential to do this before cooking.

2 Place rinsed grains in saucepan. Add 2 cups / 480 ml vegetable stock. Bring to a boil and reduce. Let simmer, covered, until all liquid has been absorbed.

Method for Vegetables

1 With a vegetable peeler, peel strips of green zucchini skin. Don't use white center part of zucchini. (You can use it later in a soup or stew.)

2 Peel strips from the carrots until you have reached the core. Don't use the core. (Again, use it later in a soup or stew.)

3 Heat remaining olive oil in skillet. Stir-fry red pepper, scallions, zucchini and carrots in batches.

4 Once all veggies have been stir-fried, season with lime juice, sesame seeds, sesame oil, ground ginger and tamari. Serve with scallops hot over quinoa and garnish with zest.

Nutritional Value Per Serving:

Calories: 460 | Calories from Fat: 159 | Protein: 29g | Carbs: 48g | Total Fat: 18g | Saturated Fat: 2g | Trans Fat: 0g | Fiber: 8g | Sodium: 516mg | Cholesterol: 37mg | Sugar: 8g

Thai Basil
Chicken Fried Rice

4 servings
2 cups / 480 ml per servings

20 minutes

45 minutes

Thai basil chicken fried rice, or Khao Pad Kra Prao Gai as it's known in Thailand, is a staple in Thai cooking. You can adjust the spices to make it as spicy or mild as you like. Mix it up it with beef strips or shrimp instead of chicken, and serve with chopsticks for authentic flair.

Note: This dish asks for cooked rice. If you have some on hand it makes the cooking time so much faster. Otherwise cook up a batch and you are ready to go.

Ingredients

4 Tbsp / 60 ml coconut butter (if unavailable, use
    olive oil)

2 shallots, peeled and finely chopped

2 scallions, whites and greens, sliced

4 cloves garlic, passed through a garlic press

2 boneless, skinless chicken breasts,
    cut into ¼-inch strips

2 Thai red peppers, cut into ribbons

2 Tbsp / 30 ml fish sauce

3 Tbsp / 45 ml oyster sauce

½ tsp / 2.5 ml sea salt

½ cup / 120 ml chopped fresh Thai basil

2 cups / 480 ml cooked brown rice

1 handful fresh cilantro, coarsely chopped

Pinch red pepper flakes

Method

1 Heat coconut butter in large wok over medium-high heat. Add shallots and scallions and stir-fry for a few minutes until fragrant.

2 Add garlic, chicken meat and red peppers. Stir-fry for four or five minutes.

3 Add fish and oyster sauces and sea salt. Stir-fry into mixture. Reduce heat slightly if too hot.

4 Add basil and rice. Stir-fry until heated through.

5 Serve hot, garnished with cilantro and a pinch of red pepper flakes.

TIP You can use leftover chicken in this salad – just make sure to cut down on the cooking time to avoid drying out the chicken.

Nutritional Value Per Serving:
Calories: 390 | Calories from Fat: 137 | Protein: 31g | Carbs: 30g |
Total Fat: 15g | Saturated Fat: 12g | Trans Fat: 0g | Fiber: 3g |
Sodium: 1341mg | Cholesterol: 69mg | Sugar: 2g

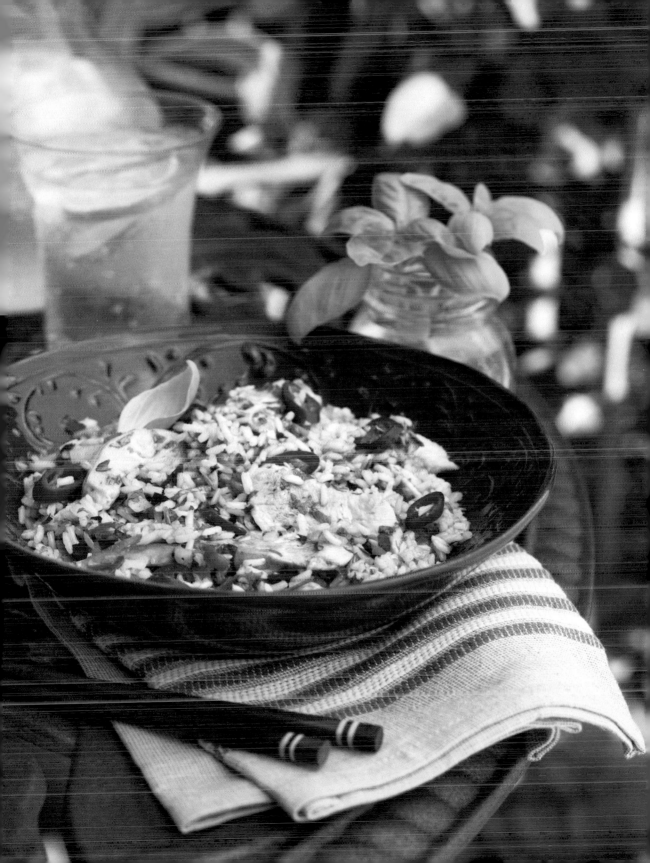

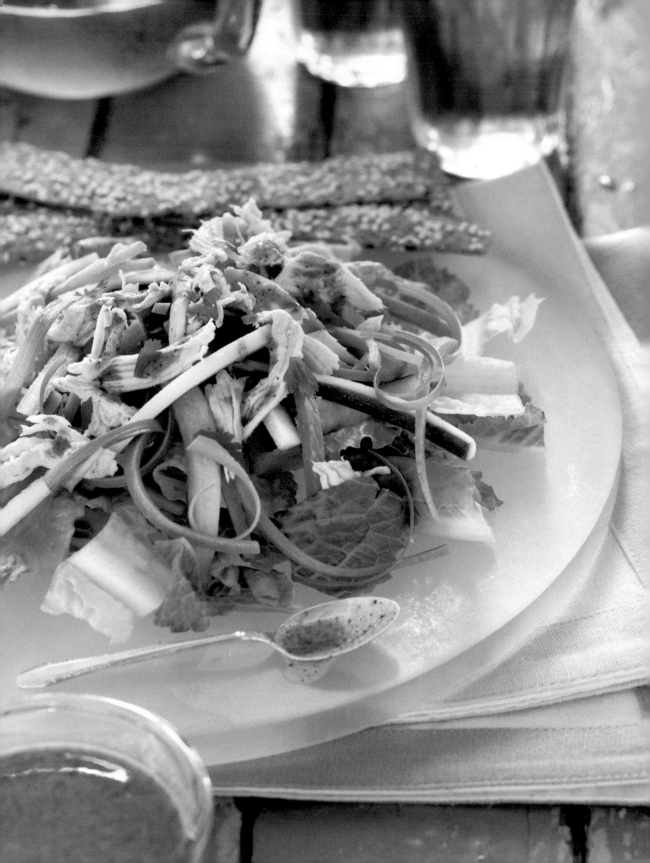

Chicken Explosion

The vibrant flavor of this dish gives it its name and disguises its healthy personality. It's easy to make so keep the Planned Leftovers strategy in mind – you can take extras for lunch the next day.

Ingredients

4 cups / 960 ml low-sodium chicken or
  vegetable stock

1 x 1-inch piece of fresh ginger, chopped

2 boneless, skinless chicken breasts

2 Tbsp / 30 ml natural nut butter (peanut, cashew
  or almond)

1 Tbsp / 15 ml natural honey

1 Tbsp / 15 ml coconut butter, melted (if unavailable,
  use olive oil)

1 dash hot chili oil

1 English cucumber, cut into matchsticks

1 bunch spring onions (about 4 or 5),
  sliced lengthwise into thin ribbons

1 firm zucchini, cut into matchsticks

2 carrots, cut into matchsticks (about 2 cups)

2 bunches Romaine lettuce, inner tender green and
  white parts only (save the dark green leaves for
  a salad), chopped

¼ cup / 60 ml coarsely chopped fresh cilantro

Method

1 Place stock in medium saucepan and bring to a boil. Add ginger. Add chicken breasts and let them cook over low heat until they are no longer pink inside, about 10 minutes.

2 Remove from heat. Using a slotted spoon, remove chicken from pan and let cool. Reserve cooking liquid for use in dressing.

3 To make dressing, combine nut butter, honey, melted coconut butter and hot chili oil in food processor or jar with tight fitting lid. Add ¼ cup / 60 ml cooking liquid. Process or shake well.

4 Combine cucumber, onions, zucchini and carrots with lettuce and toss well in large salad bowl.

5 Divide the salad among four plates. Shred cooked chicken over each salad.

6 Drizzle dressing over salad, garnish with cilantro and serve.

Nutritional Value Per Serving:
Calories: 381 | Calories from Fat: 105 | Protein: 37g | Carbs: 31g |
Total Fat: 13g | Saturated Fat: 3g | Trans Fat: 0g | Fiber: 10g |
Sodium: 610mg | Cholesterol: 69mg | Sugar: 13g

TIP Prepare the same dish with lean turkey breast!

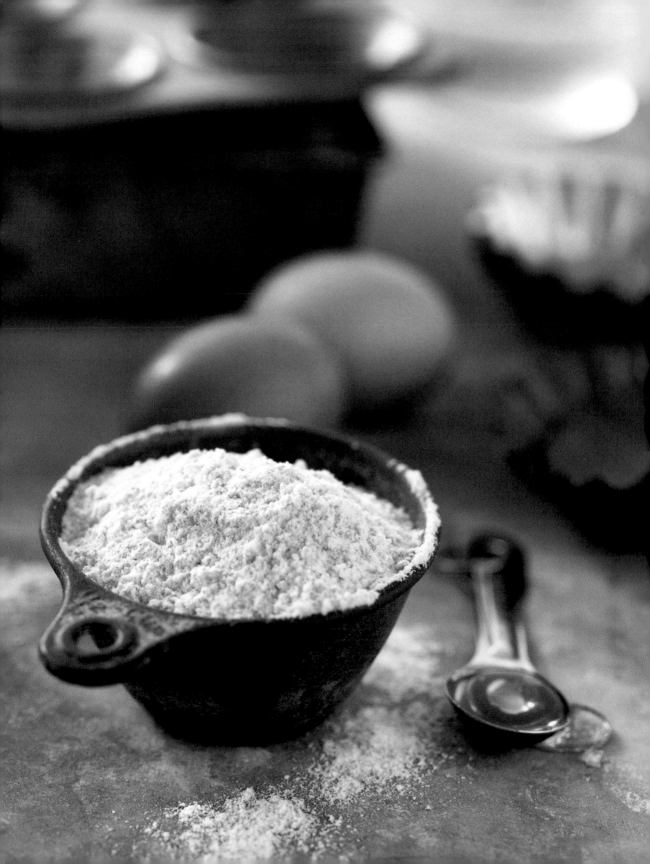

DESSERTS

8

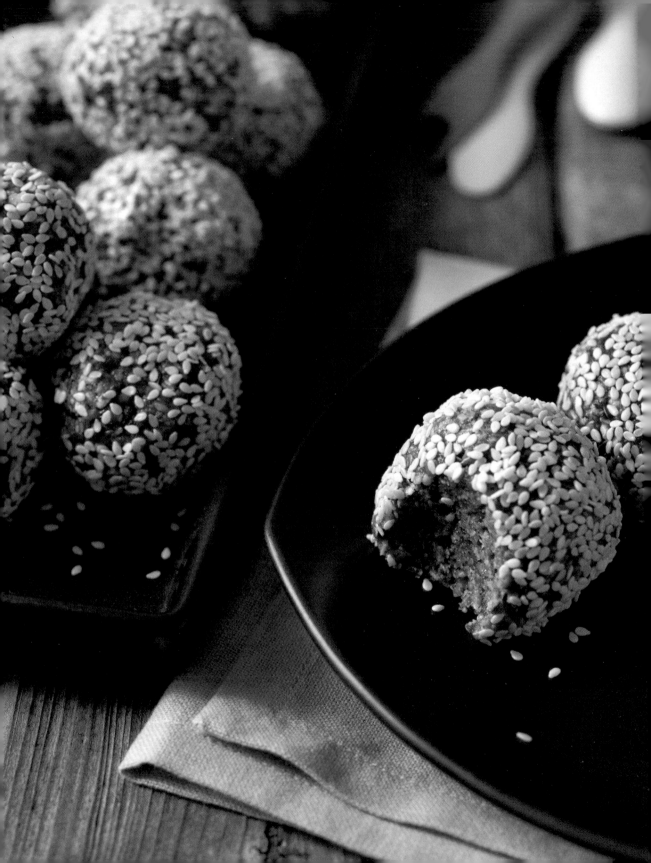

Power Balls

The quest for a pop-in-your-mouth hunger fix has waged long and wide in my home. The easier the better, and the gooier they are, the faster they disappear! These little dynamos require no cooking and are sure to be a family favorite. Anyone can make them — even your kids. Power up!

Ingredients

¾ cup / 180 ml dried apricots

¾ cup / 180 ml pitted dates

½ cup / 120 ml sunflower seeds

½ cup / 120 ml pumpkin seeds

¼ cup / 60 ml flaxseeds

4 plain brown rice cakes (spelt works too)

½ cup / 120 ml rolled oats

1 cup / 240 ml agave nectar

½ cup / 120 ml almond butter, slightly warmed

$1/3$ cup / 80 ml sesame seeds

Method

1 Place dried fruit and all seeds (except sesame seeds) in food processor. Process until crumbly.

2 Add remaining ingredients (except sesame seeds) and process until mixture is of even consistency.

3 Using a tablespoon scoop out mixture and shape into balls. Be sure to compact each ball so the mixture sticks together well.

4 Roll each ball in sesame seeds. Set on a platter and cover with plastic food wrap. Place in refrigerator.

Power Flour

Power Flour can be used in any recipe that calls for flour. Turn the page to see one!

Mix all ingredients together in an airtight container and store in the refrigerator.

¼ cup / 60 ml barley flour

¼ cup / 60 ml brown rice flour

¼ cup / 60 ml amaranth flour

¼ cup / 60 ml spelt flour

¼ cup / 60 ml kamut flour

¼ cup / 60 ml unbleached whole-wheat flour

Nutritional Value Per Serving:

Calories: 121 | Calories from Fat: 56 | Protein: 3g | Carbs: 14g | Total Fat: 7g | Saturated Fat: 1g | Trans Fat: 0g | Fiber: 3g | Sodium: 8mg | Cholesterol: 0mg | Sugar: 5g

Chamomile Tea Biscotti

22 cookies

20 minutes

50 minutes

Biscotti are hard-working cookies that double as dessert and can be part of your Eat-Clean meal as long as they are partnered with a few nuts. I love biscotti with a skim-milk latte.

Ingredients

2¼ cups / 540 ml Power Flour (see recipe page 385)

1 tsp / 5 ml baking powder

½ tsp / 2.5 ml baking soda

Pinch finely ground sea salt

⅛ tsp / 0.6 ml ground cardamom

3 egg whites and 1 whole egg

¼ cup / 60 ml fruit sugar

2 Tbsp / 30 ml natural honey

½ tsp / 2.5 ml best quality vanilla extract

2 Tbsp / 30 ml orange zest

1 Tbsp / 15 ml chamomile tea

½ cup / 120 ml dried currants

1 Tbsp / 15 ml coconut butter or olive oil

Method

1 Preheat oven to 350°F / 180°C. Prepare baking sheet by lining with parchment paper.

2 In medium mixing bowl combine dry ingredients: flour, baking powder, baking soda, sea salt and cardamom.

3 In another mixing bowl combine eggs and sugar. Using a wire whisk beat ingredients well. Add honey, vanilla extract, zest and tea. Whisk well.

4 Combine wet and dry ingredients. Add dried currants. Mix until combined.

5 Divide batter into two. Coat hands with coconut butter or olive oil and shape batter into two logs. Lay them on the baking sheet, giving each one room for expansion during baking.

6 Bake for 35 minutes. Remove from oven and let sit for about 10 minutes.

7 Reduce oven heat to 325°F / 162°C. Cut the cooled logs on the diagonal into 1-inch thick slices and arrange on baking sheet cut side down. Return to oven and bake again (that is what biscotti means – bake twice) for several minutes. Flip each cookie over to brown the other side for several minutes.

8 Remove from oven. Let cool and store in cool dry place.

What is Fruit Sugar?

Fruit sugar, also called fructose, is a simple sugar also found in honey and in some parts of plants. It is two times sweeter than regular sugar and has a lower Glycemic Index. Fructose can be found at better grocery stores and in health food stores.

Nutritional Value Per Serving:
Calories: 69 | Calories from Fat: 9 | Protein: 3g | Carbs: 13g |
Total Fat: 1g | Saturated Fat: 0.5g | Trans Fat: 0g | Fiber: 1.5g |
Sodium: 84mg | Cholesterol: 10mg | Sugar: 4g

When using tea for cooking it can be considered a spice. The same applies to coffee. Tea imparts a wonderful flavor to foods and should not be overlooked as a possible "flavor add" to foods. Brew a cup of tea and leave the tea bag in until you are ready to use it in the recipe, at least 15 minutes. Remove the tea bag and use as called for in recipe.

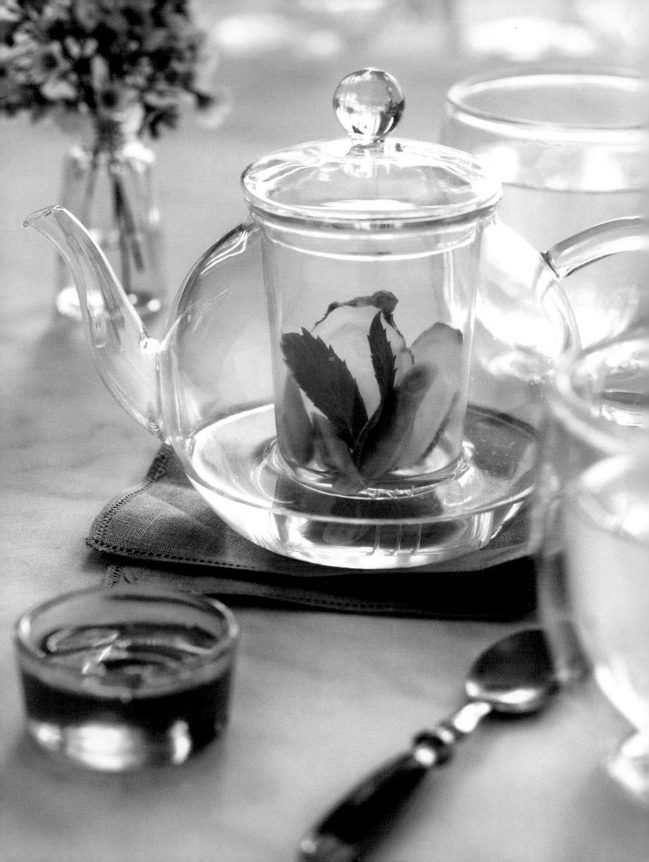

Lemongrass-Gingermint Infusion Tea

1 serving

5 minutes

5 minutes

There is no better way to relax than with a mug of your favorite tea. This infusion will not only calm you down, it will also aid your digestive system. Aaaah…

Ingredients

2 tsp / 10 ml dried lemongrass

3-5 fresh mint leaves

3 slices fresh ginger, thinly sliced

1 cup / 240 ml boiling water

Juice of ½ fresh lemon

2 tsp / 10 ml honey (optional)

Method

1 Spoon the lemongrass, mint and ginger into a mug. Pour hot water over the mix and let sit for five minutes.

2 Strain out the lemongrass, mint and ginger.

3 Squeeze lemon juice into the infusion and add honey if you need a sweet kick. Now sit back, relax and enjoy!

TIP 1 For a dramatic flavor combination, add lemongrass to your favorite flavor of tea. I like to combine it with chamomile or jasmine tea.

TIP 2 Chill in the fridge and serve over ice for a refreshing summer beverage.

Nutritional Value Per Serving with Honey:
Calories: 46.3 | Calories from Fat: 1 | Protein: 1g | Carbs: 14g |
Total Fat: 0g | Saturated Fat: 0g | Trans Fat: 0g | Fiber: 1g |
Sodium: 3mg | Cholesterol: 0mg | Sugar: 3g

Honey Almond Cookies

Sweetening treats with honey (instead of refined sugar) is popular in Europe – and a much healthier way to combat your cravings. Perfect with a hot cup of tea or a cold glass of milk, these delights will satisfy cookie monsters of all ages.

Ingredients

1 cup / 240 ml raw unsalted whole almonds, lightly toasted

1¼ cups / 300 ml unbleached whole-wheat pastry flour, fluffed with a fork

1 cup / 240 ml unbleached all-purpose flour

1 tsp / 5 ml baking powder

½ tsp / 2.5 ml sea salt

⅔ cup / 160 ml natural, organic liquid honey

¼ cup / 60 ml agave nectar

⅓ cup / 80 ml coconut butter, melted

¼ cup / 60 ml unsweetened applesauce

¼ cup / 60 ml ground flaxseed

1 large egg

1 tsp / 5 ml best quality vanilla extract

¼ cup / 60 ml sliced almonds, toasted (for garnish)

Method

1 Place almonds in food processor and process until well ground. Remove from processor and dump into large mixing bowl. Add flours, baking powder and salt. Mix well to combine.

2 In another medium-sized bowl combine honey, agave nectar, coconut butter, applesauce, flaxseed, egg and vanilla. Mix well with a mixer.

3 Combine wet and dry ingredients in larger bowl. Use clean hands to mix or mix well with wooden spoon.

4 Place, covered, in refrigerator for one hour to allow dough to set.

5 When ready to bake, preheat oven to 350°F / 180°C.

6 Prepare baking sheet by lining with parchment paper.

7 Using a 1 Tbsp / 15 ml measure, scoop out dough and shape into balls. Place on cookie sheet and press middle of dough down with your thumb to make a little well. Here is where you will place the almond slivers.

8 Bake each sheet of cookies for 12 to 15 minutes. Watch the last few minutes of baking so the cookies don't burn.

9 Remove from oven and let cool on a wire rack before storing.

10 Garnish with toasted almonds – be creative with your designs!

Nutritional Value Per Serving:
Calories: 107 | Calories from Fat: 44 | Protein: 2g | Carbs: 14g | Total Fat: 5g | Saturated Fat: 2g | Trans Fat: 0g | Fiber: 2g | Sodium: 41mg | Cholesterol: 7mg | Sugar: 7g

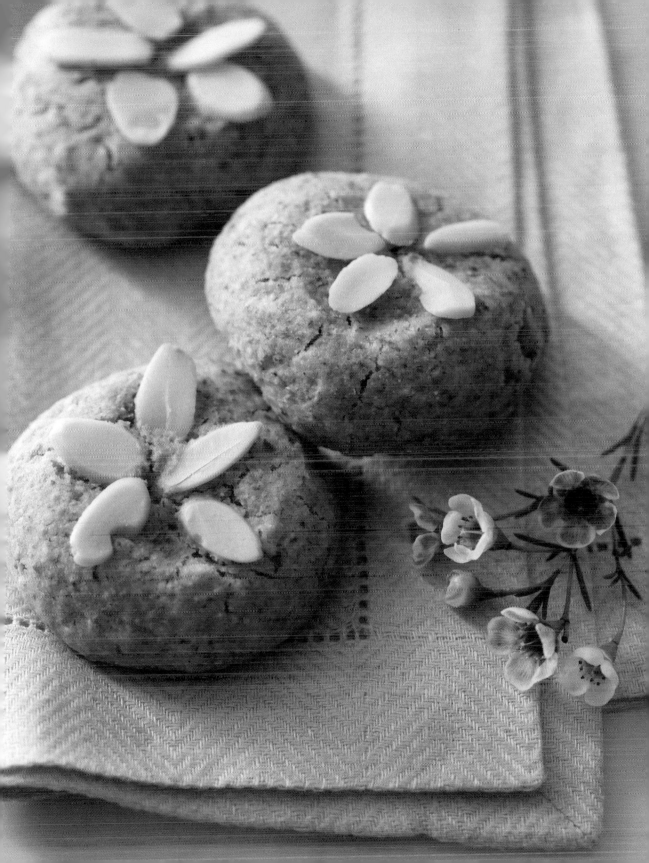

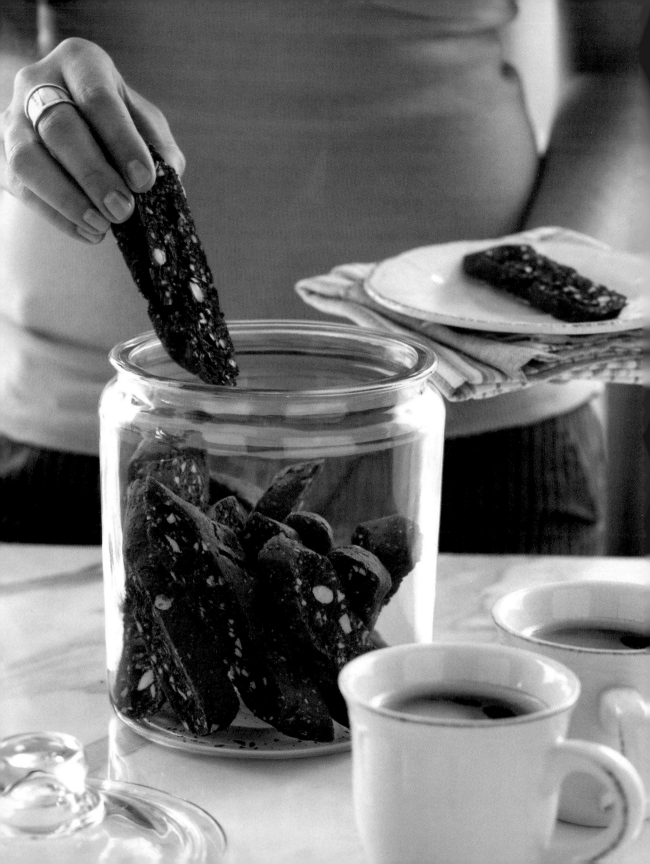

Chocolate Almond Biscotti

15 servings

30 minutes

40 minutes

Biscotti are wonderful Eat-Clean cookies to have on hand when you need a little something with your coffee. The dryness is nicely offset with a good crunch and the intense flavor of chocolate and almonds.

Ingredients

½ cup / 120 ml raw unsalted whole almonds,
    toasted and coarsely chopped, divided

½ cup / 120 ml unbleached all-purpose flour

1/3 cup / 80 ml whole-wheat flour

½ cup / 120 ml unsweetened dark cocoa powder

2 tsp / 10 ml instant coffee crystals

½ tsp / 2.5 ml baking soda

1/8 tsp / 0.6 ml sea salt

½ cup / 120 ml Sucanat or rapadura sugar

1 whole egg

1 egg white

1 tsp / 5 ml best quality vanilla extract

1 tsp / 5 ml almond extract

1 tsp / 5 ml grated lemon zest

Method

1 Preheat the oven to 350°F / 180 °C.

2 Line a baking sheet with parchment paper.

3 Put ¼ cup / 60 ml of the almonds, both flours, cocoa powder, coffee crystals, baking soda and salt in a food processor. Process for a few minutes until the almonds are finely ground. Put mixture in large mixing bowl. Set aside.

4 Combine Sucanat, egg, egg white, both extracts and lemon zest in a blender and process until mixture is foamy – three or four minutes.

5 Pour wet ingredients into flour mixture. Add remaining coarsely chopped almonds. Mix well.

6 Divide dough into two. Shape each half into a log and place logs on baking sheet.

7 Place baking sheet in the oven and bake for 15 minutes. Remove from oven and let cool for at least 10 minutes. Reduce heat to 300°F / 148°C.

8 Cut each log into ten ½-inch pieces. I like to cut mine on the diagonal.

9 Return the biscotti slices to the baking sheet and bake for about 20 minutes. Cookies should be dry and lightly browned.

10 Remove from heat and place on wire rack to cool. Only when completely cool and dry should you place the biscotti in an airtight container.

Nutritional Value Per Serving:
Calories: 94 | Calories from Fat: 28 | Protein: 3g | Carbs: 15g | Total Fat: 3g | Saturated Fat: 1g | Trans Fat: 0g | Fiber: 2g | Sodium: 63mg | Cholesterol: 14mg | Sugar: 8g

Chocolate-Coated Frozen Bananas

8 servings

10 minutes

5 minutes

This easy-to-make recipe tastes like a gourmet banana split – but it won't split your pants! Serve as a refreshing summer treat or at the end of a dinner party. I promise your guests will go bananas!

Ingredients

4 medium bananas, no brown spots

8 bamboo skewers

4 oz good-quality chocolate, 70% cocoa or darker

1½ Tbsp / 22.5 ml coconut butter (if unavailable, use olive oil)

2 Tbsp / 30 ml walnuts, chopped (the pieces should be small enough to stick to the chocolate)

Optional

1 Tbsp / 15 ml crystallized ginger, finely chopped

Method

1 Prepare small baking sheet by lining with parchment paper.

2 Peel each banana. Discard peels and cut tips off each banana. Cut each banana in half.

3 Insert a bamboo skewer into each piece of banana.

4 Lay pieces on baking sheet. Lay a piece of parchment paper gently over the bananas and place in freezer. Freeze for a few hours until banana is well frozen.

5 Before serving, melt chocolate and coconut butter gently in a double boiler. Add nuts and ginger (if using it). Mix well.

6 Dip each frozen banana piece into the chocolate mixture and return to baking sheet (or decorative platter lined with parchment paper) when done. Serve immediately.

Nutritional Value Per Serving:
Calories: 172 | Calories from Fat: 89 | Protein: 2g | Carbs: 20g |
Total Fat: 10g | Saturated Fat: 5g | Trans Fat: 0g | Fiber: 3g |
Sodium: 3mg | Cholesterol: 0mg | Sugar: 10g

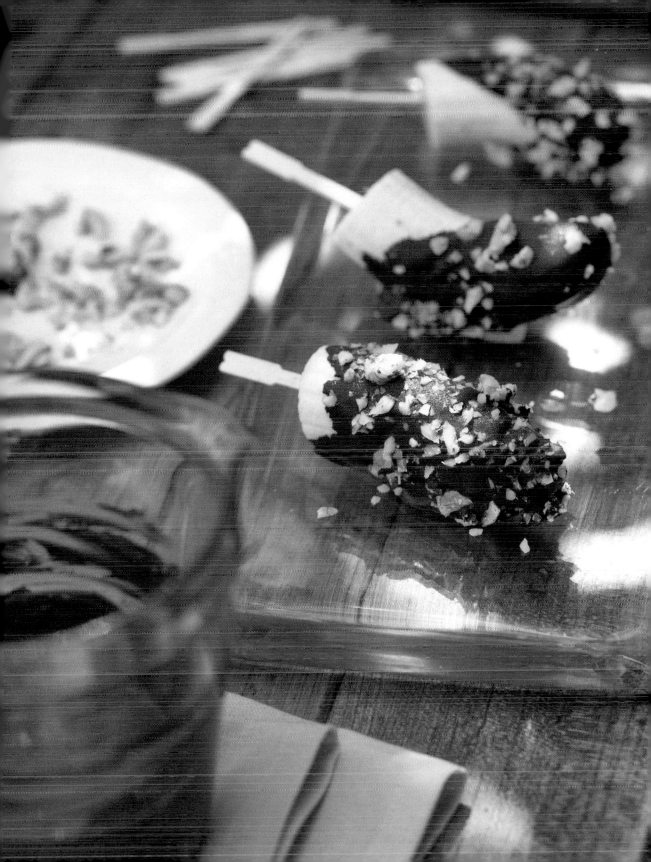

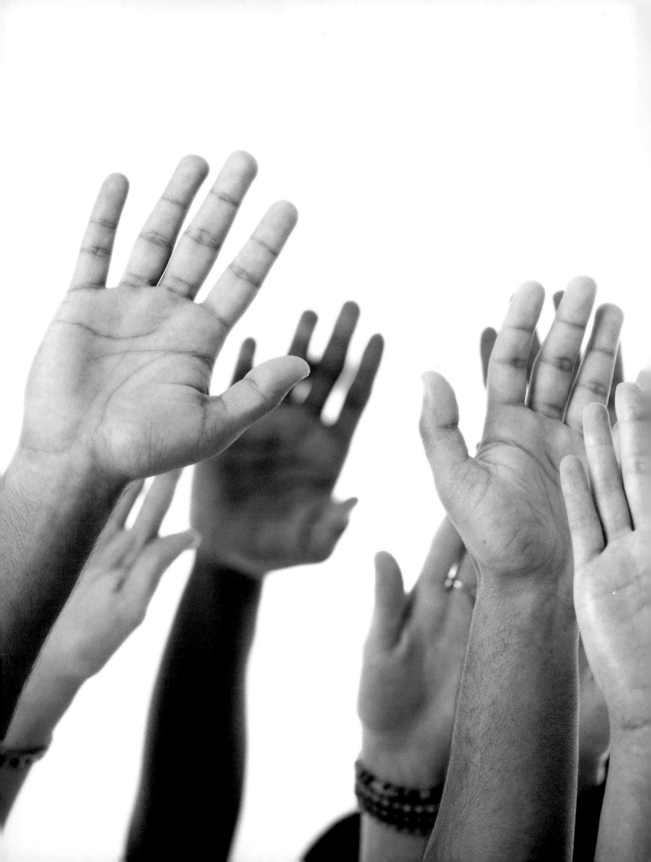

FREQUENTLY ASKED QUESTIONS

16

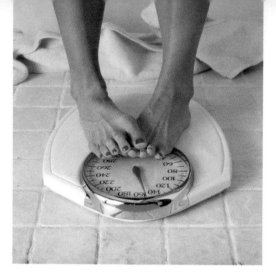

FREQUENTLY ASKED QUESTIONS

Q **HOW LONG WILL IT TAKE UNTIL I SEE RESULTS?**

A When you begin to follow the Eat-Clean life-style, you will find almost immediately you have more energy and your skin and hair become lustrous and healthy looking. This is the first sign that you are making a positive change to your health.

Each person will experience a different rate of weight loss. This is due to a number of different factors such as starting weight, genetics, the implementation of exercise and how much you dedicate yourself to Eating Clean.

Healthy weight loss occurs at a rate of two to three pounds per week. Some weeks you'll lose more, some weeks you'll lose less and some weeks you might not see any movement at all. (But don't let that discourage you! Have faith that a stall is temporary and that other positive changes are taking place inside your body.)

Losing weight at a healthy rate has numerous positive benefits. It helps your skin adjust, which mini-mizes any excess skin you might have after you fin-ish losing. Your heart, lungs and muscles also need a chance to catch up.

Q **CAN I FOLLOW THE EAT-CLEAN LIFESTYLE IF I HAVE AN ALLERGY AND/OR DIETARY RESTRICTIONS?**

A Yes, the Eat-Clean lifestyle is very flexible and can be adapted to work with any dietary issues. Just follow the Eat-Clean Principles and consume the foods you can. If you are allergic to gluten or can't eat seafood, then no worries – just don't eat them!

Q **CAN I FOLLOW THE EAT-CLEAN LIFESTYLE IF I AM A VEGETARIAN/VEGAN?**

A You do not have to eat meat, eggs or any other animal product to Eat Clean. You just have to make sure you consume protein along with complex car-bohydrates at every meal.

For meat-free Eat-Clean recipes, I use a lot of soy products such as tempeh, miso and tofu. You can also use lentils, beans and quinoa. I add edamame to soup, stews and pilafs. I also use textured vegetable protein, which works as a replacement for ground meat in any recipe. I add natural protein powder to my oatmeal and, of course, make protein shakes as well.

I have included many vegetarian recipes in all of my books in the *Eat-Clean* series, including this one.

Q CAN I FOLLOW THE EAT-CLEAN LIFESTYLE IF I HAVE DIABETES?

A If you are thinking of following the Eat-Clean lifestyle, I urge you to discuss this program with your doctor. However, many health care professionals have told me Eating Clean is exactly how they think diabetics should eat. I am certainly aware of many diabetics who use this program and whom it has helped.

Eating Clean helps to regulate blood sugar, which is one of the reasons this plan is so effective. That's why I don't suffer from the effects of hypoglycemia anymore. However, I want to reiterate that I am not a doctor, so make sure to show the program to your doctor for approval.

Q AM I TOO OLD TO SEE RESULTS?

A It is never too late to make a change for the better. Regardless of age, the Eat-Clean lifestyle can help you improve your health and physique. In fact, as I mentioned earlier in this book, I once received a wonderful letter from a woman in her 70s who had lost 75 pounds and went on to become a fitness instructor.

Q HOW MANY CALORIES SHOULD I BE EATING EACH DAY? HOW MANY CALORIES AM I EATING ON THIS PROGRAM?

A Calorie counting is not part of the Eat-Clean lifestyle. I never count calories. We now realize that different foods react in different ways in our body. Whereas we may lose weight on 2,000 calories per day of Clean food, we may gain weight on 1,600 calories per day of junk. Many, many people have messed up their metabolisms by worrying too much about calories and not enough about getting proper nutrition.

I promise that if you stick to the portion sizes I describe in the Eat-Clean Principles (on page 38), you will see results and meet your body's nutritional needs.

Q I DON'T THINK I CAN EAT THIS MUCH FOOD. IS EATING THIS WAY GOING TO MAKE ME GAIN WEIGHT?

A While it may seem like a lot of food, it's all Clean-burning fuel your body needs. Your metabolism requires constant maintenance to stay steady throughout the day. It's like putting good-quality gas in your car to ensure it runs at its best.

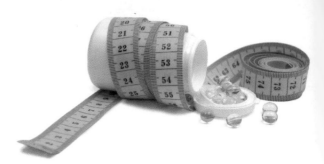

That being said, if you find you are not hungry within three hours of your last meal, you can try decreasing your portion sizes slightly.

Whatever you do, don't skip meals. Just one skipped meal instructs your body to slow down its metabolism.

Q CAN I FOLLOW THE EAT-CLEAN LIFESTYLE IF I WORK THE NIGHT SHIFT?

A The great thing about *The Eat-Clean Diet* is that it can be easily adapted to any lifestyle. Plan to eat six meals a day, every two-and-a-half to three hours. This goes for every day, whether you are working or not, no matter what time you wake up and go to bed.

For example, if you wake up at 2 pm and have your first meal of the day at 3 pm, then your next meals would follow at approximately 6 pm, 9 pm, 12 am, and 3 am. Just try not to eat within about four hours of your bedtime, whenever that is, unless you are truly hungry. Eat breakfast soon after you wake to start your day feeling energized and to get your metabolism humming!

Q DO YOU USE FAT BURNERS? CAN YOU RECOMMEND A BRAND?

A While I know many women who achieve results with fat burners, I have never taken them, so I'm not sure which ones are safe or effective. I was able to achieve my body through Eating Clean and lifting weights regularly, along with cardio. If you continue to Eat Clean, then the results will come. Fat burners alone won't cause you to lose weight. They may help you lose a little faster or a little more, but really the key is diet and exercise.

Q I AM OFTEN AWAY FROM HOME. DO YOU HAVE ANY ADVICE ON HOW I CAN EAT CLEAN WHEN I'M TRAVELING?

A I bring food with me to airports, always. Here is my emergency kit: raw almonds, apples, other hard fruit or fruit with a peel, hardboiled eggs, oatmeal and protein powder. What else I pack depends on when I might get a chance to eat it. I might pack chicken breast wraps and eat them before my flight. If they go straight from the fridge to my cooler, I know they'll be okay for a few hours, even without an ice pack.

It's inevitable that at some point I have to eat out when traveling, and when that happens I get food I know is Clean. Every airport restaurant has a salad, for example. It might not be the very best meal, but it beats French fries.

If you have to do a lot of driving for extended periods of time, your best investment is a cooler that plugs into your car. You can keep anything in there that you would in a normal fridge, and it will likely come with an adapter so you can plug it in at your hotel/motel as well.

Be creative, follow the Eat-Clean Principles, and success will follow.

Q **I'VE JUST STARTED EATING CLEAN AND I'M REALLY GASSY AND BLOATED. IS THIS NORMAL?**

A Yes, I'm afraid that reaction is quite common until you get used to this new way of eating. It's all the extra fiber and protein. However, you can help the problem by doing the following:

1. **Chew!** Whatever isn't broken down in your mouth must be broken down in your stomach, creating extra gas.
2. **Drink tons of water.**
3. **Take digestive enzymes or add kefir to your diet.** Both are inexpensive and natural ways to add healthful bacteria to your digestive system.

Once your body gets used to fibrous, healthy food, your gas problem should calm down.

Q **CAN I FOLLOW THE EAT-CLEAN LIFESTYLE IF I AM PREGNANT?**

A Eating Clean during your pregnancy is safe, but you should check with your health-care profes-

sional to ensure that you are getting everything you need for you and your baby.

You will need to pay attention to your calcium intake and avoid any supplements or foods that are not recommended during pregnancy.

Q **WHAT TYPE OF PROTEIN POWDER/PROTEIN BARS SHOULD I USE?**

A I do not recommend any brand of protein powder. However I do recommend you purchase it from a reputable company. Avoid products with fake sweeteners, sugars and other added chemicals.

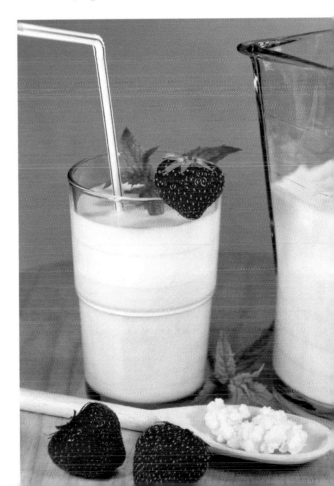

For the most part you should get your nutrition from real food. I do have smoothies quite often, but I load them up with lots of wholesome ingredients such as fresh fruit, flaxseed, plain yogurt, even tofu and oatmeal!

As for protein bars, unless I've made them myself I likely have fewer than two a year. Protein bars are great for times when you are caught with no food, but that should not happen very often if you plan ahead by packing a cooler. I've included recipes for protein bars in *The Eat-Clean Diet Cookbook* and *The Eat-Clean Diet for Family & Kids*. Creating your own protein bars is by far the best solution to this problem – this way you know exactly what you are getting.

ⓠ DO I HAVE TO FOLLOW THE MENU PLANS EXACTLY? I DON'T LIKE SOME OF THE ITEMS. CAN I USE DIFFERENT FOODS?

ⓐ The menu plans in *The Eat-Clean Diet* book series are merely suggestions. You don't have to eat something you don't like just because I've included it in the plan. Replace any of the foods, so long as you replace a complex carbohydrate with a complex carbohydrate and a lean protein with a lean protein. You can also switch foods, or move different meals to different parts of the day. Just remember to stick to the Eat-Clean Principles and you'll be fine.

ⓠ DO I HAVE TO COOK TO EAT CLEAN?

ⓐ You don't have to cook to follow the Eat-Clean lifestyle, although I like to prepare my own food –that way I can ensure it is 100% Clean. If you plan and prepare in advance, cooking will be quick and easy.

Here are some easy tips:

→ **Keep raw, unsalted nuts and nut butter around.** You can grab a piece of fruit and pair it with nuts for a complete Eat-Clean meal.

→ **Have whole-grain or Ezekiel wraps on hand.** Throw some cooked chicken breast, vegetables and hummus in a wrap and you've got a quick Clean meal.

→ **Cook large batches of food at one time.** Bake enough chicken breasts and boil enough eggs for a few days and keep leftovers in the fridge. My daughter makes large batches of turkey meatballs to use in wraps, with salad and vegetables and on whole-grain pasta.

→ **Keep vegetables and fruits washed and ready in the fridge.** These can be tossed into a salad, used for wraps or eaten with hummus or yogurt cheese. Buy prepackaged salads and keep them in your fridge.

→ **For breakfast have hardboiled egg whites with fruit, Clean granola or oatmeal with yogurt and fresh or frozen berries.**

> "Keep veggies and fruits washed and ready in the fridge."

A Lap band surgery and gastric bypass are both severe steps and should not be taken lightly. I hear from many people who have had gastric bypass who can never eat a normal-sized (not huge) meal again. Gastric-bypass patients have a hard time getting enough nutrients in their diet. They also often have a difficult time losing their last 50 pounds or so, because they can't eat enough food to keep their metabolism running high enough. The lap band procedure is adjustable and is better for getting enough nutrients once weight has been lost.

There are risks associated with both surgeries and the real key to success is not the surgery itself, but rather the change in eating habits, exercise and the way you view food. I always feel that the natural way is best – in other words, using nutrition and exercise to lose excess weight. And you must keep in mind that these operations are no magic bullet. Weight loss takes hard work and perseverance.

FOR MORE FREQUENTLY ASKED QUESTIONS, VISIT

www.eatcleandiet.com.

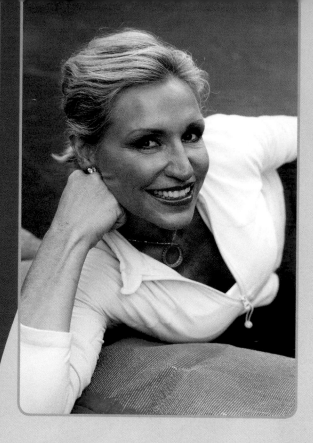

17

THE EAT-CLEAN DIET AT A GLANCE

YOU'RE READY!

After reading this book from cover to cover, you're ready to Eat Clean and watch the magic happen. I have no doubt that you are excited about starting this new phase in your life – a phase that includes a leaner physique, a healthier body and an even more sound mind.

Use these pages as a handy referral guide throughout your journey. If you find your weight loss has stalled or just need to refocus, look no further for solutions to your problems and answers to your questions.

BODY BEAUTIFUL/ BODY HEALTHY FORMULA

80% NUTRITION + 10% TRAINING + 10% GENETICS

= BODY BEAUTIFUL/BODY HEALTHY

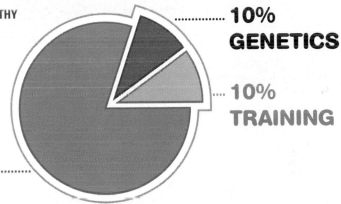

.... **10%
GENETICS**

.... **10%
TRAINING**

**80%
NUTRITION** ....

THE EAT-CLEAN PRINCIPLES

1. Eat six small meals a day. Eat every two-and-a-half to three hours.
2. Eat breakfast every day, within an hour of rising.
3. Eat a combination of lean protein and complex carbohydrates at each meal.
4. Eat sufficient (two or three servings) of healthy fats every day.
5. Drink two to three liters of water each day.
6. Carry a cooler packed with Clean foods.
7. Depend on fresh fruits and vegetables for fiber, vitamins, nutrients and enzymes. Limit your starchy complex carbohydrates to two to four servings each day.
8. Adhere to proper portion sizes.

PORTION GUIDELINES

PROTEIN: palm of one hand.

STARCHY COMPLEX CARBOHYDRATES: what can fit into one cupped hand.

COMPLEX CARBOHYDRATES FROM FRUITS & VEGETABLES: what can fit into two hands cupped together.

HEALTHY FATS: one scant handful of nuts, 1 to 2 Tbsp (15 to 30 ml) of oil.

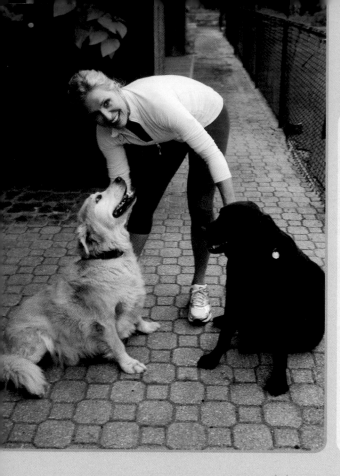

TOP TEN THINGS TO AVOID

1. Sugar, white flour and over-processed foods.
2. Artificial sugars.
3. Sugar-loaded beverages such as soda and juice.
4. Super-sizing your meals or portions.
5. Alcohol (try your best to limit alcohol).
6. Chemically charged foods.
7. Foods containing preservatives.
8. Artificial foods such as processed cheese slices.
9. Saturated and trans fats.
10. Anti-foods (calorie-dense foods with no nutritional value).

TOP FIVE WAYS TO MAKE EATING CLEAN EASIER FOR YOU

1. Pack a cooler each day.
2. Carry a water bottle everywhere.
3. Make a shopping list and stick to it.
4. Prepare planned leftovers.
5. Keep your pantry stocked with staples.

TOP FIVE EXERCISE TIPS

1. Set realistic goals for yourself – weekly, monthly and yearly.
2. Train all of your major muscle groups: arms, shoulders, chest, back, legs and abs.
3. Challenge yourself – vary your routine every few weeks.
4. Keep cardio fun – try new activities.
5. Stay focused – put your mind into your muscle.

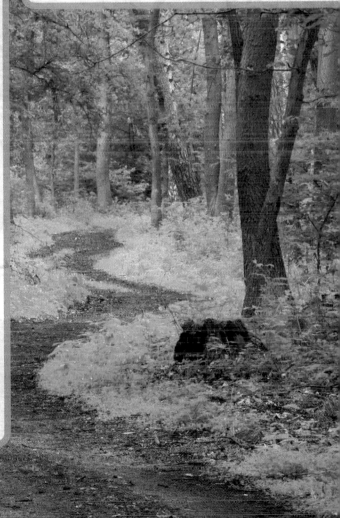

A NOTE ON MOTIVATION

Getting motivated is easy – it's staying motivated that is the hard part. Motivation has got to come from within you. Either you want to become healthier, lose weight and look great enough to stick with the program, or you don't. It's as simple as that. I can try to motivate you until I'm blue in the face but unless you are willing to make the necessary changes I'll never be able to convince you that Eating Clean for life is the way to go.

The truth is that there are many busy people out there. It seems like everyone has more obligations than they can handle – school, work, children and relationships … the list goes on! If you want to lose weight you'll have to make diet and exercise a real priority in your life. You are going to have to make a choice. You can either continue to make excuses and stay how you are forever, or decide that you really want to change and be determined to do what it takes.

Also, if you are struggling with Eating Clean, it's a good idea to constantly remind yourself of your goals and why you have made the decision to Eat Clean in the first place. Write down your goals and put them in spots where you can see them several times each day – in your car, on the refrigerator door, on the bathroom mirror, etc. When you have a clear picture of your goals in mind, it can be easier to stay focused.

VISIT EATCLEANDIET.COM FOR:

→ Motivational stories
→ Recipes
→ Fitness tips
→ Tools and support
→ Tosca's blog and forum
→ And lots more!

Make sure to stop by The Kitchen Table to post your own blogs, photos, meal plans and recipes.

CREDITS & ACKNOWLEDGMENTS

FRONT COVER PHOTO:
Paul Buceta

RECIPE PHOTOS (Chapter 15):
Donna Griffith

Marianne Wren (Food styling)

Martha Snyder (Photo assistant)

OTHER TOSCA RENO PHOTOS:
Robert Kennedy (pages 12, 15, 25, 39, 47, 51, 64, 70, 76, 81, 98, 111, 115, 143, 174, 186, 190, 203, 213, 234, 240, 404, 406)

Donna Griffith - Tosca and Garden Shots (pages 73, 132, 136, 137, 151, 173, 229, 237, 255, 256, 257, 403)

Paul Buceta (pages 7, 9, 22, 46, 109, 118, 192)

OTHER PHOTOS
Paul Buceta pages 166 and 178 (model: Linda Minard)

Stewart Volland page 43 and 238 (model: Leigh Hickombottom)

All other photos from istockphoto.com

PROP-STYLING FOR RECIPE PHOTOS (Chapter 15):
Jessica Pensabene and **Rachel Corradetti**

· ·

ACKNOWLEDGMENTS

Here we go again with another exciting book to add to our ever-growing series. *The Eat-Clean Diet Recharged* is my ninth book on a subject people can't seem to get enough of — Eating Clean! I have so many individuals to thank.

My *Eat-Clean Diet* Team Extraordinaire has spent countless hours making my words sing, with their collective graphic art and editing talents. Jessica Pensabene, who envisions "the book," lifts my ideas into reality and adds plenty of her own. Ellie Jeon and Brian Ross are two of the most talented creative people I know. Who else would be able to make oatmeal look exciting? Brian, thank you for holding your own among so many strong-minded women as you flex your significant creative muscle. Ellie, thank you for soldiering on in what has been a challenging year for you personally. Kiersten, thank you for assisting me with research — you dug up the good dirt! Rachel, I can't thank you enough for creating such delicious menu plans. It's a valuable tool that helps those who Eat Clean make sense of the process. I am also indebted to you for your creative style talents, which are evident in the resulting photos. I thank you for your dedication and support. Vinita Persaud, where would I be without your consistent edginess and talent in writing, both on the page and for the websites? Cali Hoffman, you came through with brilliant copyediting skills, for which I am grateful. Wendy Morley continues to make sense of the mayhem that is book publishing. Thank you for your strength and belief in me. I am indebted to you all.

With each successive project our intrepid photographer, Donna Griffith, perfects her craft. We have high expectations and she never fails us. Thank you once again for producing such brilliant photographs to accompany our recipes. Marianne Wren, our food stylist, is gifted with both torch and knife! Scary thought, but the food looks fabulous. I thank you.

Paul Buceta, an incredibly talented photographer, took my cover shot and several others. Every time we work together you find something more to bring out of me and into the lens of your camera. Your energy and skill at your craft dazzle me and I am so lucky to be part of your creative process. Your team Elle, Val, Sabrina and Rachel are part of my family now. It is a joy to work with you all.

A big thank you to James De Medeiros, who proofed and indexed the book. No easy task! Terry Snow and Ashif Tejani, I am grateful for your recipe-testing skills. I am proud to say that all of our recipes are completely tested before they are set out in my books. Thank you for manning up in the kitchen, boys!

I want to thank Robert Kennedy, my husband, and the man behind the idea of Eating Clean. I always knew how to eat but now I know how to do it Clean! Without this transformational idea I would still be digging into gallons of ice cream with a fork. Your dedication to my career is inspirational. I thank you. Our family is another year older. Rachel, Kiersten and Kelsey-Lynn have worked on numerous book projects, bringing that special energy only the young have. Rachel knows what's in my mind before I write it, so her translation efforts are much appreciated. Kiersten is a beam of light spreading her sparkle on all we do. Hand Kelsey a pot and a pan and she is happy making delicious food in the Eat-Clean kitchen. Chelsea sparkles with enthusiasm if you hand her a camera. No technology defeats her. Braden, Bailey and Davidson simply stand by as we rush about "creating." Thanks to all of you for being there. I am truly blessed.

None of this would be possible or worth doing if it weren't for you, the readers of my books and columns. I have learned so much through your probing questions and the result is this book. I thank you for your support. I really am always listening.

INDEX

OTHER TITLES IN THE EAT-CLEAN DIET SERIES BY TOSCA RENO

The Eat-Clean Diet Cookbook

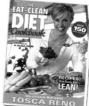

A perfect follow-up, this best-selling cookbook is bound to be your go-to guide for Clean meals, with over 150 recipes and gorgeous color photos throughout. From soups and sauces to main courses and desserts, Tosca touches on every food group, combining them into easy-to-prepare, delicious meals that are crowd favorites. Bonus info pages explain the Eat-Clean Principles, protein facts, sugar substitutes and more. Grab your apron and heat up the oven because delicious, healthy food is on the menu tonight!

The Eat-Clean Diet Workout

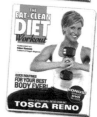

Eating Clean is a big part of the puzzle, but exercise is the missing piece. As a seasoned competitor and fitness columnist, Tosca shares her wealth of knowledge with you, including her own workout routines and secret tips from the best in the business. There are chapters devoted to each bodypart, tried-and-true equipment, training plans and nutrition. Whether you're a pro or a beginner, there is something for you in *The Eat-Clean Diet Workout*. Bonus 30-minute DVD!

The Eat-Clean Diet Workout Journal

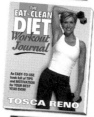

The perfect companion to your workout, *The Eat-Clean Diet Workout Journal* contains daily journal space for reps, sets, weights, exercises, cardio and goal setting. Additionally, motivational tips, quotes and photos, help guarantee you'll be in your best shape ever. Journaling increases success by as much as 50 percent!

The Eat-Clean Diet for Family & Kids

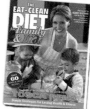

Tosca Reno has changed the face of health, diet and fitness with her Eat-Clean revolution, and now she's delivering that message to the family. In her foreword, cosmetics icon, CEO and mother-of-three Bobbi Brown says, "Tosca Reno's newest book could not have come at a better time … Healthy eating needs to start at home and it is our obligation as parents to set the right example for our kids." With tons of tips, tricks and advice, in addition to 60 kid-friendly recipes, this book is sure to become your biggest resource.

The Eat-Clean Diet for Men

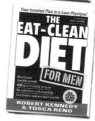

When men saw the results their wives and girlfriends were getting with *The Eat-Clean Diet*, many of them wanted to know if they could Eat Clean too. The answer? A resounding yes! In fact, Eating Clean was originally developed by, and for, men. So when men Eat Clean they are assured of getting the foods they love, and in quantities that feed their manly muscles. Along with her husband Robert Kennedy, Tosca Reno shows men the way to take care of their specific health problems and their sexual health while creating their optimal physiques, and the best news? They never have to count calories or eat like rabbits while doing so.

The Eat-Clean Diet Companion

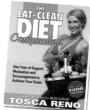

The Eat-Clean Diet Companion is the friendly support you need to make a lifestyle change and lose that extra fat for good. This food journal, personal motivator and resource tool in one contains space to track your Eat-Clean meals and goals, as well as convenient shopping lists, inspirational quotes and photos and food tips from Tosca herself. It's a proven fact that keeping a written log of what you eat can help you make positive changes to your diet, so take control of your life and start today.

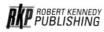
RKP ROBERT KENNEDY PUBLISHING